CHOCOLATE

A MEDICAL DICTIONARY, BIBLIOGRAPHY,
AND ANNOTATED RESEARCH GUIDE TO
INTERNET REFERENCES

JAMES N. PARKER, M.D.
AND PHILIP M. PARKER, PH.D., EDITORS

ICON Health Publications
ICON Group International, Inc.
4370 La Jolla Village Drive, 4th Floor
San Diego, CA 92122 USA

Printed in the United States of America.

Last digit indicates print number: 10 9 8 7 6 4 5 3 2 1

Publisher, Health Care: Philip Parker, Ph.D.
Editor(s): James Parker, M.D., Philip Parker, Ph.D.

Publisher's note: The ideas, procedures, and suggestions contained in this book are not intended for the diagnosis or treatment of a health problem. As new medical or scientific information becomes available from academic and clinical research, recommended treatments and drug therapies may undergo changes. The authors, editors, and publisher have attempted to make the information in this book up to date and accurate in accord with accepted standards at the time of publication. The authors, editors, and publisher are not responsible for errors or omissions or for consequences from application of the book, and make no warranty, expressed or implied, in regard to the contents of this book. Any practice described in this book should be applied by the reader in accordance with professional standards of care used in regard to the unique circumstances that may apply in each situation. The reader is advised to always check product information (package inserts) for changes and new information regarding dosage and contraindications before prescribing any drug or pharmacological product. Caution is especially urged when using new or infrequently ordered drugs, herbal remedies, vitamins and supplements, alternative therapies, complementary therapies and medicines, and integrative medical treatments.

Cataloging-in-Publication Data

Parker, James N., 1961-
Parker, Philip M., 1960-

Chocolate: A Medical Dictionary, Bibliography, and Annotated Research Guide to Internet References / James N. Parker and Philip M. Parker, editors
            p.   cm.
Includes bibliographical references, glossary, and index.
ISBN: 0-597-83581-0
1. Chocolate-Popular works. I. Title.

Disclaimer

This publication is not intended to be used for the diagnosis or treatment of a health problem. It is sold with the understanding that the publisher, editors, and authors are not engaging in the rendering of medical, psychological, financial, legal, or other professional services.

References to any entity, product, service, or source of information that may be contained in this publication should not be considered an endorsement, either direct or implied, by the publisher, editors, or authors. ICON Group International, Inc., the editors, and the authors are not responsible for the content of any Web pages or publications referenced in this publication.

Copyright Notice

Acknowledgements

The collective knowledge generated from academic and applied research summarized in various references has been critical in the creation of this book which is best viewed as a comprehensive compilation and collection of information prepared by various official agencies which produce publications on chocolate. Books in this series draw from various agencies and institutions associated with the United States Department of Health and Human Services, and in particular, the Office of the Secretary of Health and Human Services (OS), the Administration for Children and Families (ACF), the Administration on Aging (AOA), the Agency for Healthcare Research and Quality (AHRQ), the Agency for Toxic Substances and Disease Registry (ATSDR), the Centers for Disease Control and Prevention (CDC), the Food and Drug Administration (FDA), the Healthcare Financing Administration (HCFA), the Health Resources and Services Administration (HRSA), the Indian Health Service (IHS), the institutions of the National Institutes of Health (NIH), the Program Support Center (PSC), and the Substance Abuse and Mental Health Services Administration (SAMHSA). In addition to these sources, information gathered from the National Library of Medicine, the United States Patent Office, the European Union, and their related organizations has been invaluable in the creation of this book. Some of the work represented was financially supported by the Research and Development Committee at INSEAD. This support is gratefully acknowledged. Finally, special thanks are owed to Tiffany Freeman for her excellent editorial support.

About the Editors

James N. Parker, M.D.

Dr. James N. Parker received his Bachelor of Science degree in Psychobiology from the University of California, Riverside and his M.D. from the University of California, San Diego. In addition to authoring numerous research publications, he has lectured at various academic institutions. Dr. Parker is the medical editor for health books by ICON Health Publications.

Philip M. Parker, Ph.D.

Philip M. Parker is the Eli Lilly Chair Professor of Innovation, Business and Society at INSEAD (Fontainebleau, France and Singapore). Dr. Parker has also been Professor at the University of California, San Diego and has taught courses at Harvard University, the Hong Kong University of Science and Technology, the Massachusetts Institute of Technology, Stanford University, and UCLA. Dr. Parker is the associate editor for ICON Health Publications.

About ICON Health Publications

To discover more about ICON Health Publications, simply check with your preferred online booksellers, including Barnes & Noble.com and Amazon.com which currently carry all of our titles. Or, feel free to contact us directly for bulk purchases or institutional discounts:

ICON Group International, Inc.
4370 La Jolla Village Drive, Fourth Floor
San Diego, CA 92122 USA
Fax: 858-546-4341
Web site: **www.icongrouponline.com/health**

Table of Contents

FORWARD

In March 2001, the National Institutes of Health issued the following warning: "The number of Web sites offering health-related resources grows every day. Many sites provide valuable information, while others may have information that is unreliable or misleading."[1] Furthermore, because of the rapid increase in Internet-based information, many hours can be wasted searching, selecting, and printing. Since only the smallest fraction of information dealing with chocolate is indexed in search engines, such as **www.google.com** or others, a non-systematic approach to Internet research can be not only time consuming, but also incomplete. This book was created for medical professionals, students, and members of the general public who want to know as much as possible about chocolate, using the most advanced research tools available and spending the least amount of time doing so.

In addition to offering a structured and comprehensive bibliography, the pages that follow will tell you where and how to find reliable information covering virtually all topics related to chocolate, from the essentials to the most advanced areas of research. Public, academic, government, and peer-reviewed research studies are emphasized. Various abstracts are reproduced to give you some of the latest official information available to date on chocolate. Abundant guidance is given on how to obtain free-of-charge primary research results via the Internet. **While this book focuses on the field of medicine, when some sources provide access to non-medical information relating to chocolate, these are noted in the text.**

E-book and electronic versions of this book are fully interactive with each of the Internet sites mentioned (clicking on a hyperlink automatically opens your browser to the site indicated). If you are using the hard copy version of this book, you can access a cited Web site by typing the provided Web address directly into your Internet browser. You may find it useful to refer to synonyms or related terms when accessing these Internet databases. **NOTE:** At the time of publication, the Web addresses were functional. However, some links may fail due to URL address changes, which is a common occurrence on the Internet.

For readers unfamiliar with the Internet, detailed instructions are offered on how to access electronic resources. For readers unfamiliar with medical terminology, a comprehensive glossary is provided. For readers without access to Internet resources, a directory of medical libraries, that have or can locate references cited here, is given. We hope these resources will prove useful to the widest possible audience seeking information on chocolate.

The Editors

---

[1] From the NIH, National Cancer Institute (NCI): **http://www.cancer.gov/cancerinfo/ten-things-to-know**.

CHAPTER 1. STUDIES ON CHOCOLATE

Overview

In this chapter, we will show you how to locate peer-reviewed references and studies on chocolate.

The Combined Health Information Database

The Combined Health Information Database summarizes studies across numerous federal agencies. To limit your investigation to research studies and chocolate, you will need to use the advanced search options. First, go to **http://chid.nih.gov/index.html**. From there, select the "Detailed Search" option (or go directly to that page with the following hyperlink: **http://chid.nih.gov/detail/detail.html**). The trick in extracting studies is found in the drop boxes at the bottom of the search page where "You may refine your search by." Select the dates and language you prefer, and the format option "Journal Article." At the top of the search form, select the number of records you would like to see (we recommend 100) and check the box to display "whole records." We recommend that you type "chocolate" (or synonyms) into the "For these words:" box. Consider using the option "anywhere in record" to make your search as broad as possible. If you want to limit the search to only a particular field, such as the title of the journal, then select this option in the "Search in these fields" drop box. The following is what you can expect from this type of search:

- **Bittersweet Truth About Chocolate**

  Source: Renalife. 9(1): 11. 1994.

  Contact: Available from American Association of Kidney Patients. 100 South Ashley Drive, Suite 280, Tampa, FL 33602. (800) 749-2257 or (813) 233-7099.

  Summary: This brief article discusses the possibility of people on renal diets incorporating small amounts of chocolate into their diet. The author discusses the origins of chocolate; why chocolate intake must be limited (high in phosphorus and potassium); and how to wisely use chocolate treats. One recipe for Chocolate Cookie Balls is included.

- **Evaluation of a Dental Preventive Program for Danish Chocolate Workers**

  Source: Community Dentistry and Oral Epidemiology. 17(2):53-59, April 1989.

  Summary: A study evaluated the development of a program to control oral occupational diseases at two Danish chocolate factories. Eighty-nine persons (80 percent of the employees) ages 19 to 61 years, participated in a 2-year study. A dental hygienist offered preventive care to the workers. Subjects received clinical prophylaxis at four visits the first year and two visits the second year. Evaluation of program outcome consisted of clinical recordings of visible plaque index (VPI), gingival bleeding (GB), calculus index (CI), and DMFS. The study recorded data on dental conditions at baseline, as well as after 12 and 24 months. After each visit, workers completed questionnaires on dental knowledge, attitudes, dental health behavior, social network activities, and perceptions of the process. The mean GB decreased from 36 percent of the teeth scored at baseline to 9 percent at 24 months and mean DS decreased from 2.3 to 0.7 percent. The proportion of workers reporting daily tooth brushing at work increased from 6 percent to 24 percent during the program and the proportion of workers using dental floss regularly increased from 24 percent to 47 percent. Network activities in terms of involvement of family members and working group members in discussions about dental diseases and prevention tended to increase, but not with statistical significance. The majority of the workers (73 percent to 81 percent) were satisfied with scaling of their teeth, fluoride treatment, instructions and advice in preventive care, and regular control of dental health status. 8 tables, 1 figure, 24 references.

- **Three Cheers for Chocolate**

  Source: Health. 11(2):30,32,34; March 1997.

  Summary: This article discusses recent research into the components of chocolate. Studies have found that the fat in chocolate is stearic acid and oleic acid, neither of which raises cholesterol levels. However, the author says, most chocolate candy contains little cocoa butter, the source of the "good" fats. In general, the darker the chocolate, the healthier it is. It is also important to remember, though, that candy bars contain ingredients other than chocolate, and chocolate itself is high in calories.

Federally Funded Research on Chocolate

The U.S. Government supports a variety of research studies relating to chocolate. These studies are tracked by the Office of Extramural Research at the National Institutes of Health.[2] CRISP (Computerized Retrieval of Information on Scientific Projects) is a searchable database of federally funded biomedical research projects conducted at universities, hospitals, and other institutions.

Search the CRISP Web site at **http://crisp.cit.nih.gov/crisp/crisp_query.generate_screen**. You will have the option to perform targeted searches by various criteria, including geography, date, and topics related to chocolate.

---

[2] Healthcare projects are funded by the National Institutes of Health (NIH), Substance Abuse and Mental Health Services (SAMHSA), Health Resources and Services Administration (HRSA), Food and Drug Administration (FDA), Centers for Disease Control and Prevention (CDCP), Agency for Healthcare Research and Quality (AHRQ), and Office of Assistant Secretary of Health (OASH).

For most of the studies, the agencies reporting into CRISP provide summaries or abstracts. As opposed to clinical trial research using patients, many federally funded studies use animals or simulated models to explore chocolate. The following is typical of the type of information found when searching the CRISP database for chocolate:

- **Project Title: DOPAMINE POLYMORPHISMS AND SMOKING CUE-REACTIVITY**

  Principal Investigator & Institution: Erblich, Joel; Ruttenberg Cancer Center; Mount Sinai School of Medicine of Nyu of New York University New York, NY 10029

  Timing: Fiscal Year 2002; Project Start 19-SEP-2002; Project End 30-JUN-2007

  Summary: (provided by applicant): This 5-year K07 award application is designed to provide the applicant, whose formal training has been in clinical psychology, with the mentoring and "protected" time to pursue multidisciplinary research training spanning basic biology, genetics, behavioral sciences, epidemiology, and biostatistics. At the end of this training, the applicant will have developed sufficient expertise to be a fully established, independent investigator at the forefront of research exploring the biobehavioral links between genetic factors and smoking behavior. The proposed training includes both formal and informal didactics, as well as a complementary program of innovative research. Didactics will include completion of an MPH degree, other selected graduate course work in biology, and informal colloquia. The research project, which explores genetic factors in persistent smoking, will serve as a hands-on model of biobehavioral investigations of clinically relevant hypotheses grounded in the basic sciences. Most smokers express a strong interest in quitting, but only a small minority are successful. Accumulating evidence suggests that genetic factors play a role in this persistent smoking. In particular, research has demonstrated that smokers who carry specific polymorphisms that confer increased sensitivity to dopamine have higher levels of persistent smoking behavior. The underlying biobehavioral mechanisms linking these polymorphisms to persistent smoking are not yet known. Based on several independent lines of research, we propose to test the possibility that smokers with these polymorphisms display greater craving reactions to specific smoking cues, and perhaps appetitive cues generally, than smokers without, which may account for their higher levels of persistent smoking. To that end, a 4 year, laboratory-based study with 448 smokers (50 percent male, 50 percent female), is proposed. These healthy participants will be tested for specific polymorphisms, and their reactions to smoking cues, **chocolate** cues, and neutral cues will be assessed by self report and cardiovascular monitoring. In addition, they will complete questionnaires about their smoking patterns. Statistical analyses will examine relations between genotype, cue reactivity, and persistent smoking, behavior. Based on the results et that study, the applicant will begin developing and pilot testing interventions to reduce heightened reactivity among smokers with genetic vulnerability. The award is viewed as instrumental to the applicant in achieving his short-term goal of becoming an independent biobehavioral cancer control researcher, as well as his longer-term objective- to "bridge the gap" between the basic sciences and clinical applications by becoming competent in developing and testing clinically relevant "multidisciplinary" hypotheses informed by the basic biological and biobehavioral sciences.

  Website: http://crisp.cit.nih.gov/crisp/Crisp_Query.Generate_Screen

E-Journals: PubMed Central[3]

PubMed Central (PMC) is a digital archive of life sciences journal literature developed and managed by the National Center for Biotechnology Information (NCBI) at the U.S. National Library of Medicine (NLM).[4] Access to this growing archive of ejournals is free and unrestricted.[5] To search, go to **http://www.ncbi.nlm.nih.gov/entrez/query.fcgi?db=Pmc**, and type "chocolate" (or synonyms) into the search box. This search gives you access to full-text articles. The following is a sample of items found for chocolate in the PubMed Central database:

- **Characterization of a protease produced by a Trichoderma harzianum isolate which controls cocoa plant witches' broom disease.** by De Marco JL, Felix CR. 2002; http://www.pubmedcentral.gov/articlerender.fcgi?tool=pmcentrez&artid=65675

- **Cocoa Fermentations Conducted with a Defined Microbial Cocktail Inoculum.** by Schwan RF. 1998 Apr; http://www.pubmedcentral.gov/articlerender.fcgi?tool=pmcentrez&rendertype=external&artid=106173

- **Mutation of melanosome protein RAB38 in chocolate mice.** by Loftus SK, Larson DM, Baxter LL, Antonellis A, Chen Y, Wu X, Jiang Y, Bittner M, Hammer JA III, Pavan WJ. 2002 Apr 2; http://www.pubmedcentral.gov/articlerender.fcgi?tool=pmcentrez&artid=123672

- **Rate of Dehydration and Cumulative Desiccation Stress Interacted to Modulate Desiccation Tolerance of Recalcitrant Cocoa and Ginkgo Embryonic Tissues.** by Liang Y, Sun WQ. 2002 Apr 1; http://www.pubmedcentral.gov/articlerender.fcgi?tool=pmcentrez&artid=154260

- **Use of pulsed-field gel electrophoresis to link sporadic cases of invasive listeriosis with recalled chocolate milk..** by Proctor ME, Brosch R, Mellen JW, Garrett LA, Kaspar CW, Luchansky JB. 1995 Aug; http://www.pubmedcentral.gov/articlerender.fcgi?tool=pmcentrez&rendertype=external&artid=167594

The National Library of Medicine: PubMed

One of the quickest and most comprehensive ways to find academic studies in both English and other languages is to use PubMed, maintained by the National Library of Medicine.[6] The advantage of PubMed over previously mentioned sources is that it covers a greater number of domestic and foreign references. It is also free to use. If the publisher has a Web

---

[3] Adapted from the National Library of Medicine: **http://www.pubmedcentral.nih.gov/about/intro.html**.

[4] With PubMed Central, NCBI is taking the lead in preservation and maintenance of open access to electronic literature, just as NLM has done for decades with printed biomedical literature. PubMed Central aims to become a world-class library of the digital age.

[5] The value of PubMed Central, in addition to its role as an archive, lies in the availability of data from diverse sources stored in a common format in a single repository. Many journals already have online publishing operations, and there is a growing tendency to publish material online only, to the exclusion of print.

[6] PubMed was developed by the National Center for Biotechnology Information (NCBI) at the National Library of Medicine (NLM) at the National Institutes of Health (NIH). The PubMed database was developed in conjunction with publishers of biomedical literature as a search tool for accessing literature citations and linking to full-text journal articles at Web sites of participating publishers. Publishers that participate in PubMed supply NLM with their citations electronically prior to or at the time of publication.

site that offers full text of its journals, PubMed will provide links to that site, as well as to sites offering other related data. User registration, a subscription fee, or some other type of fee may be required to access the full text of articles in some journals.

To generate your own bibliography of studies dealing with chocolate, simply go to the PubMed Web site at **http://www.ncbi.nlm.nih.gov/pubmed**. Type "chocolate" (or synonyms) into the search box, and click "Go." The following is the type of output you can expect from PubMed for "chocolate" (hyperlinks lead to article summaries):

- **"Chocolate addiction": a preliminary study of its description and its relationship to problem eating.**
  Author(s): Hetherington MM, MacDiarmid JI.
  Source: Appetite. 1993 December; 21(3): 233-46.
  http://www.ncbi.nlm.nih.gov:80/entrez/query.fcgi?cmd=Retrieve&db=PubMed&list_uids=8141595&dopt=Abstract

- **A comparison of the performance of bacitracin-incorporated chocolate blood agar with chocolate blood agar plus a bacitracin disk in the isolation of Haemophilus influenzae from sputum.**
  Author(s): Nye KJ, Fallon D, Gee B, Howe S, Messer S, Turner T, Warren RE; PHLS (Midlands) Bacterial Methods Evaluation Group.
  Source: Journal of Medical Microbiology. 2001 May; 50(5): 472-5.
  http://www.ncbi.nlm.nih.gov:80/entrez/query.fcgi?cmd=Retrieve&db=PubMed&list_uids=11339257&dopt=Abstract

- **A dose-response effect from chocolate consumption on plasma epicatechin and oxidative damage.**
  Author(s): Wang JF, Schramm DD, Holt RR, Ensunsa JL, Fraga CG, Schmitz HH, Keen CL.
  Source: The Journal of Nutrition. 2000 August; 130(8S Suppl): 2115S-9S.
  http://www.ncbi.nlm.nih.gov:80/entrez/query.fcgi?cmd=Retrieve&db=PubMed&list_uids=10917932&dopt=Abstract

- **A double-blind provocative study of chocolate as a trigger of headache.**
  Author(s): Marcus DA, Scharff L, Turk D, Gourley LM.
  Source: Cephalalgia : an International Journal of Headache. 1997 December; 17(8): 855-62; Discussion 800.
  http://www.ncbi.nlm.nih.gov:80/entrez/query.fcgi?cmd=Retrieve&db=PubMed&list_uids=9453274&dopt=Abstract

- **Absorption rate of methylxanthines following capsules, cola and chocolate.**
  Author(s): Mumford GK, Benowitz NL, Evans SM, Kaminski BJ, Preston KL, Sannerud CA, Silverman K, Griffiths RR.
  Source: European Journal of Clinical Pharmacology. 1996; 51(3-4): 319-25.
  http://www.ncbi.nlm.nih.gov:80/entrez/query.fcgi?cmd=Retrieve&db=PubMed&list_uids=9010706&dopt=Abstract

- **Acceptability of fruit purees in peanut butter, oatmeal, and chocolate chip reduced-fat cookies.**
  Author(s): Swanson RB, Munsayac LJ.
  Source: Journal of the American Dietetic Association. 1999 March; 99(3): 343-5.
  http://www.ncbi.nlm.nih.gov:80/entrez/query.fcgi?cmd=Retrieve&db=PubMed&list_uids=10076588&dopt=Abstract

- **Acceptability of oatmeal chocolate chip cookies prepared using pureed white beans as a fat ingredient substitute.**
  Author(s): Rankin LL, Bingham M.
  Source: Journal of the American Dietetic Association. 2000 July; 100(7): 831-3.
  http://www.ncbi.nlm.nih.gov:80/entrez/query.fcgi?cmd=Retrieve&db=PubMed&list_uids=10916524&dopt=Abstract

- **All that chocolate--but where did it come from?**
  Author(s): Redwine DB.
  Source: Fertility and Sterility. 2000 June; 73(6): 1264-6.
  http://www.ncbi.nlm.nih.gov:80/entrez/query.fcgi?cmd=Retrieve&db=PubMed&list_uids=10856498&dopt=Abstract

- **Allergic reactions to chocolate.**
  Author(s): Ghosh JS.
  Source: The American Journal of Clinical Nutrition. 1977 June; 30(6): 834-5.
  http://www.ncbi.nlm.nih.gov:80/entrez/query.fcgi?cmd=Retrieve&db=PubMed&list_uids=868778&dopt=Abstract

- **An evaluation of the gram stain and chocolate agar culture as part of a routine urine culture set-up.**
  Author(s): Boyd DE, Flournoy DJ, Hussain Qadri SM.
  Source: Medical Microbiology and Immunology. 1980; 169(1): 63-6.
  http://www.ncbi.nlm.nih.gov:80/entrez/query.fcgi?cmd=Retrieve&db=PubMed&list_uids=6162084&dopt=Abstract

- **An investigation of the relationship of monsepecific urethritis corynebacteria to the other micoorganisms found in the urogenital tract by means of modified chocolate agar medium.**
  Author(s): Furness G, Kamat MH, Kaminski Z, Seebode JJ.
  Source: Invest Urol. 1973 March; 10(5): 387-91. No Abstract Available.
  http://www.ncbi.nlm.nih.gov:80/entrez/query.fcgi?cmd=Retrieve&db=PubMed&list_uids=4577525&dopt=Abstract

- **An investigation of the relationship of nonspecific urethritis corynebacteria to the other microorganisms found in the urogenital tract by means of a modified chocolate agar medium.**
  Author(s): Furness G, Kamat MH, Kaminski Z, Seebode JJ.
  Source: Invest Ophthalmol. 1973 March; 10(5): 387-91. No Abstract Available.
  http://www.ncbi.nlm.nih.gov:80/entrez/query.fcgi?cmd=Retrieve&db=PubMed&list_uids=4570466&dopt=Abstract

- **Antioxidant effects of polyphenols in chocolate on low-density lipoprotein both in vitro and ex vivo.**
  Author(s): Hirano R, Osakabe N, Iwamoto A, Matsumoto A, Natsume M, Takizawa T, Igarashi O, Itakura H, Kondo K.
  Source: J Nutr Sci Vitaminol (Tokyo). 2000 August; 46(4): 199-204.
  http://www.ncbi.nlm.nih.gov:80/entrez/query.fcgi?cmd=Retrieve&db=PubMed&list_uids=11185658&dopt=Abstract

- **Antioxidants in chocolate.**
  Author(s): Waterhouse AL, Shirley JR, Donovan JL.
  Source: Lancet. 1996 September 21; 348(9030): 834.
  http://www.ncbi.nlm.nih.gov:80/entrez/query.fcgi?cmd=Retrieve&db=PubMed&list_uids=8814019&dopt=Abstract

- **Barium-impregnated chocolate fudge for the study of chewing mechanism in children.**
  Author(s): Morgan JA, Gyepes MT, Jones MH, Desilets DT.
  Source: Radiology. 1970 February; 94(2): 432-3.
  http://www.ncbi.nlm.nih.gov:80/entrez/query.fcgi?cmd=Retrieve&db=PubMed&list_uids=5412818&dopt=Abstract

- **Bioavailability of (-)-epicatechin upon intake of chocolate and cocoa in human volunteers.**
  Author(s): Baba S, Osakabe N, Yasuda A, Natsume M, Takizawa T, Nakamura T, Terao J.
  Source: Free Radical Research. 2000 November; 33(5): 635-41.
  http://www.ncbi.nlm.nih.gov:80/entrez/query.fcgi?cmd=Retrieve&db=PubMed&list_uids=11200094&dopt=Abstract

- **Bitemarks in chocolate: a case report.**
  Author(s): McKenna CJ, Haron MI, Brown KA, Jones AJ.
  Source: J Forensic Odontostomatol. 2000 June; 18(1): 10-4.
  http://www.ncbi.nlm.nih.gov:80/entrez/query.fcgi?cmd=Retrieve&db=PubMed&list_uids=11324087&dopt=Abstract

- **Black holes and the chocolate cake concept.**
  Author(s): Allen A.
  Source: J Post Anesth Nurs. 1994 October; 9(5): 311-2.
  http://www.ncbi.nlm.nih.gov:80/entrez/query.fcgi?cmd=Retrieve&db=PubMed&list uids=7807411&dopt=Abstract

- **Breast milk distribution of theobromine from chocolate.**
  Author(s): Resman BH, Blumenthal P, Jusko WJ.
  Source: The Journal of Pediatrics. 1977 September; 91(3): 477-80.
  http://www.ncbi.nlm.nih.gov:80/entrez/query.fcgi?cmd=Retrieve&db=PubMed&list_uids=894424&dopt=Abstract

- **Breath hydrogen after ingestion of the bulk sweeteners sorbitol, isomalt and sucrose in chocolate.**
  Author(s): Lee A, Zumbe A, Storey D.
  Source: The British Journal of Nutrition. 1994 May; 71(5): 731-7.
  http://www.ncbi.nlm.nih.gov:80/entrez/query.fcgi?cmd=Retrieve&db=PubMed&list_uids=8054328&dopt=Abstract

- **CA 125 concentrations in ovarian 'chocolate' cyst fluid can differentiate an endometriotic cyst from a cystic corpus luteum.**
  Author(s): Koninckx PR, Muyldermans M, Moerman P, Meuleman C, Deprest J, Cornillie F.
  Source: Human Reproduction (Oxford, England). 1992 October; 7(9): 1314-7.
  http://www.ncbi.nlm.nih.gov:80/entrez/query.fcgi?cmd=Retrieve&db=PubMed&list_uids=1479017&dopt=Abstract

- **Caffeine and theobromine contents of ready-to-eat chocolate cereals.**
  Author(s): Caudle AG, Bell LN.
  Source: Journal of the American Dietetic Association. 2000 June; 100(6): 690-2.
  http://www.ncbi.nlm.nih.gov:80/entrez/query.fcgi?cmd=Retrieve&db=PubMed&list_uids=10863572&dopt=Abstract

- **Calcium supplementation of chocolate: effect on cocoa butter digestibility and blood lipids in humans.**
  Author(s): Shahkhalili Y, Murset C, Meirim I, Duruz E, Guinchard S, Cavadini C, Acheson K.
  Source: The American Journal of Clinical Nutrition. 2001 February; 73(2): 246-52.
  http://www.ncbi.nlm.nih.gov:80/entrez/query.fcgi?cmd=Retrieve&db=PubMed&list_uids=11157320&dopt=Abstract

- **Cannabinoid mimics in chocolate utilized as an argument in court.**
  Author(s): Tytgat J, Van Boven M, Daenens P.
  Source: International Journal of Legal Medicine. 2000; 113(3): 137-9.
  http://www.ncbi.nlm.nih.gov:80/entrez/query.fcgi?cmd=Retrieve&db=PubMed&list_uids=10876983&dopt=Abstract

- **Catechin contents of foods commonly consumed in The Netherlands. 2. Tea, wine, fruit juices, and chocolate milk.**
  Author(s): Arts IC, van De Putte B, Hollman PC.
  Source: Journal of Agricultural and Food Chemistry. 2000 May; 48(5): 1752-7.
  http://www.ncbi.nlm.nih.gov:80/entrez/query.fcgi?cmd=Retrieve&db=PubMed&list_uids=10820090&dopt=Abstract

- **Cefsulodin chocolate blood agar: a selective medium for the recovery of Haemophilus influenzae from the respiratory secretions of patients with cystic fibrosis.**
  Author(s): Smith A, Baker M.
  Source: Journal of Medical Microbiology. 1997 October; 46(10): 883-5.
  http://www.ncbi.nlm.nih.gov:80/entrez/query.fcgi?cmd=Retrieve&db=PubMed&list_uids=9364146&dopt=Abstract

- **Changes in brain activity related to eating chocolate: from pleasure to aversion.**
  Author(s): Small DM, Zatorre RJ, Dagher A, Evans AC, Jones-Gotman M.
  Source: Brain; a Journal of Neurology. 2001 September; 124(Pt 9): 1720-33.
  http://www.ncbi.nlm.nih.gov:80/entrez/query.fcgi?cmd=Retrieve&db=PubMed&list_uids=11522575&dopt=Abstract

- **Characterization and fat migration of palm kernel stearin as affected by addition of desiccated coconut used as base filling centre in dark chocolate.**
  Author(s): Ali A, Selamat J, Man YB, Suria AM.
  Source: International Journal of Food Sciences and Nutrition. 2001 May; 52(3): 251-61.
  http://www.ncbi.nlm.nih.gov:80/entrez/query.fcgi?cmd=Retrieve&db=PubMed&list_uids=11400474&dopt=Abstract

- **Charlotte's chocolate ice cream soda.**
  Author(s): Lutter LD.
  Source: Foot & Ankle International / American Orthopaedic Foot and Ankle Society [and] Swiss Foot and Ankle Society. 2000 March; 21(3): 181.
  http://www.ncbi.nlm.nih.gov:80/entrez/query.fcgi?cmd=Retrieve&db=PubMed&list_uids=10739147&dopt=Abstract

- **Chocolate allergy: a double-blind study.**
  Author(s): Maslansky L, Wein G.
  Source: Conn Med. 1971 January; 35(1): 5-9. No Abstract Available.
  http://www.ncbi.nlm.nih.gov:80/entrez/query.fcgi?cmd=Retrieve&db=PubMed&list_uids=5545287&dopt=Abstract

- **Chocolate and acne.**
  Author(s): Mackie BS, Mackie LE.
  Source: The Australasian Journal of Dermatology. 1974 December; 15(3): 103-9.
  http://www.ncbi.nlm.nih.gov:80/entrez/query.fcgi?cmd=Retrieve&db=PubMed&list_uids=4281299&dopt=Abstract

- **Chocolate and blood pressure in elderly individuals with isolated systolic hypertension.**
  Author(s): Taubert D, Berkels R, Roesen R, Klaus W.
  Source: Jama : the Journal of the American Medical Association. 2003 August 27; 290(8): 1029-30.
  http://www.ncbi.nlm.nih.gov:80/entrez/query.fcgi?cmd=Retrieve&db=PubMed&list_uids=12941673&dopt=Abstract

- **Chocolate and coronary disease.**
  Author(s): Kohn LA.
  Source: The American Journal of Clinical Nutrition. 1970 January; 23(1): 2-3.
  http://www.ncbi.nlm.nih.gov:80/entrez/query.fcgi?cmd=Retrieve&db=PubMed&list_uids=5412647&dopt=Abstract

- **Chocolate and heartburn: evidence of increased esophageal acid exposure after chocolate ingestion.**
  Author(s): Murphy DW, Castell DO.
  Source: The American Journal of Gastroenterology. 1988 June; 83(6): 633-6.
  http://www.ncbi.nlm.nih.gov:80/entrez/query.fcgi?cmd=Retrieve&db=PubMed&list_uids=3376917&dopt=Abstract

- **Chocolate and the auto-brewery syndrome.**
  Author(s): van Lieshout A.
  Source: Lancet. 1990 November 3; 336(8723): 1131.
  http://www.ncbi.nlm.nih.gov:80/entrez/query.fcgi?cmd=Retrieve&db=PubMed&list_uids=1978005&dopt=Abstract

- **Chocolate as a source of tea flavonoids.**
  Author(s): Arts IC, Hollman PC, Kromhout D.
  Source: Lancet. 1999 August 7; 354(9177): 488.
  http://www.ncbi.nlm.nih.gov:80/entrez/query.fcgi?cmd=Retrieve&db=PubMed&list_uids=10465183&dopt=Abstract

- **Chocolate bars contaminated with Salmonella napoli: an infectivity study.**
  Author(s): Greenwood MH, Hooper WL.
  Source: British Medical Journal (Clinical Research Ed.). 1983 April 30; 286(6375): 1394.
  http://www.ncbi.nlm.nih.gov:80/entrez/query.fcgi?cmd=Retrieve&db=PubMed&list_uids=6404474&dopt=Abstract

- **Chocolate bars in eye.**
  Author(s): Scott CM, Singh J.
  Source: Bmj (Clinical Research Ed.). 1994 December 24-31; 309(6970): 1748.
  http://www.ncbi.nlm.nih.gov:80/entrez/query.fcgi?cmd=Retrieve&db=PubMed&list_uids=7820015&dopt=Abstract

- **Chocolate biscuits are poisonous and should be banned by the year 2000.**
  Author(s): Mackay M.
  Source: N Z Med J. 1988 November 23; 101(858): 804. No Abstract Available.
  http://www.ncbi.nlm.nih.gov:80/entrez/query.fcgi?cmd=Retrieve&db=PubMed&list_uids=3194087&dopt=Abstract

- **Chocolate buttons.**
  Author(s): Holford IM.
  Source: Health Visit. 1976 January; 49(1): 7-9. No Abstract Available.
  http://www.ncbi.nlm.nih.gov:80/entrez/query.fcgi?cmd=Retrieve&db=PubMed&list_uids=1043861&dopt=Abstract

- **Chocolate cigarettes "recruit" children to smoking.**
  Author(s): Ferriman A.
  Source: Bmj (Clinical Research Ed.). 2003 February 8; 326(7384): 302.
  http://www.ncbi.nlm.nih.gov:80/entrez/query.fcgi?cmd=Retrieve&db=PubMed&list_uids=12574033&dopt=Abstract

- **Chocolate consumption and platelet function.**
  Author(s): Holt RR, Schramm DD, Keen CL, Lazarus SA, Schmitz HH.
  Source: Jama : the Journal of the American Medical Association. 2002 May 1; 287(17): 2212-3.
  http://www.ncbi.nlm.nih.gov:80/entrez/query.fcgi?cmd=Retrieve&db=PubMed&list_uids=11980520&dopt=Abstract

- **Chocolate contains additional flavonoids not found in tea.**
  Author(s): Lazarus SA, Hammerstone JF, Schmitz HH.
  Source: Lancet. 1999 November 20; 354(9192): 1825.
  http://www.ncbi.nlm.nih.gov:80/entrez/query.fcgi?cmd=Retrieve&db=PubMed&list_uids=10577676&dopt=Abstract

- **Chocolate craving and hunger state: implications for the acquisition and expression of appetite and food choice.**
  Author(s): Gibson EL, Desmond E.
  Source: Appetite. 1999 April; 32(2): 219-40.
  http://www.ncbi.nlm.nih.gov:80/entrez/query.fcgi?cmd=Retrieve&db=PubMed&list_uids=10097027&dopt=Abstract

- **Chocolate craving and liking.**
  Author(s): Rozin P, Levine E, Stoess C.
  Source: Appetite. 1991 December; 17(3): 199-212.
  http://www.ncbi.nlm.nih.gov:80/entrez/query.fcgi?cmd=Retrieve&db=PubMed&list_uids=1799282&dopt=Abstract

- **Chocolate cysts from ovarian follicles.**
  Author(s): Jain S, Dalton ME.
  Source: Fertility and Sterility. 1999 November; 72(5): 852-6.
  http://www.ncbi.nlm.nih.gov:80/entrez/query.fcgi?cmd=Retrieve&db=PubMed&list_uids=10560989&dopt=Abstract

- **Chocolate cysts of the orbit.**
  Author(s): Eiferman RA, Gushard RH.
  Source: Ann Ophthalmol. 1986 April; 18(4): 156-7.
  http://www.ncbi.nlm.nih.gov:80/entrez/query.fcgi?cmd=Retrieve&db=PubMed&list_uids=3592473&dopt=Abstract

- **Chocolate eating in healthy men during experimentally induced sadness and joy.**
  Author(s): Macht M, Roth S, Ellgring H.
  Source: Appetite. 2002 October; 39(2): 147-58.
  http://www.ncbi.nlm.nih.gov:80/entrez/query.fcgi?cmd=Retrieve&db=PubMed&list_uids=12354683&dopt=Abstract

- **Chocolate feeding studies: a novel approach for evaluating the plasma lipid effects of stearic acid.**
  Author(s): Kris-Etherton PM, Mustad VA.
  Source: The American Journal of Clinical Nutrition. 1994 December; 60(6 Suppl): 1029S-1036S.
  http://www.ncbi.nlm.nih.gov:80/entrez/query.fcgi?cmd=Retrieve&db=PubMed&list_uids=7977145&dopt=Abstract

- **Chocolate intake increases urinary excretion of polyphenol-derived phenolic acids in healthy human subjects.**
  Author(s): Rios LY, Gonthier MP, Remesy C, Mila I, Lapierre C, Lazarus SA, Williamson G, Scalbert A.
  Source: The American Journal of Clinical Nutrition. 2003 April; 77(4): 912-8.
  http://www.ncbi.nlm.nih.gov:80/entrez/query.fcgi?cmd=Retrieve&db=PubMed&list_uids=12663291&dopt=Abstract

- **Chocolate is a migraine-provoking agent.**
  Author(s): Gibb CM, Davies PT, Glover V, Steiner TJ, Clifford Rose F, Sandler M.
  Source: Cephalalgia : an International Journal of Headache. 1991 May; 11(2): 93-5.
  http://www.ncbi.nlm.nih.gov:80/entrez/query.fcgi?cmd=Retrieve&db=PubMed&list_uids=1860135&dopt=Abstract

- **Chocolate procyanidins decrease the leukotriene-prostacyclin ratio in humans and human aortic endothelial cells.**
  Author(s): Schramm DD, Wang JF, Holt RR, Ensunsa JL, Gonsalves JL, Lazarus SA, Schmitz HH, German JB, Keen CL.
  Source: The American Journal of Clinical Nutrition. 2001 January; 73(1): 36-40.
  http://www.ncbi.nlm.nih.gov:80/entrez/query.fcgi?cmd=Retrieve&db=PubMed&list_uids=11124747&dopt=Abstract

- **Chocolate, eating disorders, and affective syndromes.**
  Author(s): Zimmer B, Szekely B, Price W.
  Source: Journal of Clinical Psychopharmacology. 1986 February; 6(1): 56-7.
  http://www.ncbi.nlm.nih.gov:80/entrez/query.fcgi?cmd=Retrieve&db=PubMed&list_uids=3456358&dopt=Abstract

- **Chocolate: a flavor and texture unlike any other.**
  Author(s): Morgan J.
  Source: The American Journal of Clinical Nutrition. 1994 December; 60(6 Suppl): 1065S-1067S.
  http://www.ncbi.nlm.nih.gov:80/entrez/query.fcgi?cmd=Retrieve&db=PubMed&list_uids=7977153&dopt=Abstract

- **Chocolate: food as medicine/medicine as food.**
  Author(s): Keen CL.
  Source: Journal of the American College of Nutrition. 2001 October; 20(5 Suppl): 436S-439S; Discussion 440S-442S. Review.
  http://www.ncbi.nlm.nih.gov:80/entrez/query.fcgi?cmd=Retrieve&db=PubMed&list_uids=11603654&dopt=Abstract

- **Chocolate: food or drug?**
  Author(s): Bruinsma K, Taren DL.
  Source: Journal of the American Dietetic Association. 1999 October; 99(10): 1249-56. Review.
  http://www.ncbi.nlm.nih.gov:80/entrez/query.fcgi?cmd=Retrieve&db=PubMed&list_uids=10524390&dopt=Abstract

- **Chocolate: healing 'food of the gods'?**
  Author(s): Lee R, Balick MJ.
  Source: Alternative Therapies in Health and Medicine. 2001 September-October; 7(5): 120-2.
  http://www.ncbi.nlm.nih.gov:80/entrez/query.fcgi?cmd=Retrieve&db=PubMed&list_uids=11565391&dopt=Abstract

- **Chocolate: pleasure or pain?**
  Author(s): Rakatansky H.
  Source: R I Med. 1995 July; 78(7): 179. No Abstract Available.
  http://www.ncbi.nlm.nih.gov:80/entrez/query.fcgi?cmd=Retrieve&db=PubMed&list_uids=7655093&dopt=Abstract

- **Chocolate: pleasure or pain?**
  Author(s): Rakatansky H.
  Source: The American Journal of Psychiatry. 1989 August; 146(8): 1089.
  http://www.ncbi.nlm.nih.gov:80/entrez/query.fcgi?cmd=Retrieve&db=PubMed&list_uids=2502034&dopt=Abstract

- **Chocolate--divine food, fattening junk or nutritious supplementation?**
  Author(s): Rossner S.
  Source: European Journal of Clinical Nutrition. 1997 June; 51(6): 341-5. Review.
  http://www.ncbi.nlm.nih.gov:80/entrez/query.fcgi?cmd=Retrieve&db=PubMed&list_uids=9192189&dopt=Abstract

- **Cocoa and chocolate flavonoids: implications for cardiovascular health.**
  Author(s): Steinberg FM, Bearden MM, Keen CL.
  Source: Journal of the American Dietetic Association. 2003 February; 103(2): 215-23. Review.
  http://www.ncbi.nlm.nih.gov:80/entrez/query.fcgi?cmd=Retrieve&db=PubMed&list_uids=12589329&dopt=Abstract

- **Comparative gastrointestinal tolerance of sucrose, lactitol, or D-tagatose in chocolate.**
  Author(s): Lee A, Storey DM.
  Source: Regulatory Toxicology and Pharmacology : Rtp. 1999 April; 29(2 Pt 2): S78-82.
  http://www.ncbi.nlm.nih.gov:80/entrez/query.fcgi?cmd=Retrieve&db=PubMed&list_uids=10341165&dopt=Abstract

- **Comparative studies of gastrointestinal tolerance and acceptability of milk chocolate containing either sucrose, isomalt or sorbitol in healthy consumers and type II diabetics.**
  Author(s): Zumbe A, Brinkworth RA.
  Source: Zeitschrift Fur Ernahrungswissenschaft. 1992 March; 31(1): 40-8.
  http://www.ncbi.nlm.nih.gov:80/entrez/query.fcgi?cmd=Retrieve&db=PubMed&list_uids=1585682&dopt=Abstract

- **Comparison of epidemiological marker methods for identification of Salmonella typhimurium isolates from an outbreak caused by contaminated chocolate.**
  Author(s): Kapperud G, Lassen J, Dommarsnes K, Kristiansen BE, Caugant DA, Ask E, Jahkola M.
  Source: Journal of Clinical Microbiology. 1989 September; 27(9): 2019-24.
  http://www.ncbi.nlm.nih.gov:80/entrez/query.fcgi?cmd=Retrieve&db=PubMed&list_uids=2674198&dopt=Abstract

- **Comparison of ultrastructure adenomyotic glandular epithelium with that of attached epithelium of inner wall of chocolate cyst, with particular reference to histogenesis of endometriosis.**
  Author(s): Berduo F, Hayata T, Kawashima Y.
  Source: Nippon Sanka Fujinka Gakkai Zasshi. 1990 December; 42(12): 1697-701.
  http://www.ncbi.nlm.nih.gov:80/entrez/query.fcgi?cmd=Retrieve&db=PubMed&list_uids=2277210&dopt=Abstract

- **Consumption of tall oil-derived phytosterols in a chocolate matrix significantly decreases plasma total and low-density lipoprotein-cholesterol levels.**
  Author(s): De Graaf J, De Sauvage Nolting PR, Van Dam M, Belsey EM, Kastelein JJ, Haydn Pritchard P, Stalenhoef AF.
  Source: The British Journal of Nutrition. 2002 November; 88(5): 479-88.
  http://www.ncbi.nlm.nih.gov:80/entrez/query.fcgi?cmd=Retrieve&db=PubMed&list_uids=12425728&dopt=Abstract

- **DARPP chocolate: a caffeinated morsel of striatal signaling.**
  Author(s): Bastia E, Schwarzschild MA.
  Source: Science's Stke [electronic Resource] : Signal Transduction Knowledge Environment. 2003 January 14; 2003(165): Pe2. Review.
  http://www.ncbi.nlm.nih.gov:80/entrez/query.fcgi?cmd=Retrieve&db=PubMed&list_uids=12527819&dopt=Abstract

- **Death by chocolate?**
  Author(s): Viken R.
  Source: Tex Med. 2000 September; 96(9): 32. No Abstract Available.
  http://www.ncbi.nlm.nih.gov:80/entrez/query.fcgi?cmd=Retrieve&db=PubMed&list_uids=11004899&dopt=Abstract

- **Delayed chocolate cyst after blow-out fracture.**
  Author(s): Sutula FC, Palu RN.
  Source: Ophthalmic Plastic and Reconstructive Surgery. 1991; 7(4): 267-8.
  http://www.ncbi.nlm.nih.gov:80/entrez/query.fcgi?cmd=Retrieve&db=PubMed&list_
  uids=1764424&dopt=Abstract

- **Dental health among workers at a Danish chocolate factory.**
  Author(s): Petersen PE.
  Source: Community Dentistry and Oral Epidemiology. 1983 December; 11(6): 337-41.
  http://www.ncbi.nlm.nih.gov:80/entrez/query.fcgi?cmd=Retrieve&db=PubMed&list_
  uids=6580997&dopt=Abstract

- **Detection of trace amounts of hidden allergens: hazelnut and almond proteins in chocolate.**
  Author(s): Scheibe B, Weiss W, Rueff F, Przybilla B, Gorg A.
  Source: J Chromatogr B Biomed Sci Appl. 2001 May 25; 756(1-2): 229-37.
  http://www.ncbi.nlm.nih.gov:80/entrez/query.fcgi?cmd=Retrieve&db=PubMed&list_
  uids=11419715&dopt=Abstract

- **Digestibility of cocoa butter from chocolate in humans: a comparison with corn-oil.**
  Author(s): Shahkhalili Y, Duruz E, Acheson K.
  Source: European Journal of Clinical Nutrition. 2000 February; 54(2): 120-5.
  http://www.ncbi.nlm.nih.gov:80/entrez/query.fcgi?cmd=Retrieve&db=PubMed&list_
  uids=10694782&dopt=Abstract

- **Do we need to know how it works? Or doesn't chocolate just taste great?**
  Author(s): Rotchford JK.
  Source: Journal of Alternative and Complementary Medicine (New York, N.Y.). 2000 December; 6(6): 481-2.
  http://www.ncbi.nlm.nih.gov:80/entrez/query.fcgi?cmd=Retrieve&db=PubMed&list_
  uids=11152050&dopt=Abstract

- **Dose-related gastrointestinal response to the ingestion of either isomalt, lactitol or maltitol in milk chocolate.**
  Author(s): Koutsou GA, Storey DM, Lee A, Zumbe A, Flourie B, leBot Y, Olivier P.
  Source: European Journal of Clinical Nutrition. 1996 January; 50(1): 17-21.
  http://www.ncbi.nlm.nih.gov:80/entrez/query.fcgi?cmd=Retrieve&db=PubMed&list_
  uids=8617186&dopt=Abstract

- **Effect of bupropion on chocolate craving.**
  Author(s): Michell GF, Mebane AH, Billings CK.
  Source: The American Journal of Psychiatry. 1989 January; 146(1): 119-20.
  http://www.ncbi.nlm.nih.gov:80/entrez/query.fcgi?cmd=Retrieve&db=PubMed&list_
  uids=2492163&dopt=Abstract

- **Effect of chocolate in migraine: a double-blind study.**
  Author(s): Moffett AM, Swash M, Scott DF.
  Source: Journal of Neurology, Neurosurgery, and Psychiatry. 1974 April; 37(4): 445-8.
  http://www.ncbi.nlm.nih.gov:80/entrez/query.fcgi?cmd=Retrieve&db=PubMed&list_uids=4838915&dopt=Abstract

- **Effect of chocolate on acne vulgaris.**
  Author(s): Minkin W, Cohen HJ.
  Source: Jama : the Journal of the American Medical Association. 1970 March 16; 211(11): 1856.
  http://www.ncbi.nlm.nih.gov:80/entrez/query.fcgi?cmd=Retrieve&db=PubMed&list_uids=4244376&dopt=Abstract

- **Effect of chocolate on acne vulgaris.**
  Author(s): Maslansky L, Wein G.
  Source: Jama : the Journal of the American Medical Association. 1970 March 16; 211(11): 1856.
  http://www.ncbi.nlm.nih.gov:80/entrez/query.fcgi?cmd=Retrieve&db=PubMed&list_uids=4244375&dopt=Abstract

- **Effect of chocolate on acne vulgaris.**
  Author(s): Fulton JE Jr, Plewig G, Kligman AM.
  Source: Jama : the Journal of the American Medical Association. 1969 December 15; 210(11): 2071-4.
  http://www.ncbi.nlm.nih.gov:80/entrez/query.fcgi?cmd=Retrieve&db=PubMed&list_uids=4243053&dopt=Abstract

- **Effect of fat content and chocolate flavoring of milk on meal consumption and acceptability by schoolchildren.**
  Author(s): Garey JG, Chan MM, Parlia SR.
  Source: Journal of the American Dietetic Association. 1990 May; 90(5): 719-21.
  http://www.ncbi.nlm.nih.gov:80/entrez/query.fcgi?cmd=Retrieve&db=PubMed&list_uids=2335690&dopt=Abstract

- **Effect of fat replacement on sensory attributes of chocolate chip cookies.**
  Author(s): Charlton O, Sawyer-Morse MK.
  Source: Journal of the American Dietetic Association. 1996 December; 96(12): 1288-90.
  http://www.ncbi.nlm.nih.gov:80/entrez/query.fcgi?cmd=Retrieve&db=PubMed&list_uids=8948395&dopt=Abstract

- **Effect of isocaloric substitution of chocolate cake for potato in type I diabetic patients.**
  Author(s): Peters AL, Davidson MB, Eisenberg K.
  Source: Diabetes Care. 1990 August; 13(8): 888-92.
  http://www.ncbi.nlm.nih.gov:80/entrez/query.fcgi?cmd=Retrieve&db=PubMed&list_uids=2209326&dopt=Abstract

- **Effect of milk fat, cocoa butter, and whey protein fat replacers on the sensory properties of lowfat and nonfat chocolate ice cream.**
  Author(s): Prindiville EA, Marshall RT, Heymann H.
  Source: Journal of Dairy Science. 2000 October; 83(10): 2216-23.
  http://www.ncbi.nlm.nih.gov:80/entrez/query.fcgi?cmd=Retrieve&db=PubMed&list_uids=11049061&dopt=Abstract

- **Effect on human longevity of added dietary chocolate.**
  Author(s): Kirschbaum J.
  Source: Nutrition (Burbank, Los Angeles County, Calif.). 1998 November-December; 14(11-12): 869.
  http://www.ncbi.nlm.nih.gov:80/entrez/query.fcgi?cmd=Retrieve&db=PubMed&list_uids=9834932&dopt=Abstract

- **Effects of a milk chocolate bar per day substituted for a high-carbohydrate snack in young men on an NCEP/AHA Step 1 Diet.**
  Author(s): Kris-Etherton PM, Derr JA, Mustad VA, Seligson FH, Pearson TA.
  Source: The American Journal of Clinical Nutrition. 1994 December; 60(6 Suppl): 1037S-1042S.
  http://www.ncbi.nlm.nih.gov:80/entrez/query.fcgi?cmd=Retrieve&db=PubMed&list_uids=7977146&dopt=Abstract

- **Effects of a skimmed milk and chocolate diet on serum and skin lipids.**
  Author(s): Macdonald I.
  Source: J Sci Food Agric. 1968 May; 19(5): 270-2. No Abstract Available.
  http://www.ncbi.nlm.nih.gov:80/entrez/query.fcgi?cmd=Retrieve&db=PubMed&list_uids=5694856&dopt=Abstract

- **Effects of chocolate cystfluid on endometrioma cell growth in culture.**
  Author(s): Badawy SZ, Cuenca V, Kumar S, Holland J.
  Source: Fertility and Sterility. 1998 November; 70(5): 827-30.
  http://www.ncbi.nlm.nih.gov:80/entrez/query.fcgi?cmd=Retrieve&db=PubMed&list_uids=9806561&dopt=Abstract

- **Effects of cocoa powder and dark chocolate on LDL oxidative susceptibility and prostaglandin concentrations in humans.**
  Author(s): Wan Y, Vinson JA, Etherton TD, Proch J, Lazarus SA, Kris-Etherton PM.
  Source: The American Journal of Clinical Nutrition. 2001 November; 74(5): 596-602.
  http://www.ncbi.nlm.nih.gov:80/entrez/query.fcgi?cmd=Retrieve&db=PubMed&list_uids=11684527&dopt=Abstract

- **Endoscopic exploration and classification of the chocolate cysts.**
  Author(s): Brosens IA.
  Source: Human Reproduction (Oxford, England). 1994 December; 9(12): 2213-4.
  http://www.ncbi.nlm.nih.gov:80/entrez/query.fcgi?cmd=Retrieve&db=PubMed&list_uids=7714132&dopt=Abstract

- **Epicatechin in human plasma: in vivo determination and effect of chocolate consumption on plasma oxidation status.**
  Author(s): Rein D, Lotito S, Holt RR, Keen CL, Schmitz HH, Fraga CG.
  Source: The Journal of Nutrition. 2000 August; 130(8S Suppl): 2109S-14S.
  http://www.ncbi.nlm.nih.gov:80/entrez/query.fcgi?cmd=Retrieve&db=PubMed&list_uids=10917931&dopt=Abstract

- **Epidemic Yersinia enterocolitica infection due to contaminated chocolate milk.**
  Author(s): Black RE, Jackson RJ, Tsai T, Medvesky M, Shayegani M, Feeley JC, MacLeod KI, Wakelee AM.
  Source: The New England Journal of Medicine. 1978 January 12; 298(2): 76-9.
  http://www.ncbi.nlm.nih.gov:80/entrez/query.fcgi?cmd=Retrieve&db=PubMed&list_uids=579433&dopt=Abstract

- **Estimation of human dose of staphylococcal enterotoxin A from a large outbreak of staphylococcal food poisoning involving chocolate milk.**
  Author(s): Evenson ML, Hinds MW, Bernstein RS, Bergdoll MS.
  Source: International Journal of Food Microbiology. 1988 December 31; 7(4): 311-6.
  http://www.ncbi.nlm.nih.gov:80/entrez/query.fcgi?cmd=Retrieve&db=PubMed&list_uids=3275329&dopt=Abstract

- **Evaluation of a dental preventive program for Danish chocolate workers.**
  Author(s): Petersen PE.
  Source: Community Dentistry and Oral Epidemiology. 1989 April; 17(2): 53-9.
  http://www.ncbi.nlm.nih.gov:80/entrez/query.fcgi?cmd=Retrieve&db=PubMed&list_uids=2920539&dopt=Abstract

- **Evaluation of aluminium concentrations in samples of chocolate and beverages by electrothermal atomic absorption spectrometry.**
  Author(s): Sepe A, Costantini S, Ciaralli L, Ciprotti M, Giordano R.
  Source: Food Additives and Contaminants. 2001 September; 18(9): 788-96.
  http://www.ncbi.nlm.nih.gov:80/entrez/query.fcgi?cmd=Retrieve&db=PubMed&list_uids=11552746&dopt=Abstract

- **Factors affecting consumer preference for chocolate-flavored milks.**
  Author(s): Hampton O, Langlois BE, Tichenor D, Rudnick AW.
  Source: Journal of Dairy Science. 1969 September; 52(9): 1479-84.
  http://www.ncbi.nlm.nih.gov:80/entrez/query.fcgi?cmd=Retrieve&db=PubMed&list_uids=5395645&dopt=Abstract

- **Ferrous fumarate fortification of a chocolate drink powder.**
  Author(s): Hurrell RF, Reddy MB, Dassenko SA, Cook JD.
  Source: The British Journal of Nutrition. 1991 March; 65(2): 271-83.
  http://www.ncbi.nlm.nih.gov:80/entrez/query.fcgi?cmd=Retrieve&db=PubMed&list_uids=1645995&dopt=Abstract

- **Flavanols and procyanidins of cocoa and chocolate inhibit growth and polyamine biosynthesis of human colonic cancer cells.**
  Author(s): Carnesecchi S, Schneider Y, Lazarus SA, Coehlo D, Gosse F, Raul F.
  Source: Cancer Letters. 2002 January 25; 175(2): 147-55.
  http://www.ncbi.nlm.nih.gov:80/entrez/query.fcgi?cmd=Retrieve&db=PubMed&list_uids=11741742&dopt=Abstract

- **Flavor threshold for acetaldehyde in milk, chocolate milk, and spring water using solid phase microextraction gas chromatography for quantification.**
  Author(s): van Aardt M, Duncan SE, Bourne D, Marcy JE, Long TE, Hackney CR, Heisey C.
  Source: Journal of Agricultural and Food Chemistry. 2001 March; 49(3): 1377-81.
  http://www.ncbi.nlm.nih.gov:80/entrez/query.fcgi?cmd=Retrieve&db=PubMed&list_uids=11312867&dopt=Abstract

- **Food of the gods: cure for humanity? A cultural history of the medicinal and ritual use of chocolate.**
  Author(s): Dillinger TL, Barriga P, Escarcega S, Jimenez M, Salazar Lowe D, Grivetti LE.
  Source: The Journal of Nutrition. 2000 August; 130(8S Suppl): 2057S-72S.
  http://www.ncbi.nlm.nih.gov:80/entrez/query.fcgi?cmd=Retrieve&db=PubMed&list_uids=10917925&dopt=Abstract

- **Giving credit where it's due: chocolate chip cookies.**
  Author(s): Sharts-Hopko NC.
  Source: Mcn. the American Journal of Maternal Child Nursing. 1994 November-December; 19(6): 312.
  http://www.ncbi.nlm.nih.gov:80/entrez/query.fcgi?cmd=Retrieve&db=PubMed&list_uids=7880300&dopt=Abstract

- **Glycaemic effect and satiating capacity of potato chips and milk chocolate bar as snacks in teenagers with diabetes.**
  Author(s): Cedermark G, Selenius M, Tullus K.
  Source: European Journal of Pediatrics. 1993 August; 152(8): 635-9.
  http://www.ncbi.nlm.nih.gov:80/entrez/query.fcgi?cmd=Retrieve&db=PubMed&list_uids=8404965&dopt=Abstract

- **Happy Holidays! Power down—the chocolate chip versus the microchip. A maieutic attempt towards change.**
  Author(s): Weinstein J.
  Source: Spine. 2000 December 1; 25(23): 2973-4.
  http://www.ncbi.nlm.nih.gov:80/entrez/query.fcgi?cmd=Retrieve&db=PubMed&list_uids=11145806&dopt=Abstract

- **Harbingers of coronary heart disease: dietary saturated fatty acids and cholesterol. Is chocolate benign because of its stearic acid content?**
  Author(s): Connor WE.
  Source: The American Journal of Clinical Nutrition. 1999 December; 70(6): 951-2.
  http://www.ncbi.nlm.nih.gov:80/entrez/query.fcgi?cmd=Retrieve&db=PubMed&list_uids=10584037&dopt=Abstract

- **Hemodynamic and electrophysiologic effects of acute chocolate ingestion in young adults.**
  Author(s): Baron AM, Donnerstein RL, Samson RA, Baron JA, Padnick JN, Goldberg SJ.
  Source: The American Journal of Cardiology. 1999 August 1; 84(3): 370-3, A10.
  http://www.ncbi.nlm.nih.gov:80/entrez/query.fcgi?cmd=Retrieve&db=PubMed&list_uids=10496460&dopt=Abstract

- **High levels of methylxanthines in chocolate do not alter theobromine disposition.**
  Author(s): Shively CA, Tarka SM Jr, Arnaud MJ, Dvorchik BH, Passananti GT, Vesell ES.
  Source: Clinical Pharmacology and Therapeutics. 1985 April; 37(4): 415-24.
  http://www.ncbi.nlm.nih.gov:80/entrez/query.fcgi?cmd=Retrieve&db=PubMed&list_uids=3979003&dopt=Abstract

- **How good is chocolate?**
  Author(s): Nestel PJ.
  Source: The American Journal of Clinical Nutrition. 2001 November; 74(5): 563-4.
  http://www.ncbi.nlm.nih.gov:80/entrez/query.fcgi?cmd=Retrieve&db=PubMed&list_uids=11684518&dopt=Abstract

- **HPLC method for the quantification of procyanidins in cocoa and chocolate samples and correlation to total antioxidant capacity.**
  Author(s): Adamson GE, Lazarus SA, Mitchell AE, Prior RL, Cao G, Jacobs PH, Kremers BG, Hammerstone JF, Rucker RB, Ritter KA, Schmitz HH.
  Source: Journal of Agricultural and Food Chemistry. 1999 October; 47(10): 4184-8.
  http://www.ncbi.nlm.nih.gov:80/entrez/query.fcgi?cmd=Retrieve&db=PubMed&list_uids=10552788&dopt=Abstract

- **Immunoreactive beta-endorphin increases after an aspartame chocolate drink in healthy human subjects.**
  Author(s): Melchior JC, Rigaud D, Colas-Linhart N, Petiet A, Girard A, Apfelbaum M.
  Source: Physiology & Behavior. 1991 November; 50(5): 941-4.
  http://www.ncbi.nlm.nih.gov:80/entrez/query.fcgi?cmd=Retrieve&db=PubMed&list_uids=1805284&dopt=Abstract

- **In the land of chocolate, excitement about sugars!**
  Author(s): Stanley P.
  Source: Trends in Cell Biology. 1998 March; 8(3): 128-30. Review.
  http://www.ncbi.nlm.nih.gov:80/entrez/query.fcgi?cmd=Retrieve&db=PubMed&list_uids=9695824&dopt=Abstract

- **Increase in calciuria and oxaluria after a single chocolate bar load.**
  Author(s): Nguyen NU, Henriet MT, Dumoulin G, Widmer A, Regnard J.
  Source: Hormone and Metabolic Research. Hormon- Und Stoffwechselforschung. Hormones Et Metabolisme. 1994 August; 26(8): 383-6.
  http://www.ncbi.nlm.nih.gov:80/entrez/query.fcgi?cmd=Retrieve&db=PubMed&list_uids=7806135&dopt=Abstract

- **Influence of ascorbic acid on iron absorption from an iron-fortified, chocolate-flavored milk drink in Jamaican children.**
  Author(s): Davidsson L, Walczyk T, Morris A, Hurrell RF.
  Source: The American Journal of Clinical Nutrition. 1998 May; 67(5): 873-7.
  http://www.ncbi.nlm.nih.gov:80/entrez/query.fcgi?cmd=Retrieve&db=PubMed&list_uids=9583844&dopt=Abstract

- **Influence of the consumption frequency of filled chocolate products on the demineralization of human enamel in vivo. A microhardness and microradiographic investigation.**
  Author(s): van Herpen BP, Arends HJ.
  Source: Caries Research. 1986; 20(6): 529-33.
  http://www.ncbi.nlm.nih.gov:80/entrez/query.fcgi?cmd=Retrieve&db=PubMed&list_uids=3465446&dopt=Abstract

- **Inhibition of in vitro low-density lipoprotein oxidation by oligomeric procyanidins present in chocolate and cocoas.**
  Author(s): Pearson DA, Schmitz HH, Lazarus SA, Keen CL.
  Source: Methods Enzymol. 2001; 335: 350-60. No Abstract Available.
  http://www.ncbi.nlm.nih.gov:80/entrez/query.fcgi?cmd=Retrieve&db=PubMed&list_uids=11400384&dopt=Abstract

- **International outbreak of Salmonella Eastbourne infection traced to contaminated chocolate.**
  Author(s): Craven PC, Mackel DC, Baine WB, Barker WH, Gangarosa EJ.
  Source: Lancet. 1975 April 5; 1(7910): 788-92.
  http://www.ncbi.nlm.nih.gov:80/entrez/query.fcgi?cmd=Retrieve&db=PubMed&list_uids=48010&dopt=Abstract

- **Isolation of Helicobacter pylori after transport from a regional laboratory of gastric biopsy specimens in saline, Portagerm pylori or cultured on chocolate agar.**
  Author(s): Grove DI, McLeay RA, Byron KE, Koutsouridis G.
  Source: Pathology. 2001 August; 33(3): 362-4.
  http://www.ncbi.nlm.nih.gov:80/entrez/query.fcgi?cmd=Retrieve&db=PubMed&list_uids=11523941&dopt=Abstract

- **Lactose malabsorption as influenced by chocolate milk, skim milk, sucrose, whole milk, and lactic cultures.**
  Author(s): Dehkordi N, Rao DR, Warren AP, Chawan CB.
  Source: Journal of the American Dietetic Association. 1995 April; 95(4): 484-6.
  http://www.ncbi.nlm.nih.gov:80/entrez/query.fcgi?cmd=Retrieve&db=PubMed&list_uids=7699193&dopt=Abstract

- **Letter: Chocolate, beta-phenethylamine and migraine re-examined.**
  Author(s): Schweitzer JW, Friedhoff AJ, Schwartz R.
  Source: Nature. 1975 September 18; 257(5523): 256.
  http://www.ncbi.nlm.nih.gov:80/entrez/query.fcgi?cmd=Retrieve&db=PubMed&list_uids=1167288&dopt=Abstract

- **Letter: Contaminated chocolate balls.**
  Author(s): Dickinson PC.
  Source: Can Med Assoc J. 1974 May 4; 110(9): 1018-9. No Abstract Available.
  http://www.ncbi.nlm.nih.gov:80/entrez/query.fcgi?cmd=Retrieve&db=PubMed&list_uids=4823106&dopt=Abstract

- **Like drugs for chocolate: separate rewards modulated by common mechanisms?**
  Author(s): Grigson PS.
  Source: Physiology & Behavior. 2002 July; 76(3): 389-95. Review.
  http://www.ncbi.nlm.nih.gov:80/entrez/query.fcgi?cmd=Retrieve&db=PubMed&list_uids=12117575&dopt=Abstract

- **Liking for chocolate, depression, and suicidal preoccupation.**
  Author(s): Lester D, Bernard D.
  Source: Psychological Reports. 1991 October; 69(2): 570.
  http://www.ncbi.nlm.nih.gov:80/entrez/query.fcgi?cmd=Retrieve&db=PubMed&list_uids=1763170&dopt=Abstract

- **Low cariogenic potential of mixtures of sucrose and chocolate, cocoa or confectionery coatings.**
  Author(s): Yankell SL, Emling RC, Shi X, Greco MR.
  Source: J Clin Dent. 1988 Summer; 1(1): 28-30. No Abstract Available.
  http://www.ncbi.nlm.nih.gov:80/entrez/query.fcgi?cmd=Retrieve&db=PubMed&list_uids=3254705&dopt=Abstract

- **Low-fat chocolate gingerbread.**
  Author(s): Efanoff DA.
  Source: Journal of the American Dietetic Association. 1975 February; 66(2): 168.
  http://www.ncbi.nlm.nih.gov:80/entrez/query.fcgi?cmd=Retrieve&db=PubMed&list_uids=1112960&dopt=Abstract

- **Malevolent chocolate frosting.**
  Author(s): Scoggin C.
  Source: The New England Journal of Medicine. 1977 January 27; 296(4): 233.
  http://www.ncbi.nlm.nih.gov:80/entrez/query.fcgi?cmd=Retrieve&db=PubMed&list_uids=831102&dopt=Abstract

- **Marijuana and chocolate.**
  Author(s): James JS.
  Source: Aids Treat News. 1996 October 18; (No 257): 3-4.
  http://www.ncbi.nlm.nih.gov:80/entrez/query.fcgi?cmd=Retrieve&db=PubMed&list_uids=11363932&dopt=Abstract

- **MDMA ("ecstasy") abuse: psychopathological features and craving for chocolate: a case series.**
  Author(s): Schifano F, Magni G.
  Source: Biological Psychiatry. 1994 December 1; 36(11): 763-7.
  http://www.ncbi.nlm.nih.gov:80/entrez/query.fcgi?cmd=Retrieve&db=PubMed&list_uids=7858073&dopt=Abstract

- **Melting chocolate and melting snowmen: analogical reasoning and causal relations.**
  Author(s): Goswami U, Brown AL.
  Source: Cognition. 1990 April; 35(1): 69-95.
  http://www.ncbi.nlm.nih.gov:80/entrez/query.fcgi?cmd=Retrieve&db=PubMed&list_uids=2340713&dopt=Abstract

- **Methylxanthine composition and consumption patterns of cocoa and chocolate products.**
  Author(s): Shively CA, Tarka SM Jr.
  Source: Prog Clin Biol Res. 1984; 158: 149-78. Review.
  http://www.ncbi.nlm.nih.gov:80/entrez/query.fcgi?cmd=Retrieve&db=PubMed&list_uids=6396642&dopt=Abstract

- **Milk chocolate as the fatty meal in oral cholecystography.**
  Author(s): Harvey IC.
  Source: Clinical Radiology. 1977 November; 28(6): 635-6.
  http://www.ncbi.nlm.nih.gov:80/entrez/query.fcgi?cmd=Retrieve&db=PubMed&list_uids=589919&dopt=Abstract

- **Mood modulation by food: an exploration of affect and cravings in 'chocolate addicts'.**
  Author(s): Macdiarmid JI, Hetherington MM.
  Source: The British Journal of Clinical Psychology / the British Psychological Society. 1995 February; 34 (Pt 1): 129-38.
  http://www.ncbi.nlm.nih.gov:80/entrez/query.fcgi?cmd=Retrieve&db=PubMed&list_uids=7757035&dopt=Abstract

- **Mutation of melanosome protein RAB38 in chocolate mice.**
  Author(s): Loftus SK, Larson DM, Baxter LL, Antonellis A, Chen Y, Wu X, Jiang Y, Bittner M, Hammer JA 3rd, Pavan WJ.
  Source: Proceedings of the National Academy of Sciences of the United States of America. 2002 April 2; 99(7): 4471-6. Epub 2002 March 26.
  http://www.ncbi.nlm.nih.gov:80/entrez/query.fcgi?cmd=Retrieve&db=PubMed&list_uids=11917121&dopt=Abstract

- **Natural rubber latex allergy to adhesive in chocolate bar wrappers.**
  Author(s): Hughes TM.
  Source: Contact Dermatitis. 2001 January; 44(1): 46-7.
  http://www.ncbi.nlm.nih.gov:80/entrez/query.fcgi?cmd=Retrieve&db=PubMed&list_uids=11156021&dopt=Abstract

- **No evidence for a link between consumption of chocolate and coronary heart disease.**
  Author(s): Kris-Etherton PM, Pelkman CL, Zhao G, Wang Y.
  Source: The American Journal of Clinical Nutrition. 2000 October; 72(4): 1059-61.
  http://www.ncbi.nlm.nih.gov:80/entrez/query.fcgi?cmd=Retrieve&db=PubMed&list_uids=11010953&dopt=Abstract

- **On flavouring barium sulphate: use of an instant chocolate mixture.**
  Author(s): Neaman MP.
  Source: J Can Assoc Radiol. 1966 December; 17(4): 231. No Abstract Available.
  http://www.ncbi.nlm.nih.gov:80/entrez/query.fcgi?cmd=Retrieve&db=PubMed&list_uids=5957557&dopt=Abstract

- **Outbreak of Salmonella napoli infection caused by contaminated chocolate bars.**
  Author(s): Gill ON, Sockett PN, Bartlett CL, Vaile MS, Rowe B, Gilbert RJ, Dulake C, Murrell HC, Salmaso S.
  Source: Lancet. 1983 March 12; 1(8324): 574-7.
  http://www.ncbi.nlm.nih.gov:80/entrez/query.fcgi?cmd=Retrieve&db=PubMed&list_uids=6131266&dopt=Abstract

- **Outbreak of Salmonella typhimurium infection traced to contaminated chocolate and caused by a strain lacking the 60-megadalton virulence plasmid.**
  Author(s): Kapperud G, Gustavsen S, Hellesnes I, Hansen AH, Lassen J, Hirn J, Jahkola M, Montenegro MA, Helmuth R.
  Source: Journal of Clinical Microbiology. 1990 December; 28(12): 2597-601.
  http://www.ncbi.nlm.nih.gov:80/entrez/query.fcgi?cmd=Retrieve&db=PubMed&list_uids=2279988&dopt=Abstract

- **Ovarian chocolate cyst with markedly elevated serum CA19-9 level: a case report.**
  Author(s): Takemori M, Sugimura K.
  Source: European Journal of Obstetrics, Gynecology, and Reproductive Biology. 1991 December 13; 42(3): 241-4.
  http://www.ncbi.nlm.nih.gov:80/entrez/query.fcgi?cmd=Retrieve&db=PubMed&list_uids=1773881&dopt=Abstract

- **Passover matzoh and chocolate Easter eggs.**
  Author(s): Imperato PJ.
  Source: N Y State J Med. 1990 April; 90(4): 196-200. No Abstract Available.
  http://www.ncbi.nlm.nih.gov:80/entrez/query.fcgi?cmd=Retrieve&db=PubMed&list_uids=2333163&dopt=Abstract

- **Patterns of chocolate consumption.**
  Author(s): Seligson FH, Krummel DA, Apgar JL.
  Source: The American Journal of Clinical Nutrition. 1994 December; 60(6 Suppl): 1060S-1064S.
  http://www.ncbi.nlm.nih.gov:80/entrez/query.fcgi?cmd=Retrieve&db=PubMed&list_uids=7977152&dopt=Abstract

- **Perception of sweetness intensity determines women's hedonic and other perceptual responsiveness to chocolate food.**
  Author(s): Geiselman PJ, Smith CF, Williamson DA, Champagne CM, Bray GA, Ryan DH.
  Source: Appetite. 1998 August; 31(1): 37-48.
  http://www.ncbi.nlm.nih.gov:80/entrez/query.fcgi?cmd=Retrieve&db=PubMed&list_uids=9716434&dopt=Abstract

- **Pharmacological versus sensory factors in the satiation of chocolate craving.**
  Author(s): Michener W, Rozin P.
  Source: Physiology & Behavior. 1994 September; 56(3): 419-22.
  http://www.ncbi.nlm.nih.gov:80/entrez/query.fcgi?cmd=Retrieve&db=PubMed&list_uids=7972390&dopt=Abstract

- **Phenol antioxidant quantity and quality in foods: cocoa, dark chocolate, and milk chocolate.**
  Author(s): Vinson JA, Proch J, Zubik L.
  Source: Journal of Agricultural and Food Chemistry. 1999 December; 47(12): 4821-4.
  http://www.ncbi.nlm.nih.gov:80/entrez/query.fcgi?cmd=Retrieve&db=PubMed&list_uids=10606537&dopt=Abstract

- **Plasma kinetics in man of epicatechin from black chocolate.**
  Author(s): Richelle M, Tavazzi I, Enslen M, Offord EA.
  Source: European Journal of Clinical Nutrition. 1999 January; 53(1): 22-6.
  http://www.ncbi.nlm.nih.gov:80/entrez/query.fcgi?cmd=Retrieve&db=PubMed&list_uids=10048796&dopt=Abstract

- **Pleasure and excess: liking for and overconsumption of chocolate.**
  Author(s): Hetherington MM, Macdiarmid JI.
  Source: Physiology & Behavior. 1995 January; 57(1): 27-35.
  http://www.ncbi.nlm.nih.gov:80/entrez/query.fcgi?cmd=Retrieve&db=PubMed&list_uids=7878121&dopt=Abstract

- **Polyphenols in chocolate, which have antioxidant activity, modulate immune functions in humans in vitro.**
  Author(s): Sanbongi C, Suzuki N, Sakane T.
  Source: Cellular Immunology. 1997 May 1; 177(2): 129-36.
  http://www.ncbi.nlm.nih.gov:80/entrez/query.fcgi?cmd=Retrieve&db=PubMed&list_uids=9178639&dopt=Abstract

- **Preschool children maintain intake of other foods at a meal including sugared chocolate milk.**
  Author(s): Wilson JF.
  Source: Appetite. 1991 February; 16(1): 61-7.
  http://www.ncbi.nlm.nih.gov:80/entrez/query.fcgi?cmd=Retrieve&db=PubMed&list_uids=2018405&dopt=Abstract

- **PROP (6-n-Propylthiouracil) tasting and sensory responses to caffeine, sucrose, neohesperidin dihydrochalcone and chocolate.**
  Author(s): Ly A, Drewnowski A.
  Source: Chemical Senses. 2001 January; 26(1): 41-7.
  http://www.ncbi.nlm.nih.gov:80/entrez/query.fcgi?cmd=Retrieve&db=PubMed&list_uids=11124214&dopt=Abstract

- **Recurrence of chocolate cysts after laparoscopic ablation.**
  Author(s): Jones KD, Sutton CJ.
  Source: The Journal of the American Association of Gynecologic Laparoscopists. 2002 August; 9(3): 315-20.
  http://www.ncbi.nlm.nih.gov:80/entrez/query.fcgi?cmd=Retrieve&db=PubMed&list_uids=12101328&dopt=Abstract

- **Salsolinol in urine following chocolate consumption by social drinkers.**
  Author(s): Hirst M, Evans DR, Gowdey CW.
  Source: Alcohol Drug Res. 1987; 7(5-6): 493-501.
  http://www.ncbi.nlm.nih.gov:80/entrez/query.fcgi?cmd=Retrieve&db=PubMed&list_uids=3620015&dopt=Abstract

- **Scientists say chocolate might be sweet for hearts.**
  Author(s): Spake A.
  Source: U.S. News & World Report. 2000 February 28; 128(8): 78.
  http://www.ncbi.nlm.nih.gov:80/entrez/query.fcgi?cmd=Retrieve&db=PubMed&list_uids=11184123&dopt=Abstract

- **Self-administered use of fluoride among Danish chocolate workers.**
  Author(s): Petersen PE.
  Source: Scand J Dent Res. 1990 April; 98(2): 189-91.
  http://www.ncbi.nlm.nih.gov:80/entrez/query.fcgi?cmd=Retrieve&db=PubMed&list_uids=2343278&dopt=Abstract

- **Sensory analysis of polystyrene packaging material taint in cocoa powder for drinks and chocolate flakes.**
  Author(s): Linssen JP, Janssens JL, Reitsma JC, Roozen JP.
  Source: Food Additives and Contaminants. 1991 January-February; 8(1): 1-7.
  http://www.ncbi.nlm.nih.gov:80/entrez/query.fcgi?cmd=Retrieve&db=PubMed&list_uids=2015928&dopt=Abstract

- **Sensory properties of chocolate and their development.**
  Author(s): Hoskin JC.
  Source: The American Journal of Clinical Nutrition. 1994 December; 60(6 Suppl): 1068S-1070S. Review.
  http://www.ncbi.nlm.nih.gov:80/entrez/query.fcgi?cmd=Retrieve&db=PubMed&list_uids=7977154&dopt=Abstract

- **Small toys contained in chocolate eggs--good or bad surprise?**
  Author(s): Kehrt R, Niggemann B, Klaue S, Wahn U.
  Source: Respiratory Medicine. 2002 November; 96(11): 955-6.
  http://www.ncbi.nlm.nih.gov:80/entrez/query.fcgi?cmd=Retrieve&db=PubMed&list_uids=12418595&dopt=Abstract

- **Solitary conjunctival hemangioma presenting as a chocolate cyst.**
  Author(s): Loya N, Kremer I, Goldenfeld M, Swetliza E.
  Source: Archives of Ophthalmology. 1988 October; 106(10): 1457.
  http://www.ncbi.nlm.nih.gov:80/entrez/query.fcgi?cmd=Retrieve&db=PubMed&list_uids=3178556&dopt=Abstract

- **Suppressing thoughts about chocolate.**
  Author(s): Johnston L, Bulik CM, Anstiss V.
  Source: The International Journal of Eating Disorders. 1999 July; 26(1): 21-7.
  http://www.ncbi.nlm.nih.gov:80/entrez/query.fcgi?cmd=Retrieve&db=PubMed&list_uids=10349580&dopt=Abstract

- **Survival of Salmonella eastbourne and Salmonella typhimurium in milk chocolate prepared with artificially contaminated milk powder.**
  Author(s): Tamminga SK, Beumer RR, Kampelmacher EH, van Leusden FM.
  Source: J Hyg (Lond). 1977 December; 79(3): 333-7. No Abstract Available.
  http://www.ncbi.nlm.nih.gov:80/entrez/query.fcgi?cmd=Retrieve&db=PubMed&list_uids=336788&dopt=Abstract

- **Sweets, chocolate, and atypical depressive traits.**
  Author(s): Schuman M, Gitlin MJ, Fairbanks L.
  Source: The Journal of Nervous and Mental Disease. 1987 August; 175(8): 491-5.
  http://www.ncbi.nlm.nih.gov:80/entrez/query.fcgi?cmd=Retrieve&db=PubMed&list_uids=3625189&dopt=Abstract

- **The "blue" people with "chocolate" blood--methemoglobinemia.**
  Author(s): Mack RB.
  Source: N C Med J. 1982 April; 43(4): 292-3. No Abstract Available.
  http://www.ncbi.nlm.nih.gov:80/entrez/query.fcgi?cmd=Retrieve&db=PubMed&list_uids=6953322&dopt=Abstract

- **The adsorption of salicylates by a milk chocolate-charcoal mixture.**
  Author(s): Eisen TF, Grbcich PA, Lacouture PG, Shannon MW, Woolf A.
  Source: Annals of Emergency Medicine. 1991 February; 20(2): 143-6.
  http://www.ncbi.nlm.nih.gov:80/entrez/query.fcgi?cmd=Retrieve&db=PubMed&list_uids=1996795&dopt=Abstract

- **The adverse effect of chocolate on lower esophageal sphincter pressure.**
  Author(s): Wright LE, Castell DO.
  Source: Am J Dig Dis. 1975 August; 20(8): 703-7.
  http://www.ncbi.nlm.nih.gov:80/entrez/query.fcgi?cmd=Retrieve&db=PubMed&list_uids=239592&dopt=Abstract

- **The deposition of dental plaque in young adults on a diet containing chocolate and skim-milk powder.**
  Author(s): Grenby TH.
  Source: Archives of Oral Biology. 1974 March; 19(3): 213-5.
  http://www.ncbi.nlm.nih.gov:80/entrez/query.fcgi?cmd=Retrieve&db=PubMed&list_uids=4135012&dopt=Abstract

- The effect of a chocolate bar supplementation on moderate exercise recovery of recreational runners.
  Author(s): Chen JD, Ai H, Shi JD, Wu YZ, Chen ZM.
  Source: Biomed Environ Sci. 1996 September; 9(2-3): 247-55.
  http://www.ncbi.nlm.nih.gov:80/entrez/query.fcgi?cmd=Retrieve&db=PubMed&list_uids=8886339&dopt=Abstract

- The effect of fluoridated chocolate-flavored milk on caries incidence in elementary school children: two and three-year studies.
  Author(s): Legett BJ Jr, Garbee WH, Gardiner JF, Lancaster DM.
  Source: Asdc J Dent Child. 1987 January-February; 54(1): 18-21.
  http://www.ncbi.nlm.nih.gov:80/entrez/query.fcgi?cmd=Retrieve&db=PubMed&list_uids=3468137&dopt=Abstract

- The endoscopic localization of endometrial implants in the ovarian chocolate cyst
  Author(s): Brosens IA, Puttemans PJ, Deprest J.
  Source: Fertility and Sterility. 1994 June; 61(6): 1034-8.
  http://www.ncbi.nlm.nih.gov:80/entrez/query.fcgi?cmd=Retrieve&db=PubMed&list_uids=8194613&dopt=Abstract

- The medical history of chocolate.
  Author(s): Binder DK.
  Source: Pharos Alpha Omega Alpha Honor Med Soc. 2001 Spring; 64(2): 22-6. No Abstract Available.
  http://www.ncbi.nlm.nih.gov:80/entrez/query.fcgi?cmd=Retrieve&db=PubMed&list_uids=12517084&dopt=Abstract

- The role of fatty acid saturation on plasma lipids, lipoproteins, and apolipoproteins: I. Effects of whole food diets high in cocoa butter, olive oil, soybean oil, dairy butter, and milk chocolate on the plasma lipids of young men.
  Author(s): Kris-Etherton PM, Derr J, Mitchell DC, Mustad VA, Russell ME, McDonnell ET, Salabsky D, Pearson TA.
  Source: Metabolism: Clinical and Experimental. 1993 January; 42(1): 121-9.
  http://www.ncbi.nlm.nih.gov:80/entrez/query.fcgi?cmd=Retrieve&db=PubMed&list_uids=8446039&dopt=Abstract

- The role of low progesterone and tension as triggers of perimenstrual chocolate and sweets craving: some negative experimental evidence.
  Author(s): Michener W, Rozin P, Freeman E, Gale L.
  Source: Physiology & Behavior. 1999 September; 67(3): 417-20.
  http://www.ncbi.nlm.nih.gov:80/entrez/query.fcgi?cmd=Retrieve&db=PubMed&list_uids=10497961&dopt=Abstract

- This and that: chocolate addiction, the dual pharmacogenetics of asparagus eaters, and the arithmetic of freedom.
  Author(s): Max B.
  Source: Trends in Pharmacological Sciences. 1989 October; 10(10): 390-3.
  http://www.ncbi.nlm.nih.gov:80/entrez/query.fcgi?cmd=Retrieve&db=PubMed&list_uids=2617661&dopt=Abstract

- **Time to B. cereus about hot chocolate.**
  Author(s): Nelms PK, Larson O, Barnes-Josiah D.
  Source: Public Health Reports (Washington, D.C. : 1974). 1997 May-June; 112(3): 240-4.
  http://www.ncbi.nlm.nih.gov:80/entrez/query.fcgi?cmd=Retrieve&db=PubMed&list_
  uids=9160059&dopt=Abstract

- **Tolerance and breath hydrogen excretion following ingestion of maltitol incorporated at two levels into milk chocolate consumed by healthy young adults with and without fasting.**
  Author(s): Storey DM, Koutsou GA, Lee A, Zumbe A, Olivier P, Le Bot Y, Flourie B.
  Source: The Journal of Nutrition. 1998 March; 128(3): 587-92.
  http://www.ncbi.nlm.nih.gov:80/entrez/query.fcgi?cmd=Retrieve&db=PubMed&list_
  uids=9482768&dopt=Abstract

- **Toys within chocolate eggs--an ingestion hazard.**
  Author(s): Weizman Z, Krugliak P.
  Source: Acta Paediatrica (Oslo, Norway : 1992). 1998 April; 87(4): 478-9.
  http://www.ncbi.nlm.nih.gov:80/entrez/query.fcgi?cmd=Retrieve&db=PubMed&list_
  uids=9628313&dopt=Abstract

- **Transient hyperoxaluria after ingestion of chocolate as a high risk factor for calcium oxalate calculi.**
  Author(s): Balcke P, Zazgornik J, Sunder-Plassmann G, Kiss A, Hauser AC, Gremmel F, Derfler K, Stockenhuber F, Schmidt P.
  Source: Nephron. 1989; 51(1): 32-4.
  http://www.ncbi.nlm.nih.gov:80/entrez/query.fcgi?cmd=Retrieve&db=PubMed&list_
  uids=2915754&dopt=Abstract

- **Treatment of recurrent chocolate cysts by transvaginal aspiration and tetracycline sclerotherapy.**
  Author(s): Aboulghar MA, Mansour RT, Serour GI, Sattar M, Ramzy AM, Amin YM.
  Source: Journal of Assisted Reproduction and Genetics. 1993 November; 10(8): 531-3.
  http://www.ncbi.nlm.nih.gov:80/entrez/query.fcgi?cmd=Retrieve&db=PubMed&list_
  uids=8081092&dopt=Abstract

- **Trigeminal herpes zoster/chocolate-vanilla tongue.**
  Author(s): Braverman I, Uri N, Greenberg E.
  Source: Otolaryngology and Head and Neck Surgery. 2000 March; 122(3): 463.
  http://www.ncbi.nlm.nih.gov:80/entrez/query.fcgi?cmd=Retrieve&db=PubMed&list_
  uids=10699831&dopt=Abstract

- **Use of pulsed-field gel electrophoresis to link sporadic cases of invasive listeriosis with recalled chocolate milk.**
  Author(s): Proctor ME, Brosch R, Mellen JW, Garrett LA, Kaspar CW, Luchansky JB.
  Source: Applied and Environmental Microbiology. 1995 August; 61(8): 3177-9.
  http://www.ncbi.nlm.nih.gov:80/entrez/query.fcgi?cmd=Retrieve&db=PubMed&list_
  uids=7487050&dopt=Abstract

- **Vascular effects of cocoa rich in flavan-3-ols.**
  Author(s): Heiss C, Dejam A, Kleinbongard P, Schewe T, Sies H, Kelm M.
  Source: Jama : the Journal of the American Medical Association. 2003 August 27; 290(8): 1030-1.
  http://www.ncbi.nlm.nih.gov:80/entrez/query.fcgi?cmd=Retrieve&db=PubMed&list_uids=12941674&dopt=Abstract

CHAPTER 2. NUTRITION AND CHOCOLATE

Overview

In this chapter, we will show you how to find studies dedicated specifically to nutrition and chocolate.

Finding Nutrition Studies on Chocolate

The National Institutes of Health's Office of Dietary Supplements (ODS) offers a searchable bibliographic database called the IBIDS (International Bibliographic Information on Dietary Supplements; National Institutes of Health, Building 31, Room 1B29, 31 Center Drive, MSC 2086, Bethesda, Maryland 20892-2086, Tel: 301-435-2920, Fax: 301-480-1845, E-mail: ods@nih.gov). The IBIDS contains over 460,000 scientific citations and summaries about dietary supplements and nutrition as well as references to published international, scientific literature on dietary supplements such as vitamins, minerals, and botanicals.[7] The IBIDS includes references and citations to both human and animal research studies.

As a service of the ODS, access to the IBIDS database is available free of charge at the following Web address: **http://ods.od.nih.gov/databases/ibids.html**. After entering the search area, you have three choices: (1) IBIDS Consumer Database, (2) Full IBIDS Database, or (3) Peer Reviewed Citations Only.

Now that you have selected a database, click on the "Advanced" tab. An advanced search allows you to retrieve up to 100 fully explained references in a comprehensive format. Type "chocolate" (or synonyms) into the search box, and click "Go." To narrow the search, you can also select the "Title" field.

---

[7] Adapted from **http://ods.od.nih.gov**. IBIDS is produced by the Office of Dietary Supplements (ODS) at the National Institutes of Health to assist the public, healthcare providers, educators, and researchers in locating credible, scientific information on dietary supplements. IBIDS was developed and will be maintained through an interagency partnership with the Food and Nutrition Information Center of the National Agricultural Library, U.S. Department of Agriculture.

The following is a typical result when searching for recently indexed consumer information on chocolate:

- **Death by chocolate: facts and myths.**
  Author(s): Medical College of Georgia, Augusta.
  Source: Feldman, E.B. Nutrition-today (USA). (May-June 1998). volume 33(3) page 106-112. chocolate cocoa beans theobroma cacao history plant products proximate composition nutritive value chemical composition food technology confectionery industry cocoa industry food consumption diet fats nutrients blood lipids cholesterol lipoproteins risk food intake nutrition physiology human behaviour nervous system diseases toxicity immunity food allergies 0029-666X

- **Oysters, chocolate, apricots as aphrodisiacs: Fact of fantasy?**
  Source: Scanlon, D. Environmental-nutrition (USA). (June 1994). volume 17(6) page 1, 6. diet weight gain weight reduction disease control risk adipose tissues 0893-4452
  Summary: regime alimentaire gain de poids regime pour reduction de poids controle de maladies risque tissu adipeux

Additional consumer oriented references include:

- **Chocolate cake and a diet soda, please.**
  Source: Tufts-University-diet-and-nutrition-letter (USA). (July 1987). volume 5(5) page 2. sweeteners therapeutic diets hunger 0747-4105

- **Chocolate.**
  Source: Anonymous Harv-Mens-Health-Watch. 2001 June; 5(11): 6-8 1089-1102

- **Chocolate. Your heart's delight?**
  Source: Anonymous Mayo-Clin-Health-Lett. 2001 February; 19(2): 7 0741-6245

- **Effect of isocaloric substitution of chocolate cake for potato in type I diabetic patients.**
  Author(s): Division of Endocrinology, Cedars-Sinai Medical Center, Los Angeles, California 90048.
  Source: Peters, A L Davidson, M B Eisenberg, K Diabetes-Care. 1990 August; 13(8): 888-92 0149-5992

- **EN surveys 18 varieties of a cold weather favorite: a steaming mug of hot chocolate.**
  Source: Lepke, J. Environmental-nutrition (USA). (January 1993). volume 16(1) page 5. chocolate trade marks nutritive value 0893-4452

- **Let them eat chocolate.**
  Source: Pi Sunyer, F.X. Veg-times. Mt. Morris, Ill. : Vegetarian Times. April 1991. (164) page 44-46. 0164-8497

- **The chocolate myth factory.**
  Source: Liebman, B. Nutr-action-health-lett. [Washington, D.C. : Center for Science in the Public Interest,. March 2001. volume 28 (2) page 7-9. 0885-7792

- **The temptation of chocolate.**
  Source: Robinson, Dick. Health. New York : Health Magazine. February 1984. volume 16 (2) page 50, 52-53. 0279-3547

Additional physician-oriented references include:

- **A double-blind provocative study of chocolate as a trigger of headache.**
  Author(s): University of Pittsburgh, Pain Evaluation and Treatment Institute, PA 15213, USA. dawn@peti.sm.upmc.edu

Source: Marcus, D A Scharff, L Turk, D Gourley, L M Cephalalgia. 1997 December; 17(8): 855-62; discussion 800 0333-1024

- **Absorption rate of methylxanthines following capsules, cola and chocolate.**
  Author(s): Department of Psychiatry and Behavioral Sciences, Johns Hopkins University School of Medicine, Baltimore, MD 21224, USA.
  Source: Mumford, G K Benowitz, N L Evans, S M Kaminski, B J Preston, K L Sannerud, C A Silverman, K Griffiths, R R Eur-J-Clin-Pharmacol. 1996; 51(3-4): 319-25 0031-6970

- **An international outbreak of Salmonella nima from imported chocolate.**
  Source: Hockin, J.C. D'Aoust, J.Y. Bowering, D. Jessop, J.H. Khanna, B. Lior, H. Milling, M.E. J-Food-Prot. Ames, Iowa : International Association of Milk, Food, and Environmental Sanitarians. January 1989. volume 52 (1) page 51-54. charts. 0362-028X

- **Biochemical effect of chocolate colouring and flavouring like substances on thyroid function and protein biosynthesis.**
  Author(s): Biochemical Department, Faculty of Agriculture, Zagazig University, Egypt.
  Source: el Saadany, S S Nahrung. 1991; 35(4): 335-43 0027-769X

- **Cannabinoid mimics in chocolate utilized as an argument in court.**
  Author(s): Laboratory of Toxicology, E, Leuven, Belgium. jan.tytgat@farm.kuleuven.ac.be
  Source: Tytgat, J Van Boven, M Daenens, P Int-J-Legal-Med. 2000; 113(3): 137-9 0937-9827

- **Characterization of cocoa butter and cocoa butter equivalents by bulk and molecular carbon isotope analyses: implications for vegetable fat quantification in chocolate.**
  Author(s): Institut de Mineralogie et Geochimie, Universite de Lausanne, Switzerland. Jorge.Spangenberg@imp.unil.ch
  Source: Spangenberg, J E Dionisi, F J-Agric-Food-Chem. 2001 September; 49(9): 4271-7 0021-8561

- **Chocolate cake and a diet soda, please.**
  Source: Tufts-University-diet-and-nutrition-letter (USA). (July 1987). volume 5(5) page 2. sweeteners therapeutic diets hunger 0747-4105

- **Chocolate procyanidins decrease the leukotriene-prostacyclin ratio in humans and human aortic endothelial cells.**
  Source: Schramm, D.D. Wang, J.F. Holt, R.R. Ensunsa, J.L. Gonsalves, J.L. Lazarus, S.A. Schmitz, H.H. German, J.B. Keen, C.L. Am-j-clin-nutr. Bethesda, Md. : American Society for Clinical Nutrition. January 2001. volume 73 (1) page 36-40. 0002-9165

- **Chocolate.**
  Source: Anonymous Harv-Mens-Health-Watch. 2001 June; 5(11): 6-8 1089-1102

- **Chocolate. Your heart's delight?**
  Source: Anonymous Mayo-Clin-Health-Lett. 2001 February; 19(2): 7 0741-6245

- **Cocoa and chocolate flavonoids: implications for cardiovascular health.**
  Author(s): Didactic Program in Dietetics, Department of Nutrition, University of California, Davis, CA, USA. fmsteinberg@ucdavis.edu
  Source: Steinberg, F M Bearden, M M Keen, C L J-Am-Diet-Assoc. 2003 February; 103(2): 215-23 0002-8223

- **Cocoa and chocolate: composition, bioavailability, and health implications.**
  Source: Borchers, A.T. Keen, C.L. Hannum, S.M. Gershwin, M.E. J-med-food. Larchmont, NY : Mary Ann Liebert, Inc., c1998-. 2000. volume 3 (2) page 77-105. 1096-620X

- **Cocoa products decrease low density lipoprotein oxidative susceptibility but do not affect biomarkers of inflammation in humans.**
  Author(s): Center for Human Nutrition, University of Texas Southwestern Medical Center, Dallas 75390-9073, USA.
  Source: Mathur, S Devaraj, S Grundy, S M Jialal, I J-Nutr. 2002 December; 132(12): 3663-7 0022-3166

- **Consumption of tall oil-derived phytosterols in a chocolate matrix significantly decreases plasma total and low-density lipoprotein-cholesterol levels.**
  Author(s): Department of General Internal Medicine, University Medical Centre Nijmegen, The Netherlands. J.deGraaf@aig.azn.nl
  Source: De Graaf, J De Sauvage Nolting, P R Van Dam, M Belsey, E M Kastelein, J J Haydn Pritchard, P Stalenhoef, A F Br-J-Nutr. 2002 November; 88(5): 479-88 0007-1145

- **Content of trans fatty acids in margarines, plant oils, fried products and chocolate spreads in Austria.**
  Source: Wagner, K.H. Auer, E. Elmadfa, I. Eur-food-res-technol. Berlin : Springer, c1999-. 2000. volume 210 (4) page 237-241. 1438-2377

- **DARPP chocolate: a caffeinated morsel of striatal signaling.**
  Author(s): Center for Aging, Genetics and Neurodegeneration, Department of Neurology, Massachusetts General Hospital, Boston, MA 02129, USA.
  Source: Bastia, E Schwarzschild, M A Sci-STKE. 2003 January 14; 2003(165): PE2 1525-8882

- **Determination of conjugated linoleic acid (CLA) concentrations in milk chocolate.**
  Author(s): Technical Center, Hershey Foods Corporation, P.O. Box 805, 1025 Reese Avenue, Hershey, PA 17033-0805, USA.
  Source: Hurst, W J Tarka, S M Dobson, G Reid, C M J-Agric-Food-Chem. 2001 March; 49(3): 1264-5 0021-8561

- **Development of a rapid method for the detection of cocoa butter equivalents in mixtures with cocoa butter.**
  Author(s): European Commission, DG Joint Research Centre, Institute for Health and Consumer Protection, Ispra, Italy.
  Source: Barcarolo, R Anklam, E J-AOAC-Int. 2001 Sep-October; 84(5): 1485-9 1060-3271

- **DSC characterisation of cocoa butter polymorphs.**
  Source: Spigno, G. Pagella, C. De Faveri, D.M. Ital-j-food-sci. Pinerolo, Italy : Chiriotti Editori, 1989-. 2001. volume 13 (3) page 275-284. 1120-1770

- **Effect of milk fat, cocoa butter, and whey protein fat replacers on the sensory properties of lowfat and nonfat chocolate ice cream.**
  Author(s): Department of Food Science and Human Nutrition University of Missouri, Columbia 65211, USA.
  Source: Prindiville, E A Marshall, R T Heymann, H J-Dairy-Sci. 2000 October; 83(10): 2216-23 0022-0302

- **Effects of alkalized cocoa powder and soy lecithin on physical characteristics of chocolate beverage powders.**
  Source: Selamat, J. Hussin, N. Zain, A.M. Che Man, Y.B. J-food-process-preserv. Trumbull, Conn. : Food & Nutrition Press Inc. August 1998. volume 22 (3) page 241-254. 0145-8892

- **Effects of cocoa powder and dark chocolate on LDL oxidative susceptibility and prostaglandin concentrations in humans.**
  Author(s): Graduate Program in Nutrition, The Pennsylvania State University, University Park.
  Source: Wan, Y Vinson, J A Etherton, T D Proch, J Lazarus, S A Kris Etherton, P M Am-J-Clin-Nutr. 2001 November; 74(5): 596-602 0002-9165

- **Effects of cocoa powder and dark chololate on LDL oxidative susceptibility and prostaglandin concentrations in humans.**
  Source: Wan, Y. Vinson, J.A. Etherton, T.D. Proch, J. Lazarus, S.A. Kris Etherton, P.M. Am-j-clin-nutr. Bethesda, Md. : American Society for Clinical Nutrition. November 2001. volume 74 (5) page 596-602. 0002-9165

- **Effects of cocoa upon the growth of weanling male Sprague-Dawley rats fed fluid whole milk diets [Chocolate, nutritional value, hematology].**
  Source: Morrissey, R.B. Burkholder, B.D. Tarka, S.M. Jr. Nutr-Rep-Int. Los Altos, Calif. : Geron-X, Inc. February 1984. volume 29 (2) page 263-271. 0029-6635

- **Effects of milk fat, cocoa butter, or selected fat replacers on flavor volatiles of chocolate ice cream.**
  Author(s): Dairy Farmers of America, Springfield, MO, USA.
  Source: Welty, W M Marshall, R T Grun, I U Ellersieck, M R J-Dairy-Sci. 2001 January; 84(1): 21-30 0022-0302

- **Effects of soy protein isolates on quality of chocolates during storage.**
  Source: Selamat, J. Hussin, N. Zain, A.M. Che Man, Y.B. J-food-process-preserv. Trumbull, Conn. : Food & Nutrition Press Inc. August 1998. volume 22 (3) page 185-197. 0145-8892

- **Emerging health benefits from cocoa and chocolate.**
  Source: Hannum, S.M. Erdman, J.W. Jr. J-med-food. Larchmont, NY : Mary Ann Liebert, Inc., c1998-. 2000. volume 3 (2) page73-75. 1096-620X

- **EN surveys 18 varieties of a cold weather favorite: a steaming mug of hot chocolate.**
  Source: Lepke, J. Environmental-nutrition (USA). (January 1993). volume 16(1) page 5. chocolate trade marks nutritive value 0893-4452

- **Evaluation of aluminium concentrations in samples of chocolate and beverages by electrothermal atomic absorption spectrometry.**
  Author(s): Istituto Superiore di Sanita, Applied Toxicology Department, Rome, Italy.
  Source: Sepe, A Costantini, S Ciaralli, L Ciprotti, M Giordano, R Food-Addit-Contam. 2001 Sep; 18(9): 788-96 0265-203X

- **Flavanols and procyanidins of cocoa and chocolate inhibit growth and polyamine biosynthesis of human colonic cancer cells.**
  Author(s): Laboratory of Nutritional Chemoprevention in Digestive Oncology, IRCAD, 1 place de l'hopital, 67091, Strasbourg, France.
  Source: Carnesecchi, Stephanie Schneider, Yann Lazarus, Sheryl A Coehlo, David Gosse, Francine Raul, Francis Cancer-Lett. 2002 January 25; 175(2): 147-55 0304-3835

- **Flavonoids of cocoa inhibit recombinant human 5-lipoxygenase.**
  Author(s): Institut fur Physiologische Chemie I, Heinrich-Heine-Universitat Dusseldorf, Germany.
  Source: Schewe, Tankred Kuhn, Hartmut Sies, Helmut J-Nutr. 2002 July; 132(7): 1825-9 0022-3166

- **Formation of guaiacol in chocolate milk by the psychrotrophic bacterium Rahnella aquatilis.**
  Author(s): Food Science Australia, PO Box 52, North Ryde, NSW 1670, Australia.
  Source: Jensen, N Varelis, P Whitfield, F B Lett-Appl-Microbiol. 2001 November; 33(5): 339-43 0266-8254

- **Harbingers of coronary heart disease: dietary saturated fatty acids and cholesterol. Is chocolate benign because of its stearic acid content.**
  Source: Connor, W.E. Am-j-clin-nutr. Bethesda, Md. : American Society for Clinical Nutrition. December 1999. volume 70 (6) page 951-952. 0002-9165

- **How good is chocolate.**
  Source: Nestel, P.J. Am-j-clin-nutr. Bethesda, Md. : American Society for Clinical Nutrition. November 2001. volume 74 (5) page 563-564. 0002-9165

- **I. Kinetics and metabolism of theobromine in male rats [Purine derivatives in cocoa, chocolate products, and tea].**
  Source: Bonati, M. Latini, R. Sadurska, B. Riva, E. Galletti, F. Toxicology. Limerick : Elsevier Biomedical. April 16, 1984. volume 30 (4) page 327-341. 0300-483X

- **II. Kinetics and metabolism of theobromine in male and female non-pregnant and pregnant rabbits [Purine derivatives in cocoa, chocolate products and tea].**
  Source: Latini, R. Bonati, M. Gaspari, F. Traina, G.L. Jiritano, L. Toxicology. Limerick : Elsevier Biomedical. April 16, 1984. volume 30 (4) page 343-354. 0300-483X

- **Improved analysis of theobromine and caffeine in chocolate food products formulated with cocoa powder.**
  Source: Caudle, A.G. Gu, Y. Bell, L.N. Food-res-int. Oxford : Elsevier Science Ltd. 2001. volume 34 (7) page 599-603. 0963-9969

- **Let them eat chocolate.**
  Source: Pi Sunyer, F.X. Veg-times. Mt. Morris, Ill. : Vegetarian Times. April 1991. (164) page 44-46. 0164-8497

- **Light-oxidized flavor development and vitamin A degradation in chocolate milk.**
  Source: Chapman, K.W. Rosenberry, L.C. Bandler, D.K. Boor, K.J. J-food-sci. Chicago, Ill. : Institute of Food Technologists. Sept/October 1998. volume 63 (5) page 930-934. 0022-1147

- **Low cariogenic potential of mixtures of sucrose and chocolate, cocoa or confectionery coatings.**
  Source: Yankell, S L Emling, R C Shi, X Greco, M R J-Clin-Dent. 1988 Summer; 1(1): 28-30 0895-8831

- **Mood modulation by food: an exploration of affect and cravings in 'chocolate addicts'.**
  Author(s): Psychology Department, University of Dundee, UK.
  Source: Macdiarmid, J I Hetherington, M M Br-J-Clin-Psychol. 1995 February; 34 (Pt 1)129-38 0144-6657

- **Polyphenols in chocolate: is there a contribution to human health.**
  Source: Wollgast, J. Anklam, E. Food-res-int. Oxford : Elsevier Science Ltd. 2000. volume 33 (6) page 449-459. 0963-9969

- **PROP (6-n-Propylthiouracil) tasting and sensory responses to caffeine,sucrose, neohesperidin dihydrochalcone and chocolate.**
  Author(s): Nutritional Sciences Program, University of Washington, Seattle, WA 98195-353410, USA.

Source: Ly, A Drewnowski, A Chem-Senses. 2001 January; 26(1): 41-7 0379-864X

- **Protection against peroxynitrite by cocoa polyphenol oligomers.**
  Author(s): Institut fur Physiologische Chemie I, Heinrich-Heine-Universitat Dusseldorf, Postfach 101007, D-40001, Dusseldorf, Germany.
  Source: Arteel, G E Sies, H FEBS-Lett. 1999 November 26; 462(1-2): 167-70 0014-5793

- **Quantification of the predominant monomeric catechins in baking chocolate standard reference material by LC/APCI-MS.**
  Author(s): Analytical Chemistry Division, National Institute of Standards and Technology (NIST), Gaithersburg, Maryland 20899-0001, USA. bryant.nelson@nist.gov
  Source: Nelson, B C Sharpless, K E J-Agric-Food-Chem. 2003 January 29; 51(3): 531-7 0021-8561

- **Review on polyphenols in Theobroma cacao: changes in composition during the manufacture of chocolate and methodology for identification and quantification.**
  Source: Wollgast, J. Anklam, E. Food-res-int. Oxford : Elsevier Science Ltd. 2000. volume 33 (6) page 423-447. 0963-9969

- **Salsolinol in urine following chocolate consumption by social drinkers.**
  Source: Hirst, M Evans, D R Gowdey, C W Alcohol-Drug-Res. 1987; 7(5-6): 493-501 0883-1386

- **Sensory and physical properties of chocolate chip cookies made with vegetable shortening or fat replacers at 50 and 75% levels.**
  Source: Armbrister, W.L. Setser, C.S. Cereal-chem. St. Paul, Minn. : American Association of Cereal Chemists, 1924-. July/August 1994. volume 71 (4) page 344-351. 0009-0352

- **The chocolate myth factory.**
  Source: Liebman, B. Nutr-action-health-lett. [Washington, D.C. : Center for Science in the Public Interest,. March 2001. volume 28 (2) page 7-9. 0885-7792

- **The temptation of chocolate.**
  Source: Robinson, Dick. Health. New York : Health Magazine. February 1984. volume 16 (2) page 50, 52-53. 0279-3547

- **Use of palm mid-fraction in white chocolate formulation.**
  Source: Samsudin, S. Rahim, M.A.A. J-sci-food-agric. Sussex : John Wiley & Sons Limited. August 1996. volume 71 (4) page 483-490. 0022-5142

- **Value assignment of nutrient concentrations in standard reference material 2384 baking chocolate.**
  Author(s): National Food Processors Association, 1350 I Street NW, Suite 300, Washington, DC 20005, USA. katherine.sharpless@nist.gov
  Source: Sharpless, K E Brown Thomas, J Nelson, B C Phinney, C S Sieber, J R Wood, L J Yen, J H Howell, D W J-Agric-Food-Chem. 2002 November 20; 50(24): 7069-75 0021-8561

Federal Resources on Nutrition

In addition to the IBIDS, the United States Department of Health and Human Services (HHS) and the United States Department of Agriculture (USDA) provide many sources of information on general nutrition and health. Recommended resources include:

- healthfinder®, HHS's gateway to health information, including diet and nutrition: **http://www.healthfinder.gov/scripts/SearchContext.asp?topic=238&page=0**

- The United States Department of Agriculture's Web site dedicated to nutrition information: **www.nutrition.gov**

- The Food and Drug Administration's Web site for federal food safety information: **www.foodsafety.gov**

- The National Action Plan on Overweight and Obesity sponsored by the United States Surgeon General: **http://www.surgeongeneral.gov/topics/obesity/**

- The Center for Food Safety and Applied Nutrition has an Internet site sponsored by the Food and Drug Administration and the Department of Health and Human Services: **http://vm.cfsan.fda.gov/**

- Center for Nutrition Policy and Promotion sponsored by the United States Department of Agriculture: **http://www.usda.gov/cnpp/**

- Food and Nutrition Information Center, National Agricultural Library sponsored by the United States Department of Agriculture: **http://www.nal.usda.gov/fnic/**

- Food and Nutrition Service sponsored by the United States Department of Agriculture: **http://www.fns.usda.gov/fns/**

Additional Web Resources

A number of additional Web sites offer encyclopedic information covering food and nutrition. The following is a representative sample:

- AOL: **http://search.aol.com/cat.adp?id=174&layer=&from=subcats**

- Family Village: **http://www.familyvillage.wisc.edu/med_nutrition.html**

- Google: **http://directory.google.com/Top/Health/Nutrition/**

- Healthnotes: **http://www.healthnotes.com/**

- Open Directory Project: **http://dmoz.org/Health/Nutrition/**

- Yahoo.com: **http://dir.yahoo.com/Health/Nutrition/**

- WebMD®Health: **http://my.webmd.com/nutrition**

- WholeHealthMD.com: **http://www.wholehealthmd.com/reflib/0,1529,,00.html**

The following is a specific Web list relating to chocolate; please note that any particular subject below may indicate either a therapeutic use, or a contraindication (potential danger), and does not reflect an official recommendation (some Web sites are subscription based):

- **Minerals**

    Biotin
    Source: Integrative Medicine Communications; www.drkoop.com

    Copper
    Source: Integrative Medicine Communications; www.drkoop.com

Magnesium
Source: Integrative Medicine Communications; www.drkoop.com

Manganese
Source: Prima Communications, Inc.www.personalhealthzone.com

Vitamin H (Biotin)
Source: Integrative Medicine Communications; www.drkoop.com

- **Food and Diet**

  Brazil Nuts
  Source: Healthnotes, Inc. www.healthnotes.com

  Cherries
  Source: Healthnotes, Inc. www.healthnotes.com

  Chocolate
  Source: Healthnotes, Inc. www.healthnotes.com

  Chocolate
  Source: WholeHealthMD.com, LLC. www.wholehealthmd.com
  Hyperlink:
  http://www.wholehealthmd.com/refshelf/foods_view/0,1523,179,00.html

  Coffee
  Source: Healthnotes, Inc. www.healthnotes.com

  Dairy-Free Diet
  Source: Healthnotes, Inc. www.healthnotes.com

  Diet Drinks
  Source: Healthnotes, Inc. www.healthnotes.com

  Diet Powders
  Source: Healthnotes, Inc. www.healthnotes.com

  Energy Bars
  Source: Healthnotes, Inc. www.healthnotes.com

  Feingold Diet
  Source: Healthnotes, Inc. www.healthnotes.com

  Frozen Yogurt
  Source: Healthnotes, Inc. www.healthnotes.com

  Gluten-Free Diet
  Source: Healthnotes, Inc. www.healthnotes.com

  Hazelnuts

Source: WholeHealthMD.com, LLC. www.wholehealthmd.com
Hyperlink:
http://www.wholehealthmd.com/refshelf/foods_view/0,1523,307,00.html

Hypertension
Source: Healthnotes, Inc. www.healthnotes.com

Ice Cream
Source: Healthnotes, Inc. www.healthnotes.com

Low-Fat Diet
Source: Healthnotes, Inc. www.healthnotes.com

Low-Fat Recipes Index
Source: Healthnotes, Inc. www.healthnotes.com

Low-Oxalate Diet
Source: Healthnotes, Inc. www.healthnotes.com

Low-Purine Diet
Source: Healthnotes, Inc. www.healthnotes.com

Macadamia Nuts
Source: Healthnotes, Inc. www.healthnotes.com

Macrobiotic Diet
Source: Healthnotes, Inc. www.healthnotes.com

Mascarpone
Source: Healthnotes, Inc. www.healthnotes.com

Muffins
Source: Healthnotes, Inc. www.healthnotes.com

Peppers, sweet
Source: WholeHealthMD.com, LLC. www.wholehealthmd.com
Hyperlink:
http://www.wholehealthmd.com/refshelf/foods_view/0,1523,31,00.html

Seeds
Source: WholeHealthMD.com, LLC. www.wholehealthmd.com
Hyperlink:
http://www.wholehealthmd.com/refshelf/foods_view/0,1523,288,00.html

Snacks and Desserts
Source: Healthnotes, Inc. www.healthnotes.com

Soy and Protein Shakes
Source: Healthnotes, Inc. www.healthnotes.com

Soy milk
Source: WholeHealthMD.com, LLC. www.wholehealthmd.com
Hyperlink:
http://www.wholehealthmd.com/refshelf/foods_view/0,1523,200,00.html

Soy Nuts
Source: Healthnotes, Inc. www.healthnotes.com

Sports Gels
Source: Healthnotes, Inc. www.healthnotes.com

Tofu
Source: Healthnotes, Inc. www.healthnotes.com

Tyramine-Free Diet
Source: Healthnotes, Inc. www.healthnotes.com

Water
Source: Healthnotes, Inc. www.healthnotes.com

CHAPTER 3. ALTERNATIVE MEDICINE AND CHOCOLATE

Overview

In this chapter, we will begin by introducing you to official information sources on complementary and alternative medicine (CAM) relating to chocolate. At the conclusion of this chapter, we will provide additional sources.

National Center for Complementary and Alternative Medicine

The National Center for Complementary and Alternative Medicine (NCCAM) of the National Institutes of Health (**http://nccam.nih.gov/**) has created a link to the National Library of Medicine's databases to facilitate research for articles that specifically relate to chocolate and complementary medicine. To search the database, go to the following Web site: **http://www.nlm.nih.gov/nccam/camonpubmed.html**. Select "CAM on PubMed." Enter "chocolate" (or synonyms) into the search box. Click "Go." The following references provide information on particular aspects of complementary and alternative medicine that are related to chocolate:

- **A dose-response effect from chocolate consumption on plasma epicatechin and oxidative damage.**
  Author(s): Wang JF, Schramm DD, Holt RR, Ensunsa JL, Fraga CG, Schmitz HH, Keen CL.
  Source: The Journal of Nutrition. 2000 August; 130(8S Suppl): 2115S-9S.
  http://www.ncbi.nlm.nih.gov:80/entrez/query.fcgi?cmd=Retrieve&db=PubMed&list_uids=10917932&dopt=Abstract

- **A pilot study on antiplaque effects of mastic chewing gum in the oral cavity.**
  Author(s): Takahashi K, Fukazawa M, Motohira H, Ochiai K, Nishikawa H, Miyata T.
  Source: J Periodontol. 2003 April; 74(4): 501-5.
  http://www.ncbi.nlm.nih.gov:80/entrez/query.fcgi?cmd=Retrieve&db=PubMed&list_uids=12747455&dopt=Abstract

- **A short history of nitroglycerine and nitric oxide in pharmacology and physiology.**
  Author(s): Marsh N, Marsh A.

Source: Clinical and Experimental Pharmacology & Physiology. 2000 April; 27(4): 313-9.
http://www.ncbi.nlm.nih.gov:80/entrez/query.fcgi?cmd=Retrieve&db=PubMed&list_
uids=10779131&dopt=Abstract

- **Acceptability of oatmeal chocolate chip cookies prepared using pureed white beans as a fat ingredient substitute.**
  Author(s): Rankin LL, Bingham M.
  Source: Journal of the American Dietetic Association. 2000 July; 100(7): 831-3.
  http://www.ncbi.nlm.nih.gov:80/entrez/query.fcgi?cmd=Retrieve&db=PubMed&list_
  uids=10916524&dopt=Abstract

- **Antioxidant polyphenols in tea, cocoa, and wine.**
  Author(s): Dreosti IE.
  Source: Nutrition (Burbank, Los Angeles County, Calif.). 2000 July-August; 16(7-8): 692-4. Review.
  http://www.ncbi.nlm.nih.gov:80/entrez/query.fcgi?cmd=Retrieve&db=PubMed&list_
  uids=10906600&dopt=Abstract

- **Applications of inulin and oligofructose in health and nutrition.**
  Author(s): Kaur N, Gupta AK.
  Source: Journal of Biosciences. 2002 December; 27(7): 703-14. Review.
  http://www.ncbi.nlm.nih.gov:80/entrez/query.fcgi?cmd=Retrieve&db=PubMed&list_
  uids=12571376&dopt=Abstract

- **Approach to the management of premenstrual syndrome.**
  Author(s): Massil HY, O'Brien PM.
  Source: Clinical Obstetrics and Gynecology. 1987 June; 30(2): 443-52.
  http://www.ncbi.nlm.nih.gov:80/entrez/query.fcgi?cmd=Retrieve&db=PubMed&list_
  uids=3608284&dopt=Abstract

- **Assessment of the palatability of vehicles for activated charcoal in pediatric volunteers.**
  Author(s): Dagnone D, Matsui D, Rieder MJ.
  Source: Pediatric Emergency Care. 2002 February; 18(1): 19-21.
  http://www.ncbi.nlm.nih.gov:80/entrez/query.fcgi?cmd=Retrieve&db=PubMed&list_
  uids=11862132&dopt=Abstract

- **Autism, an extreme challenge to integrative medicine. Part 2: medical management.**
  Author(s): Kidd PM.
  Source: Alternative Medicine Review : a Journal of Clinical Therapeutic. 2002 December; 7(6): 472-99. Review.
  http://www.ncbi.nlm.nih.gov:80/entrez/query.fcgi?cmd=Retrieve&db=PubMed&list_
  uids=12495373&dopt=Abstract

- **Bacteriology of postpartum oviducts and endometrium.**
  Author(s): Spore WW, Moskal PA, Nakamura RM, Mishell DR Jr.
  Source: American Journal of Obstetrics and Gynecology. 1970 June 15; 107(4): 572-7.
  http://www.ncbi.nlm.nih.gov:80/entrez/query.fcgi?cmd=Retrieve&db=PubMed&list_
  uids=5463700&dopt=Abstract

- **Bias and misrepresentation revisited: "perspective" on saturated fat.**
  Author(s): Keys A, Grande F, Anderson JT.
  Source: The American Journal of Clinical Nutrition. 1974 February; 27(2): 188-212. Review.
  http://www.ncbi.nlm.nih.gov:80/entrez/query.fcgi?cmd=Retrieve&db=PubMed&list_uids=4591426&dopt=Abstract

- **Biofeedback training in the therapy of flushing.**
  Author(s): Wilkin JK, Tarbox A.
  Source: Cutis; Cutaneous Medicine for the Practitioner. 1983 January; 31(1): 74-5.
  http://www.ncbi.nlm.nih.gov:80/entrez/query.fcgi?cmd=Retrieve&db=PubMed&list_uids=6825463&dopt=Abstract

- **Calcium supplementation of chocolate: effect on cocoa butter digestibility and blood lipids in humans.**
  Author(s): Shahkhalili Y, Murset C, Meirim I, Duruz E, Guinchard S, Cavadini C, Acheson K.
  Source: The American Journal of Clinical Nutrition. 2001 February; 73(2): 246-52.
  http://www.ncbi.nlm.nih.gov:80/entrez/query.fcgi?cmd=Retrieve&db=PubMed&list_uids=11157320&dopt=Abstract

- **Characterization of cocoa butter extracted from hybrid cultivars of Theobroma cacao L.**
  Author(s): Padilla FC, Liendo R, Quintana A.
  Source: Arch Latinoam Nutr. 2000 June; 50(2): 200-5.
  http://www.ncbi.nlm.nih.gov:80/entrez/query.fcgi?cmd=Retrieve&db=PubMed&list_uids=11048595&dopt=Abstract

- **Chocolate as a source of tea flavonoids.**
  Author(s): Arts IC, Hollman PC, Kromhout D.
  Source: Lancet. 1999 August 7; 354(9177): 488.
  http://www.ncbi.nlm.nih.gov:80/entrez/query.fcgi?cmd=Retrieve&db=PubMed&list_uids=10465183&dopt=Abstract

- **Chocolate: food as medicine/medicine as food.**
  Author(s): Keen CL.
  Source: Journal of the American College of Nutrition. 2001 October; 20(5 Suppl): 436S-439S; Discussion 440S-442S. Review.
  http://www.ncbi.nlm.nih.gov:80/entrez/query.fcgi?cmd=Retrieve&db=PubMed&list_uids=11603654&dopt=Abstract

- **Chocolate: healing 'food of the gods'?**
  Author(s): Lee R, Balick MJ.
  Source: Alternative Therapies in Health and Medicine. 2001 September-October; 7(5): 120-2.
  http://www.ncbi.nlm.nih.gov:80/entrez/query.fcgi?cmd=Retrieve&db=PubMed&list_uids=11565391&dopt=Abstract

- **Cocoa and chocolate flavonoids: implications for cardiovascular health.**
  Author(s): Steinberg FM, Bearden MM, Keen CL.

Source: Journal of the American Dietetic Association. 2003 February; 103(2): 215-23. Review.

http://www.ncbi.nlm.nih.gov:80/entrez/query.fcgi?cmd=Retrieve&db=PubMed&list_uids=12589329&dopt=Abstract

- **Cocoa extract protects against early alcohol-induced liver injury in the rat.**
  Author(s): McKim SE, Konno A, Gabele E, Uesugi T, Froh M, Sies H, Thurman RG, Arteel GE.
  Source: Archives of Biochemistry and Biophysics. 2002 October 1; 406(1): 40-6.
  http://www.ncbi.nlm.nih.gov:80/entrez/query.fcgi?cmd=Retrieve&db=PubMed&list_uids=12234488&dopt=Abstract

- **Cocoa products decrease low density lipoprotein oxidative susceptibility but do not affect biomarkers of inflammation in humans.**
  Author(s): Mathur S, Devaraj S, Grundy SM, Jialal I.
  Source: The Journal of Nutrition. 2002 December; 132(12): 3663-7.
  http://www.ncbi.nlm.nih.gov:80/entrez/query.fcgi?cmd=Retrieve&db=PubMed&list_uids=12468604&dopt=Abstract

- **Collaborative study of the International Office of Cocoa, Chocolate and Sugar Confectionery on Salmonella detection from cocoa and chocolate processing environmental samples.**
  Author(s): De Smedt JM, Chartron S, Cordier JL, Graff E, Hoekstra H, Lecoupeau JP, Lindblom M, Milas J, Morgan RM, Nowacki R, et al.
  Source: International Journal of Food Microbiology. 1991 August; 13(4): 301-8.
  http://www.ncbi.nlm.nih.gov:80/entrez/query.fcgi?cmd=Retrieve&db=PubMed&list_uids=1911087&dopt=Abstract

- **Comparison of the antioxidant activity of commonly consumed polyphenolic beverages (coffee, cocoa, and tea) prepared per cup serving.**
  Author(s): Richelle M, Tavazzi I, Offord E.
  Source: Journal of Agricultural and Food Chemistry. 2001 July; 49(7): 3438-42.
  http://www.ncbi.nlm.nih.gov:80/entrez/query.fcgi?cmd=Retrieve&db=PubMed&list_uids=11453788&dopt=Abstract

- **Composition of cocoa shell fat as related to cocoa butter.**
  Author(s): El-Saied HM, Morsi MK, Amer MM.
  Source: Zeitschrift Fur Ernahrungswissenschaft. 1981 June; 20(2): 145-51.
  http://www.ncbi.nlm.nih.gov:80/entrez/query.fcgi?cmd=Retrieve&db=PubMed&list_uids=7269661&dopt=Abstract

- **Consumption of tall oil-derived phytosterols in a chocolate matrix significantly decreases plasma total and low-density lipoprotein-cholesterol levels.**
  Author(s): De Graaf J, De Sauvage Nolting PR, Van Dam M, Belsey EM, Kastelein JJ, Haydn Pritchard P, Stalenhoef AF.
  Source: The British Journal of Nutrition. 2002 November; 88(5): 479-88.
  http://www.ncbi.nlm.nih.gov:80/entrez/query.fcgi?cmd=Retrieve&db=PubMed&list_uids=12425728&dopt=Abstract

- **Dietary flavanols and procyanidin oligomers from cocoa (Theobroma cacao) inhibit platelet function.**
  Author(s): Murphy KJ, Chronopoulos AK, Singh I, Francis MA, Moriarty H, Pike MJ, Turner AH, Mann NJ, Sinclair AJ.
  Source: The American Journal of Clinical Nutrition. 2003 June; 77(6): 1466-73.
  http://www.ncbi.nlm.nih.gov:80/entrez/query.fcgi?cmd=Retrieve&db=PubMed&list_uids=12791625&dopt=Abstract

- **Do we need to know how it works? Or doesn't chocolate just taste great?**
  Author(s): Rotchford JK.
  Source: Journal of Alternative and Complementary Medicine (New York, N.Y.). 2000 December; 6(6): 481-2.
  http://www.ncbi.nlm.nih.gov:80/entrez/query.fcgi?cmd=Retrieve&db=PubMed&list_uids=11152050&dopt=Abstract

- **Effect of cocoa bran on low-density lipoprotein oxidation and fecal bulking.**
  Author(s): Jenkins DJ, Kendall CW, Vuksan V, Vidgen E, Wong E, Augustin LS, Fulgoni V 3rd.
  Source: Archives of Internal Medicine. 2000 August 14-28; 160(15): 2374-9.
  http://www.ncbi.nlm.nih.gov:80/entrez/query.fcgi?cmd=Retrieve&db=PubMed&list_uids=10927737&dopt=Abstract

- **Effect on human longevity of added dietary chocolate.**
  Author(s): Kirschbaum J.
  Source: Nutrition (Burbank, Los Angeles County, Calif.). 1998 November-December; 14(11-12): 869.
  http://www.ncbi.nlm.nih.gov:80/entrez/query.fcgi?cmd=Retrieve&db=PubMed&list_uids=9834932&dopt=Abstract

- **Evidence that the antioxidant flavonoids in tea and cocoa are beneficial for cardiovascular health.**
  Author(s): Kris-Etherton PM, Keen CL.
  Source: Current Opinion in Lipidology. 2002 February; 13(1): 41-9. Review.
  http://www.ncbi.nlm.nih.gov:80/entrez/query.fcgi?cmd=Retrieve&db=PubMed&list_uids=11790962&dopt=Abstract

- **Flavanols and procyanidins of cocoa and chocolate inhibit growth and polyamine biosynthesis of human colonic cancer cells.**
  Author(s): Carnesecchi S, Schneider Y, Lazarus SA, Coehlo D, Gosse F, Raul F.
  Source: Cancer Letters. 2002 January 25; 175(2): 147-55.
  http://www.ncbi.nlm.nih.gov:80/entrez/query.fcgi?cmd=Retrieve&db=PubMed&list_uids=11741742&dopt=Abstract

- **Flavonoids of cocoa inhibit recombinant human 5-lipoxygenase.**
  Author(s): Schewe T, Kuhn H, Sies H.
  Source: The Journal of Nutrition. 2002 July; 132(7): 1825-9.
  http://www.ncbi.nlm.nih.gov:80/entrez/query.fcgi?cmd=Retrieve&db=PubMed&list_uids=12097654&dopt=Abstract

- **Food of the gods: cure for humanity? A cultural history of the medicinal and ritual use of chocolate.**
  Author(s): Dillinger TL, Barriga P, Escarcega S, Jimenez M, Salazar Lowe D, Grivetti LE.
  Source: The Journal of Nutrition. 2000 August; 130(8S Suppl): 2057S-72S.
  http://www.ncbi.nlm.nih.gov:80/entrez/query.fcgi?cmd=Retrieve&db=PubMed&list_uids=10917925&dopt=Abstract

- **In vitro pharmacological activity of the tetrahydroisoquinoline salsolinol present in products from Theobroma cacao L. like cocoa and chocolate.**
  Author(s): Melzig MF, Putscher I, Henklein P, Haber H.
  Source: Journal of Ethnopharmacology. 2000 November; 73(1-2): 153-9.
  http://www.ncbi.nlm.nih.gov:80/entrez/query.fcgi?cmd=Retrieve&db=PubMed&list_uids=11025151&dopt=Abstract

- **Liquid chromatographic/electrospray ionization tandem mass spectrometric study of the phenolic composition of cocoa (Theobroma cacao).**
  Author(s): Sanchez-Rabaneda F, Jauregui O, Casals I, Andres-Lacueva C, Izquierdo-Pulido M, Lamuela-Raventos RM.
  Source: Journal of Mass Spectrometry : Jms. 2003 January; 38(1): 35-42.
  http://www.ncbi.nlm.nih.gov:80/entrez/query.fcgi?cmd=Retrieve&db=PubMed&list_uids=12526004&dopt=Abstract

- **Rate of dehydration and cumulative desiccation stress interacted to modulate desiccation tolerance of recalcitrant cocoa and ginkgo embryonic tissues.**
  Author(s): Liang Y, Sun WQ.
  Source: Plant Physiology. 2002 April; 128(4): 1323-31.
  http://www.ncbi.nlm.nih.gov:80/entrez/query.fcgi?cmd=Retrieve&db=PubMed&list_uids=11950981&dopt=Abstract

- **Scientists say chocolate might be sweet for hearts.**
  Author(s): Spake A.
  Source: U.S. News & World Report. 2000 February 28; 128(8): 78.
  http://www.ncbi.nlm.nih.gov:80/entrez/query.fcgi?cmd=Retrieve&db=PubMed&list_uids=11184123&dopt=Abstract

- **The influence of dietary tea, coffee and cocoa on protein and energy utilization of soya-bean meal and barley in rats.**
  Author(s): Eggum BO, Pedersen B, Jacobsen I.
  Source: The British Journal of Nutrition. 1983 September; 50(2): 197-205.
  http://www.ncbi.nlm.nih.gov:80/entrez/query.fcgi?cmd=Retrieve&db=PubMed&list_uids=6684477&dopt=Abstract

- **Toxicity of jimson weed seed and cocoa shell meal to broilers.**
  Author(s): Day EJ, Dilworth BC.
  Source: Poultry Science. 1984 March; 63(3): 466-8.
  http://www.ncbi.nlm.nih.gov:80/entrez/query.fcgi?cmd=Retrieve&db=PubMed&list_uids=6718300&dopt=Abstract

- **Wholesomeness of irradiated cocoa beans. The effect of gamma irradiation on the chemical constituents of cocoa beans.**
  Author(s): Takyi EE, Amuh IK.
  Source: Journal of Agricultural and Food Chemistry. 1979 September-October; 27(5): 979-82.
  http://www.ncbi.nlm.nih.gov:80/entrez/query.fcgi?cmd=Retrieve&db=PubMed&list_uids=546960&dopt=Abstract

Additional Web Resources

A number of additional Web sites offer encyclopedic information covering CAM and related topics. The following is a representative sample:

- Alternative Medicine Foundation, Inc.: **http://www.herbmed.org/**

- AOL: **http://search.aol.com/cat.adp?id=169&layer=&from=subcats**

- Chinese Medicine: **http://www.newcenturynutrition.com/**

- drkoop.com®: **http://www.drkoop.com/InteractiveMedicine/IndexC.html**

- Family Village: **http://www.familyvillage.wisc.edu/med_altn.htm**

- Google: **http://directory.google.com/Top/Health/Alternative/**

- Healthnotes: **http://www.healthnotes.com/**

- MedWebPlus:
  http://medwebplus.com/subject/Alternative_and_Complementary_Medicine

- Open Directory Project: **http://dmoz.org/Health/Alternative/**

- HealthGate: **http://www.tnp.com/**

- WebMD®Health: **http://my.webmd.com/drugs_and_herbs**

- WholeHealthMD.com: **http://www.wholehealthmd.com/reflib/0,1529,,00.html**

- Yahoo.com: **http://dir.yahoo.com/Health/Alternative_Medicine/**

The following is a specific Web list relating to chocolate; please note that any particular subject below may indicate either a therapeutic use, or a contraindication (potential danger), and does not reflect an official recommendation (some Web sites are subscription based):

- **General Overview**

  Acne Vulgaris
  Source: Healthnotes, Inc. www.healthnotes.com

  Allergic Reaction, Angioedema
  Source: Integrative Medicine Communications; www.drkoop.com

  Allergic Rhinitis
  Source: Integrative Medicine Communications; www.drkoop.com

Allergies and Sensitivities
Source: Healthnotes, Inc. www.healthnotes.com

Alzheimer's Disease
Source: Healthnotes, Inc. www.healthnotes.com

Amenorrhea
Source: Integrative Medicine Communications; www.drkoop.com

Angioedema
Source: Integrative Medicine Communications; www.drkoop.com

Anxiety
Source: Healthnotes, Inc. www.healthnotes.com

Arthritis, Rheumatoid
Source: Integrative Medicine Communications; www.drkoop.com

Birth Defects Prevention
Source: Healthnotes, Inc. www.healthnotes.com

Breast Cancer
Source: Integrative Medicine Communications; www.drkoop.com

Burns
Source: Integrative Medicine Communications; www.drkoop.com

Cold Sores
Source: Healthnotes, Inc. www.healthnotes.com

Cold Sores
Source: Integrative Medicine Communications; www.drkoop.com

Cyclic Mastalgia
Alternative names: Cyclic Mastitis, Fibrocystic Breast Disease
Source: Prima Communications, Inc.www.personalhealthzone.com

Diarrhea
Source: Integrative Medicine Communications; www.drkoop.com

Dysmenorrhea
Source: Integrative Medicine Communications; www.drkoop.com

Endometriosis
Source: Integrative Medicine Communications; www.drkoop.com

Female Infertility
Source: Healthnotes, Inc. www.healthnotes.com

Fibrocystic Breast Disease
Source: Healthnotes, Inc. www.healthnotes.com

Gastritis
Source: Healthnotes, Inc. www.healthnotes.com

Gastroesophageal Reflux Disease
Source: Healthnotes, Inc. www.healthnotes.com

Gastroesophageal Reflux Disease
Source: Integrative Medicine Communications; www.drkoop.com

Genital Herpes
Source: Healthnotes, Inc. www.healthnotes.com

Hay Fever
Source: Integrative Medicine Communications; www.drkoop.com

Headache, Migraine
Source: Integrative Medicine Communications; www.drkoop.com

Headache, Tension
Source: Integrative Medicine Communications; www.drkoop.com

Heartburn
Source: Integrative Medicine Communications; www.drkoop.com

Herpes
Alternative names: Genital Herpes, Cold Sores
Source: Prima Communications, Inc.www.personalhealthzone.com

Herpes Simplex Virus
Source: Integrative Medicine Communications; www.drkoop.com

Hives
Source: Healthnotes, Inc. www.healthnotes.com

Hypoparathyroidism
Source: Integrative Medicine Communications; www.drkoop.com

Hypothermia
Source: Integrative Medicine Communications; www.drkoop.com

Inflammatory Bowel Disease
Source: Integrative Medicine Communications; www.drkoop.com

Insomnia
Source: Healthnotes, Inc. www.healthnotes.com

Kidney Stones
Source: Healthnotes, Inc. www.healthnotes.com

Kidney Stones
Source: Integrative Medicine Communications; www.drkoop.com

Liver Cirrhosis
Source: Healthnotes, Inc. www.healthnotes.com

Lupus
Source: Integrative Medicine Communications; www.drkoop.com

Menstrual Pain
Source: Integrative Medicine Communications; www.drkoop.com

Menstruation, Absence of
Source: Integrative Medicine Communications; www.drkoop.com

Migraine Headache
Source: Integrative Medicine Communications; www.drkoop.com

Migraine Headaches
Source: Prima Communications, Inc.www.personalhealthzone.com

Multiple Sclerosis
Source: Integrative Medicine Communications; www.drkoop.com

Osteoporosis
Source: Healthnotes, Inc. www.healthnotes.com

Parathyroid, Underactive
Source: Integrative Medicine Communications; www.drkoop.com

PMS
Source: Integrative Medicine Communications; www.drkoop.com

Post Traumatic Stress Disorder
Source: Integrative Medicine Communications; www.drkoop.com

Premenstrual Syndrome
Source: Integrative Medicine Communications; www.drkoop.com

PTSD
Source: Integrative Medicine Communications; www.drkoop.com

Rheumatoid Arthritis
Source: Integrative Medicine Communications; www.drkoop.com

Rhinitis, Allergic
Source: Integrative Medicine Communications; www.drkoop.com

Shingles and Postherpetic Neuralgia
Source: Healthnotes, Inc. www.healthnotes.com

Systemic Lupus Erythematosus
Source: Integrative Medicine Communications; www.drkoop.com

Tension Headache
Source: Integrative Medicine Communications; www.drkoop.com

Ulcerative Colitis
Source: Integrative Medicine Communications; www.drkoop.com

- **Alternative Therapy**

   Chocolate Therapy
   Source: The Canoe version of A Dictionary of Alternative-Medicine Methods, by
   Priorities for Health editor Jack Raso, M.S., R.D.
   Hyperlink: http://www.canoe.ca/AltmedDictionary/c.html

- **Herbs and Supplements**

   Arginine
   Source: Healthnotes, Inc. www.healthnotes.com

   Arginine
   Source: Prima Communications, Inc.www.personalhealthzone.com

   Carob
   Source: Healthnotes, Inc. www.healthnotes.com

   Catechins
   Source: WholeHealthMD.com, LLC. www.wholehealthmd.com
   Hyperlink:
   http://www.wholehealthmd.com/refshelf/substances_view/0,1525,1023,00.html

   Cinnamomum
   Alternative names: Cinnamon; Cinnamomum zeylanicum
   Source: Alternative Medicine Foundation, Inc. www.amfoundation.org

   Hibiscus
   Alternative names: Hibiscus, Roselle; Hibiscus sp.
   Source: Alternative Medicine Foundation, Inc. www.amfoundation.org

   Luffa
   Alternative names: Luffa sp.
   Source: Alternative Medicine Foundation, Inc. www.amfoundation.org

   Lysine
   Source: Prima Communications, Inc.www.personalhealthzone.com

   Lysine
   Source: WholeHealthMD.com, LLC. www.wholehealthmd.com
   Hyperlink:
   http://www.wholehealthmd.com/refshelf/substances_view/0,1525,862,00.html

Origanum
Alternative names: Oregano; Origanum vulgare
Source: Alternative Medicine Foundation, Inc. www.amfoundation.org

Phenylalanine
Source: Integrative Medicine Communications; www.drkoop.com

Piper nigrum
Alternative names: Black Pepper
Source: Alternative Medicine Foundation, Inc. www.amfoundation.org

Trigonella
Alternative names: Fenugreek; Trigonella foenum graecum L.
Source: Alternative Medicine Foundation, Inc. www.amfoundation.org

Yohimbe
Source: WholeHealthMD.com, LLC. www.wholehealthmd.com
Hyperlink:
http://www.wholehealthmd.com/refshelf/substances_view/0,1525,830,00.html

General References

A good place to find general background information on CAM is the National Library of Medicine. It has prepared within the MEDLINEplus system an information topic page dedicated to complementary and alternative medicine. To access this page, go to the MEDLINEplus site at **http://www.nlm.nih.gov/medlineplus/alternativemedicine.html**. This Web site provides a general overview of various topics and can lead to a number of general sources.

CHAPTER 4. DISSERTATIONS ON CHOCOLATE

Overview

In this chapter, we will give you a bibliography on recent dissertations relating to chocolate. We will also provide you with information on how to use the Internet to stay current on dissertations. **IMPORTANT NOTE:** When following the search strategy described below, you may discover <u>non-medical dissertations</u> that use the generic term "chocolate" (or a synonym) in their titles. To accurately reflect the results that you might find while conducting research on chocolate, <u>we have not necessarily excluded non-medical dissertations</u> in this bibliography.

Dissertations on Chocolate

ProQuest Digital Dissertations, the largest archive of academic dissertations available, is located at the following Web address: **http://wwwlib.umi.com/dissertations**. From this archive, we have compiled the following list covering dissertations devoted to chocolate. You will see that the information provided includes the dissertation's title, its author, and the institution with which the author is associated. The following covers recent dissertations found when using this search procedure:

- **Brazil's Chocolate Forest: Environmental and Economic Roles of Conservation in Bahia's Cocoa Agroecosystem** by Johns, Norman Denny, Jr., Phd from The University of Texas at Austin, 1996, 248 pages
  http://wwwlib.umi.com/dissertations/fullcit/9719391

- **The Influence of Surfactants and Moisture on the Colloidal and Rheological Properties of Model Chocolate Dispersions** by Garbolino, Chiara; Phd from The Pennsylvania State University, 2002, 139 pages
  http://wwwlib.umi.com/dissertations/fullcit/3064917

Keeping Current

Ask the medical librarian at your library if it has full and unlimited access to the *ProQuest Digital Dissertations* database. From the library, you should be able to do more complete searches via **http://wwwlib.umi.com/dissertations**.

CHAPTER 5. CLINICAL TRIALS AND CHOCOLATE

Overview

In this chapter, we will show you how to keep informed of the latest clinical trials concerning chocolate.

Recent Trials on Chocolate

The following is a list of recent trials dedicated to chocolate.[8] Further information on a trial is available at the Web site indicated.

- **Effects of Kava on the Body's Elimination of Caffeine and Dextromethorphan**

   Condition(s): Healthy

   Study Status: This study is completed.

   Sponsor(s): Warren G Magnuson Clinical Center (CC)

   Purpose - Excerpt: This study will examine how kava-a widely used herbal remedy-may affect the body's elimination of other medicines. Many people take kava to reduce anxiety or cause sedation. Since this product is considered a food supplement and not a drug, it is not subject to the rigorous pre-market testing required for prescription and over-the-counter (OTC) drugs. As a result, information has not been collected on possible interactions between kava and other medications. This study will look at how kava affects the elimination of caffeine-a compound commonly found in **chocolate**, coffee, tea and soft drinks-and dextromethorphan-an OTC cough suppressant. Normal healthy volunteers 21 years of age or older may be eligible for this 30-day study. Candidates will provide a medical history and undergo a physical examination and routine blood tests. Women of childbearing age will have a urine pregnancy test. Study participants will not drink alcoholic beverages or take any medications (except those given in the study) for 2 weeks prior to the study and throughout its duration. In addition, they will abstain from caffeine, grapefruit and grapefruit juice and charbroiled foods for at least 72 hours before and throughout each study day that urine is collected. On day 1 of the study, study subjects will take one dose each of caffeine and dextromethorphan at 4:00 P.M.. They will empty their bladder before the dosing and

---

[8] These are listed at **www.ClinicalTrials.gov**.

then collect all their urine after the dosing for the rest of the day and including the next mornings first urine. They will bring the urine samples to the Clinical Center when the collection is complete. This procedure will be repeated 1 week later (study day 8). After the second urine collection is completed, subjects will take 200 milligrams of kava 3 times a day for 21 days. On study day 29 (after 21 days of kava), subjects will repeat the dextromethorphan and caffeine dosing and urine collection described above, while continuing to take kava. Subjects will have an electroencephalograph (EEG) done before starting kava and again at the end of kava (study day 30). For this procedure, several electrodes (metal cups attached to wires) are secured to the scalp with a glue-like substance. A conductive gel fills the space between the electrode and the scalp to ensure good contact. The electrodes will remain in place for about 2 hours and then removed. The subject lies quietly on a bed during the EEG recording. Participation in the study will end with another physical examination and blood tests following the second EEG and urine collection.

Phase(s): Phase IV; MEDLINEplus consumer health information

Study Type: Interventional

Contact(s): see Web site below

Web Site: http://clinicaltrials.gov/ct/show/NCT00009542

Keeping Current on Clinical Trials

The U.S. National Institutes of Health, through the National Library of Medicine, has developed ClinicalTrials.gov to provide current information about clinical research across the broadest number of diseases and conditions.

The site was launched in February 2000 and currently contains approximately 5,700 clinical studies in over 59,000 locations worldwide, with most studies being conducted in the United States. ClinicalTrials.gov receives about 2 million hits per month and hosts approximately 5,400 visitors daily. To access this database, simply go to the Web site at **http://www.clinicaltrials.gov/** and search by "chocolate" (or synonyms).

While ClinicalTrials.gov is the most comprehensive listing of NIH-supported clinical trials available, not all trials are in the database. The database is updated regularly, so clinical trials are continually being added. The following is a list of specialty databases affiliated with the National Institutes of Health that offer additional information on trials:

- For clinical studies at the Warren Grant Magnuson Clinical Center located in Bethesda, Maryland, visit their Web site: **http://clinicalstudies.info.nih.gov/**

- For clinical studies conducted at the Bayview Campus in Baltimore, Maryland, visit their Web site: **http://www.jhbmc.jhu.edu/studies/index.html**

- For cancer trials, visit the National Cancer Institute: **http://cancertrials.nci.nih.gov/**

- For eye-related trials, visit and search the Web page of the National Eye Institute: **http://www.nei.nih.gov/neitrials/index.htm**

- For heart, lung and blood trials, visit the Web page of the National Heart, Lung and Blood Institute: **http://www.nhlbi.nih.gov/studies/index.htm**

- For trials on aging, visit and search the Web site of the National Institute on Aging: **http://www.grc.nia.nih.gov/studies/index.htm**

- For rare diseases, visit and search the Web site sponsored by the Office of Rare Diseases: **http://ord.aspensys.com/asp/resources/rsch_trials.asp**

- For alcoholism, visit the National Institute on Alcohol Abuse and Alcoholism: **http://www.niaaa.nih.gov/intramural/Web_dicbr_hp/particip.htm**

- For trials on infectious, immune, and allergic diseases, visit the site of the National Institute of Allergy and Infectious Diseases: **http://www.niaid.nih.gov/clintrials/**

- For trials on arthritis, musculoskeletal and skin diseases, visit newly revised site of the National Institute of Arthritis and Musculoskeletal and Skin Diseases of the National Institutes of Health: **http://www.niams.nih.gov/hi/studies/index.htm**

- For hearing-related trials, visit the National Institute on Deafness and Other Communication Disorders: **http://www.nidcd.nih.gov/health/clinical/index.htm**

- For trials on diseases of the digestive system and kidneys, and diabetes, visit the National Institute of Diabetes and Digestive and Kidney Diseases: **http://www.niddk.nih.gov/patient/patient.htm**

- For drug abuse trials, visit and search the Web site sponsored by the National Institute on Drug Abuse: **http://www.nida.nih.gov/CTN/Index.htm**

- For trials on mental disorders, visit and search the Web site of the National Institute of Mental Health: **http://www.nimh.nih.gov/studies/index.cfm**

- For trials on neurological disorders and stroke, visit and search the Web site sponsored by the National Institute of Neurological Disorders and Stroke of the NIH: **http://www.ninds.nih.gov/funding/funding_opportunities.htm#Clinical_Trials**

CHAPTER 6. PATENTS ON CHOCOLATE

Overview

Patents can be physical innovations (e.g. chemicals, pharmaceuticals, medical equipment) or processes (e.g. treatments or diagnostic procedures). The United States Patent and Trademark Office defines a patent as a grant of a property right to the inventor, issued by the Patent and Trademark Office.[9] Patents, therefore, are intellectual property. For the United States, the term of a new patent is 20 years from the date when the patent application was filed. If the inventor wishes to receive economic benefits, it is likely that the invention will become commercially available within 20 years of the initial filing. It is important to understand, therefore, that an inventor's patent does not indicate that a product or service is or will be commercially available. The patent implies only that the inventor has "the right to exclude others from making, using, offering for sale, or selling" the invention in the United States. While this relates to U.S. patents, similar rules govern foreign patents.

In this chapter, we show you how to locate information on patents and their inventors. If you find a patent that is particularly interesting to you, contact the inventor or the assignee for further information. **IMPORTANT NOTE:** When following the search strategy described below, you may discover non-medical patents that use the generic term "chocolate" (or a synonym) in their titles. To accurately reflect the results that you might find while conducting research on chocolate, we have not necessarily excluded non-medical patents in this bibliography.

Patents on Chocolate

By performing a patent search focusing on chocolate, you can obtain information such as the title of the invention, the names of the inventor(s), the assignee(s) or the company that owns or controls the patent, a short abstract that summarizes the patent, and a few excerpts from the description of the patent. The abstract of a patent tends to be more technical in nature, while the description is often written for the public. Full patent descriptions contain much more information than is presented here (e.g. claims, references, figures, diagrams, etc.). We

---

[9] Adapted from the United States Patent and Trademark Office:
http://www.uspto.gov/web/offices/pac/doc/general/whatis.htm.

will tell you how to obtain this information later in the chapter. The following is an example of the type of information that you can expect to obtain from a patent search on chocolate:

- **A blooming resistant chocolate**

  Inventor(s): Yokobori; Hideo (Tokyo, JP), Itagaki; Kazuo (Tokyo, JP), Maruzeni; Shouji (Tokyo, JP), Yasuda; Nozomi (Tokyo, JP)

  Assignee(s): Asahi Denka Kogyo Kabushiki Kaisha (Tokyo, JP)

  Patent Number: 4,847,105

  Date filed: February 25, 1987

  Abstract: A hard butter of the present invention is obtained by adding 0.05 to 20% by weight of polyglycerol fatty acid ester(s), which is prepared by binding four or more moles in average of fatty acid(s) to polyglycerol(s) having five or more in average of hydroxyl groups, to a hard butter. With the use of the hard butter of the present invention, the anti-blooming properties of a chocolate are enhanced with little limitation on the composition of the same. In particular, chocolates containing trans and lauric hard butters can be more freely compounded thereby than in the case of conventional ones.

  Excerpt(s): This invention relates to a hard butter and a chocolate of excellent qualities. More particularly, it relates to a hard butter and a chocolate highly resistant to blooming. That is, the hard butter of the present invention can remarkably enhance the antiblooming properties of chocolates and chocolate products. Thus the chocolate of the present invention which contains said hard butter is made available with a wider range of composition which can hardly be achieved with the use of conventional ones.... Conventional processes for maintaining the gloss of the surface of a chocolate include compounding of various emulsifiers or particular fats and/or oils. However there has been found no remarkable effect obtained by using any emulsifiers. On the other hand, the compounding of particular fats and/or oils and the elevation of the melting points of fats and/or oils, as described above, are somewhat effective in maintaining the gloss of the surface of a chocolate, i.e., in improving the anti-blooming properties thereof. However these processes highly restrict the composition of products, since it is required to compound a large amount of fats and/or oils in order to maintain the gloss of the surface of the products.... Further the composition of chocolate products is frequently limited from the viewpoint of the antiblooming properties. It is particularly difficult to freely compound those containing trans and lauric hard butters. Namely, it is extremely difficult to compound conventional trans hard butter in a chocolate less than 85% by weight based on the total oleaginous components thereof except milk fat. Namely, it is extremely difficult to compound more than 15% by weight of cacao butter thereto based on the total oleaginous components thereof except milk fat. Fat blooming would readily occur in the case of a product wherein cacao butter is used in an amount exceeding the above value, which damages the commercial value thereof. Further it is extremely difficult to compound conventional lauric hard butter in a chocolate less than 95% by weight based on the total oleaginous components thereof except milk fat. That is, it is extremely difficult to compound more than 5% by weight of cacao butter thereto based on the total oleaginous components thereof except milk fat. Thus conventional chocolate products usually contain 4% by weight or less of cacao butter. Fat blooming would readily occur in the case of a product wherein cacao butter is used in an amount exceeding the above value, which damages the commercial value thereof.

  Web site: http://www.delphion.com/details?pn=US04847105__

- **Anti-blooming composition, and laurin fat and chocolate containing the same**

Inventor(s): Hokuyo; Kosuke (Osaka-fu, JP), Hayashi; Miho (Osaka-fu, JP), Yamaguchi; Shuichi (Osaka-fu, JP), Izumi; Tsugio (Osaka-fu, JP)

Assignee(s): Fuji Oil Company, Limited (Osaka-fu, JP)

Patent Number: 5,609,906

Date filed: March 9, 1995

Abstract: An anti-blooming composition which comprises a fatty acid monoglyceride composed of a fatty acid having 16 carbon atoms (A) and a fatty acid monoglyceride composed of a fatty acid having 18 carbon atoms (B), a weight ratio of A/B being 30/70 or larger is disclosed. A laurin fat and laurin fat chocolate containing the above anti-blooming composition is also disclosed.

Excerpt(s): The present invention relates to an anti-blooming composition, particularly, that suitable for preventing fat blooming of laurin fats and a laurin fat and chocolate containing the same.... In general, the quality of chocolate is greatly influenced by the raw materials used and various production conditions and, in particular, sufficient care should be taken not to form fat blooming which stains the surface of a product in off-white during its storage, resulting in loss of commercial value of the product.... A laurin fat, the main constituent fatty acid of which is lauric acid having 12 carbon atoms, has been known to be a raw material fat for the production of chocolate which does not require a tempering operation and, in addition to the production of bar chocolate, it has been used for the production of chocolate for coating cakes, doughnuts, biscuits and the like by blending suitable other oils and fats. However, the problem of fat blooming is still present.

Web site: http://www.delphion.com/details?pn=US05609906__

- **Apparatus comprising a tempering column for continuous tempering of fat-containing chocolate-like masses with improved stirring**

Inventor(s): Aasted; Lars (Charlottenlund, DK)

Assignee(s): Aasted Mikroverk ApS (Farum, DK)

Patent Number: 5,899,562

Date filed: May 8, 1997

Abstract: The invention concerns an apparatus having a cylindrical tempering column comprising a cooling stage and a subsequent reheating stage for continuous tempering of a fat-containing, chocolate-like mass. A plurality of interconnected mass chambers are separated by intermediary heat exchange chambers. The mass chambers comprise mixing and stirring elements (8) with radially extending, plate shaped arms (11) comprising plate shaped mixing blades (13, 14, 15, 16; 17, 18, 19, 20). According to the invention, an opening (24) for flow of the chocolate mass therethrough is arranged in the plate shaped arm (11) at a part of the arm located between the inner mixing blade (13; 17) and the hub. Hereby is provided an axial flow of the mass close to the drive shaft, so that nests and zones of no stirring in the mass are avoided around the shaft, especially where the plate shaped arm is connected with the hub. The total surface area of the plate shaped arms (11) and of the mixing blades (13, 14, 15, 16; 17, 18, 19, 20) may decrease gradually in direction out towards the peripheral cylinder wall. Hereby is achieved a considerable more uniform stirring of the mass at all areas of the chamber followed by an enhanced heat transport in the mass than was possible with the prior temperers.

Excerpt(s): The invention concerns the field of apparatuses having a cylindrical tempering column comprising a cooling stage and a subsequent reheating stage for continuous tempering of a fat-containing, chocolate-like mass pumped therethrough, which tempering column further comprise a plurality of interconnected mass chambers, which are separated by intermediary heat exchange chambers adapted to absorb heat from the mass chambers or to submit heat to the mass chambers during flow of cooling media through the cooling stage or flow of heating media through the reheating stage, respectively. The mass chambers further comprise mixing and stirring elements, which are rotated by the action of a common, central drive shaft arranged in the column. The mixing and stirring elements further comprise at least one radially extending, plate shaped arm comprising upper and lower, essentially vertically extending, plate shaped mixing blades, and which upper mixing blades extend radially opposite to the extension of the lower mixing blades, seen in the direction of rotation of the mixing and stirring elements or in the opposite direction, respectively.... The persons skilled within the above mentioned field of apparatuses for tempering have since long been observant to the fact, that the most optimal heat exchange between the mass and the heat exchange chambers during the flow of the mass through the column, is obtained when a good and uniform stirring of the mass is achieved in all parts and zones of a mass chamber.... Though, for several decades it has been known to provide the plate shaped arms of the mixing and stirring elements with mixing blades, which extend along the radial leading or trailing edge of the plate shaped arm for the provision of forceful, radial flow of the chocolate mass in towards the centre of the mass chamber, and half a turn later again flow out towards the peripheral cylinder wall of the chamber--mass movements, which continuously shifts between an ingoing and an outgoing radial flow when the mass being pumped through the chamber in question.

Web site: http://www.delphion.com/details?pn=US05899562__

- **Apparatus for coating foods, such as sweets, baked goods and the like, with flowable coating substances, such as chocolate and other icings**

Inventor(s): Koch; Peter (Pinneberg, DE), de Koomen; Joost J. (Mechanicsburg, PA)

Assignee(s): Hosokawa Kreuter GmbH (Hamburg, DE)

Patent Number: 5,954,876

Date filed: May 4, 1998

Abstract: An apparatus for coating foods, such as sweets, baked goods and the like, with flowable coating substances, such as chocolate and other icings. The apparatus includes an endless conveyor belt for the coated goods or the goods to be coated and a run-off plate arranged underneath the conveyor belt for excess coating substance. A catch container is provided for receiving the excess coating substance from the run-off plate. A separate scraping belt for removing excess coating substance or scraping the run-off plate is provided underneath the conveyor belt and above the run-off plate.

Excerpt(s): The present invention relates to an apparatus for coating foods, such as sweets, baked goods and the like, with flowable coating substances, such as chocolate and other icings. The apparatus includes an endless conveyor belt for the coated goods or the goods to be coated and a run-off plate arranged underneath the conveyor belt for excess coating substance. A catch container is provided for receiving the excess coating substance from the run-off plate.... Various constructions of the above-described apparatus are known in the art. They are also called coating or icing machines and are used in the production of bars, pralines, waffles, ice cream, sugar products, baked goods with long shelf lives or fine baked goods, snacks or also fat-free articles. The coating usually consists, for example, of chocolate, caramel, cocoa, icings, icings of shortening or sugar. The coating process is carried out in the liquid state. Following the coating process, the coating substance is cooled and dried to reach the solid state.... In the known apparatus of the above-described type, a conveyor belt is provided which is composed of a braided material or also of belts. Preferably, they are belts of rod braiding. Devices which apply the coating substance to the goods from above and below are arranged above and below the conveyor belt and, thus, above and below the goods to be coated. An excess amount of substance is applied, i.e., more substance is applied than is required for coating the goods. This excess coating substance then drops between the goods, or the coating substance is blown off. The excess substance is collected in a catch container and is returned to be reused. A slightly inclined run-off plate leads to the catch container.

Web site: http://www.delphion.com/details?pn=US05954876__

- **Apparatus for continuous tempering of chocolate-like mass**

  Inventor(s): Haslund; Henning (Bj.ae butted.verskov, DK)

  Assignee(s): Aasted-Mikroverk ApS (Farum, DK)

  Patent Number: 6,105,489

  Date filed: March 15, 1999

  Abstract: The invention concerns an apparatus for continuously tempering a fat containing chocolate mass, whereby the mass is subjected to a primary cooling, a subsequent secondary cooling creating crystals in the mass, and a final reheating.

  Excerpt(s): The invention concerns a method of continuously tempering a fat-containing, chocolate-like mass, whereby the mass is subjected to a primary cooling, a subsequent secondary cooling creating crystals in the mass, and a final reheating.... The invention further concerns an apparatus for continuous tempering of a fat-containing, chocolate-like mass, comprising a primary cooling section, a subsequent secondary cooling section in which crystals are created in the mass, and a final reheating section.... For many years, the method has been used extensively for production of a great variety of chocolate-like masses. Before tempering, the chocolate-like mass is warmed up to around 40-60.degree. C. After tempering, the mass typically has a temperature of around 29-33.degree. C., whereafter it is being used for many purposes, such as being filled in moulds, deposited on top of other articles, etc.

  Web site: http://www.delphion.com/details?pn=US06105489__

- **Apparatus for continuous tempering of fat-containing, chocolate masses**

  Inventor(s): Aasted; Lars (Charlottenlund, DK)

  Assignee(s): Aasted Mikroverk ApS (Farum, DK)

  Patent Number: 5,850,782

  Date filed: May 8, 1997

Abstract: An apparatus having a cylindrical tempering column comprising a cooling stage and a subsequent reheating stage for continuous tempering of a fat-containing, chocolate-like mass. A plurality of Interconnected mass chambers are separated by intermediary heat exchange chambers. The mass chambers comprise mixing and stirring elements (8) with radially extending, plate shaped arms (11) comprising plate shaped mixing blades (13, 14, 15, 16; 17, 18, 19, 20). An upper or lower mixing blade (16; 20) arranged at the peripheral end of the mixing and stirring element (8) has a vertically extending end surface (27), thereby providing a shear gap between the end surface (27) and the cylinder wall (28). Thus the effect of a shear is provided at the comparatively large surface area at the cylinder wall and a considerable increase of the total area of the shear gaps is obtained. Furthermore, the total surface area of the plate shaped arms (11) and of the mixing blades (13, 14, 15, 16; 17, 18, 19, 20) may decrease gradually in direction out towards the peripheral cylinder wall. Hereby is achieved a considerable more uniform stirring of the mass at all areas of the chamber followed by an enhanced heat transport in the mass.

Excerpt(s): The invention concerns the field of apparatuses having a cylindrical tempering column comprising a cooling stage and a subsequent reheating stage for continuous tempering of a fat-containing, chocolate-like mass pumped therethrough, which tempering column further comprises a plurality of interconnected mass chambers, which are separated by intermediary heat exchange chambers adapted to absorb heat from the mass chambers or to submit heat to the mass chambers during flow of cooling media through the cooling stage or flow of heating media through the reheating stage, respectively. The mass chambers further comprise mixing and stirring elements, which are rotated by the action of a common, central drive shaft arranged in the column. The mixing and stirring elements further comprise at least one radially extending, plate shaped arm comprising upper and lower, essentially vertically extending, plate shaped mixing blades, and which upper mixing blades extend radially opposite to the extension of the lower mixing blades, seen in the direction of rotation of the mixing and stirring elements or in the opposite direction, respectively.... The persons skilled within the above mentioned field of apparatuses for tempering have since long been observant to the fact, that the most optimal heat exchange between the mass and the heat exchange chambers during the flow of the mass through the column, is obtained when a good and uniform stirring of the mass is achieved in all parts of a mass chamber.... Though, for several decades it has been known to provide the plate shaped arms of the mixing and stirring elements with mixing blades, which extends along the radial leading or trailing edge of the plate shaped arm for the provision of forceful, radial flow of the chocolate mass in towards the centre of the mass chamber, and half a turn later again flow out towards the peripheral cylinder wall of the chamber--mass movements, which continuously shift between an ingoing and an outgoing radial flow.

Web site: http://www.delphion.com/details?pn=US05850782__

- **Apparatus for continuously and automatically molding chocolate block having ornamental relief pattern**

  Inventor(s): Akutagawa; Tokuji (Tokyo, JP)

  Assignee(s): Akutagawa Confectionery Co., Ltd. (Tokyo, JP)

  Patent Number: 4,501,544

  Date filed: December 7, 1983

Abstract: An apparatus for automatically molding a chocolate block is provided according to the invention. The chocolate block includes an ornamental relief pattern made of first chocolate material of one color and a body portion carrying the relief pattern and made of a second chocolate material of different color. The chocolate block is produced by combining a first mold for molding the first chocolate material and a second mold for molding the second chocolate material. The second chocolate material adhering on the face of the first mold is cleaned by cleaner means such as a roller, scraper or a rinsing chamber.

Excerpt(s): The present invention relates to an apparatus for molding chocolate, and particularly to an apparatus for molding chocolate blocks each including an ornamental relief pattern made of a first chocolate material of one color and a body portion carrying the ornamental relief pattern and made of a second chocolate material of different color through a continuous automation system.... In a known process for molding a chocolate block having an ornamental relief pattern, a first chocolate material for forming the ornamental relief pattern is heated to be fluidized and then cast into a first or lower mold having a smooth top face and one or more engraved mold cavities forming the ornamental relief patterns, such as desired design or letters. After scraping the top face of the first mold, the first chocolate material is cooled at some extent, and a second or upper mold having one or more through-openings is placed on the first mold. Before the first chocolate material contained in the engraved mold cavities of the first mold is not yet solidified, a second chocolate material having color different from that of the first chocolate material is heated to be fluidized and then cast into the through-openings of the second mold. After he first and second chocolate materials are crystallized and solidified, the upper or second mold is separated from the lower or first mold to remove the molded chocolate block from the combined molds.... However, in the known process, the fluidized second chocolate material tends to penetrate into the gap inevitably formed at the interface between the top face of the lower mold and the bottom frace of the upper mold. The penetrating second chocolate material having the color and quality different from those of the first chocolate material adheres on the top face of the first mold, and the thus adhering second chocolate material is mixed with the first chocolate material at the scraping step of the next operation cycle, thereby to deteriorate the quality and appearance of the product chocolate block, resulting in loss of commercial value of the product. In the conventional process, the residual second chocolate material adhering on the top face of the lower mold surrounding the engraved cavities for molding he ornamental relief pattern is removed by manual operations. However, such manual operations are time consuming and ineffective.

Web site: http://www.delphion.com/details?pn=US04501544__

- **Apparatus for continuously conching chocolate mass**

  Inventor(s): Callebaut; Frans (Bambrugge, BE), Bruyland; Rudy (Herdersem/Aalst, BE)

  Assignee(s): Callebaut N.V. (Lebbeke-Wieze, BE)

  Patent Number: 5,320,427

  Date filed: September 28, 1992

  Abstract: In the continuous conching of chocolate mass in a conche (10) it is important to ensure essentially constant contents of the conche (10). For this purpose, the infeed of starting material and/or the discharge of the conched chocolate mass is monitored, namely measured, especially by means of weighing. In response to the measurement results, the infeed or the discharge is controlled, especially by means of altering the conveying capacity of a compulsory conveyor (screw conveyor 21) for discharging the conched mass. The conched chocolate mass is dry, i.e. it contains neither lecithin nor cocoa butter. Lecithin is added in the region of the screw conveyor (21) which is followed by a mixing device (22).

Excerpt(s): The invention relates to a process for continuously conching chocolate (starting) mass in a conche, into which starting material is continuously introduced and from which, correspondingly, conched chocolate mass is continuously discharged. Furthermore, the invention relates to an apparatus for conching the chocolate mass and for discharging same.... After being pretreated in the usual way, the (dry) starting material for the production of chocolate mass is intimately mixed in a mixing vessel (conche) for a longer period. Thereafter, the (conched) chocolate mass can be discharged to be further processed. A continuous conching of chocolate mass, i.e. a continuos operation of a conche with a continuous infeed of starting material and a likewise continuous extraction of conched chocolate mass is already known. DE-A-39 18 813 proposes to connect a plurality, namely three conches with one another for a continously running operation. The starting material is fed to a first conche, the partially conched material is fed to a second conche and finally to a third conche. From the latter, the ready-conched chocolate mass is discharged.... In this known proposal, screw conveyors are used as conveying means for the partially or completely conched chocolate mass. Each conche forms a lateral top overflow and each overflow is connected to a screw conveyor. The screw conveyors assigned to the first and second conche transport the chocolate mass to the (upper) inlet side of the following conche. The screw conveyor of the third or last conche serves for discharging the ready-conched chocolate mass.

Web site: http://www.delphion.com/details?pn=US05320427__

- **Apparatus for continuously molding chocolate products**

Inventor(s): Suttle; James M. (East Stroudsburg, PA), Martin; John M. (Glendale, CA), Willcocks; Neil A. (Flanders, NJ), Camporini; Alfred V. (Hackettstown, NJ), Collins; Thomas M. (Nazareth, PA)

Assignee(s): Mars, Incorporated (McLean, VA)

Patent Number: 6,302,677

Date filed: February 1, 2001

Abstract: Methods for continuously molding finished chocolate tablets, pieces and the like are disclosed. Apparatus for use with the method, comprise a chilled rotating mold having at least one recess into which liquid chocolate is deposited. Liquid chocolate, is held in place by a retaining/casting belt as the rotating mold turns. The liquid chocolate cools and partially sets while in contact with the rotating mold and retaining/casting belt, and a molded chocolate is removed from the recess. Novel finished chocolate molded products made by the methods and with the apparatus, having detailed surface design and surface gloss are also disclosed.

Excerpt(s): The invention relates to the molding of chocolate. Specifically, the disclosed method and apparatus are directed to the continuous molding of chocolate tablets, pieces and the like on a rotary mold.... Finished chocolates having a desired three-dimensional shape or having an image or design imprinted on a surface are conventionally produced by molding, and are herein referred to as "molded chocolate". The finished chocolate may be a solid block, a hollow shell, or a shell filled with a confectionery material such as fondant, fudge or soft caramel (Chocolate, Cocoa and Confectionery: Science and Technology by Bernard W. Minifie, Third Edition, page 183, herein incorporated by reference in its entirety). Whatever the particular form of the finished chocolate, all are characterized by attributes such as detailed finishes and high surface gloss. Further, these finished chocolates do not require further processing such as enrobing with chocolate, which only provides a home-made look to a product and lacks high gloss and fine surface detail.... Conventional molding typically employs very large numbers of molds, usually made of polycarbonate. These polycarbonate molds are typically flat, approximately 1 inch in height and anywhere from 1 to 2 feet long and 1 to 5 feet in width.

Web site: http://www.delphion.com/details?pn=US06302677__

- **Apparatus for continuously tempering chocolate masses and the like**

Inventor(s): Heyde; Hans (Wallenhorst, DE)

Assignee(s): Sollich GmbH & Co., KG (Bad Salzuflen, DE)

Patent Number: 6,241,377

Date filed: November 9, 1999

Abstract: An apparatus for continuously tempering chocolate masses and the like includes a plurality of tempering chambers (17) including tempering surfaces (18) and being interconnected for the flow of a tempering medium. A plurality of mass chambers (7) is interconnected for the flow of the mass to be tempered, each of the mass chambers (7) being arranged between the tempering surfaces (18) of the tempering chambers (17). A plurality of driven mixing discs (6) has a radius, a circumference, an outer diameter, an inner diameter, a top side (10) and a bottom side (11). The mixing discs (6) are arranged inside the mass chambers (7), and they include openings (22) allowing for a passage of the mass to be tempered from the bottom side (11) toward the top side (10). A majority of mixing blades (12) is arranged at the top sides (10) and at the bottom sides (11) of the mixing discs (6) without continuous channels being formed between the mixing blades (12). The mixing blades (12) have a length which is less than the radius of the mixing discs (6), and the mixing blades (12) are designed and arranged to take the mass to be tempered off the tempering surfaces (18) and to mix the mass.

Excerpt(s): This application claims the benefit of co-pending German patent application number 198 54 204.6 entitled "Vorrichtung zum kontinuierlichen Temperieren von zu verarbeitenden kakaobutterhaltigen oder ahnlichen fetthaltigen Massen", filed on Nov. 24, 1998.... The present invention generally relates to generally relates to an apparatus for continuously tempering chocolate masses and the like. Such an apparatus includes a plurality of tempering chambers and a plurality of mass chambers, each of the mass chambers being arranged between the tempering surfaces of the tempering chambers. The mass chambers are interconnected for the flow of the mass to be tempered. More particularly, the present invention relates to an apparatus for continuously tempering chocolate masses and the like including a plurality of driven mixing discs being arranged inside the mass chambers. A majority of mixing blades is arranged at the top sides and at the bottom sides of the mixing discs.... The present invention is applicable to all mass chambers no matter whether the mass chamber is part of a cooling zone, a cooling level, a crystallization zone, a crystallization level, a reheat zone, a reheat level or the like. The tempering medium may either be a cooling medium or a heating medium. Usually, the tempering medium is water. Nevertheless, the cooling medium may also be a medium different from water. The present invention is applicable no matter whether the tempering chambers adjacent to the mass chamber are connected to one and the same, or to different tempering circuits.

Web site: http://www.delphion.com/details?pn=US06241377__

- **Apparatus for controlling the temperature of flowable chocolate materials**

Inventor(s): Sollich; Helmut (Kalletal, DE)

Assignee(s): Sollich KG Spezialmaschinenfabrik (Bad Salzuflen, DE)

Patent Number: 4,178,105

Date filed: May 30, 1978

Abstract: An apparatus for the temperature control of flowable chocolate, such apparatus comprising a rotor rotating in a temperature-controlled housing and having means which bear resiliently against the housing and which wipe the chocolate away from the housing during rotation of the rotor.

Excerpt(s): The present invention relates to an apparatus for controlling the temperature of fat-containing materials, such as flowable chocolate or the like.... In order to impart a specific structure to chocolate materials having the smallest possible and regularly distributed crystals, it is known to control the temperature thereof to bring it into a viscous flowable state and to mix it by means of agitators. For this purpose it is known to carry out the temperature control or tempering in a cylindrical annular chamber between a rotor housing and a rotor rotating therein. The rotor housing is temperature-controlled so that the chocolate is in a viscously flowable state. In this manner, the crystals thus achieve their desired mini-structure. Through the rotation of the rotor the chocolate is caused to be thoroughly mixed, uniform distribution of the miniaturized crystals being achieved thereby.... In this process the chocolate must be prevented from being deposited on the inner wall of the rotor housing. If this were not to be counteracted, the inner wall of the rotor housing would rapidly become coated with a cohesive layer of chocolate. This would prevent the transfer of heat between the rotor housing and the chocolate material exteriorly of the layer adjoining the inner wall of the rotor housing, with the result that the cooling capacity would have to be increased in an attempt to discharge sufficient heat through the layer of adhering chocolate and out of the chocolate material to the outside of the layer, and this would impair the economy of the process. On the other hand, the chocolate of the adhering layer and the other chocolate material would not be admixed, and it is precisely this step which must be afforded according to the object of the process, because uniform distribution of minimum sized crystals must be achieved by the mixing operation. Finally, if the chocolate were to be subjected to too low a temperature for a long period, the crystals in the layer adhering to the inside of the housing would be stimulated into continual growth. The required minicrystals can be obtained only by means of a specific temperature acting over a specific period. An ordinary rotor rotating in a housing would therefore provide uniform distribution of minimum sized crystals in respect of the chocolate situated in the cylindrical annular chamber between the rotor and the housing, but these crystals would not be uniform.

Web site: http://www.delphion.com/details?pn=US04178105__

- **Apparatus for depositing chocolate chips and the like onto edible food products**

Inventor(s): Thompson; John M. (Alton, IL)

Assignee(s): Ralston Purina Company (St. Louis, MO)

Patent Number: 4,655,161

Date filed: December 13, 1985

Abstract: An apparatus and method are provided for depositing chips of chocolate, fudge, and the like on food products. The apparatus comprises a hopper shaped to retain the chips therein, and a depositor roll having a peripheral surface with a plurality of recessed pockets into which the chips are received. A feed plate extends from an outlet portion of the hopper to the depositor roll at an elevation substantially commensurate with the longitudinal axis of the depositor roll. The feed plate preferably has a length which is greater than twice the dimension of one of the chips to form a dynamic, free-surface reservoir in which the chips temporarily pool prior to lodging in the depositor roll pockets. When the depositor roll is rotated, the chips continuously feed from the hopper, along the feed plate, and into the depositor roll pockets. The chips are gently swept upwardly in the pockets out of the chip reservoir, and deposited onto food products conveyed under the depositor roll, without breaking or smashing the chips.

Excerpt(s): The present invention relates to the field of edible food processing, and in particular, to an apparatus and method of depositing chips of chocolate, fudge, and the like onto food products.... In the processing of certain types of edible, human food products, relatively fragile bits or chips of confection are deposited onto food articles conveyed therebelow. For example, in the manufacture of granola bars, and other similar food items, morsels or chips of chocolate or fudge (hereinafter referred to as "chips") are sprinkled on top of a continuously moving sheet or layer of granola. The chips are deposited at a predetermined flow rate, which is varied to coordinate with the speed of the overall process. The chips and the granola are subsequently pressed together, and cut to shape.... The chips are typically quite soft and fragile, such that they must be handled very gently in order to avoid breaking and/or smashing the chips, which can clog the chip depositor, and/or detract from the appearance and quality of the processed food article. Conventional depositor machines and methods that are presently used in the food processing industry tend to break up such soft chips, and smash or mash the chips into the machine, which results in food waste, and requires expensive and time consuming cleaning and repair.

Web site: http://www.delphion.com/details?pn=US04655161__

- **Apparatus for determining crystallization solidification curves of chocolate masses and similar fatty masses**

Inventor(s): Sollich; Helmut (Rabenkirchen, DE)

Assignee(s): Sollich GmbH & Co. KG (DE)

Patent Number: 4,889,434

Date filed: April 8, 1988

Abstract: An apparatus for determining crystallization solidification curves of chocolate masses and similar fatty masses is equipped with a measuring chamber 8 which is formed by a cooled wall and into which projects a temperature-measuring sensor 16.

Here, the liquid chocolate mass is brought to solidification. A device for recording the temperature pattern in the solidifying chocolate mass against time is provided. A piston/cylinder unit 6, 7 which is arranged so as to dip with its open end face 10 into the chocolate mass to be measured serves as a measuring chamber 8. A drive is provided for the stroke of the piston 7. The piston 7 carries the temperature-measuring sensor 16. A device 6 for removing the solidified sample from the piston 7 and temperature-measuring sensor 16 is also provided.

Excerpt(s): The invention relates to an apparatus for determining crystallization solidification curves of chocolate masses and similar fatty masses, with a measuring chamber which is formed by a cooled wall, into which projects a temperature-measuring sensor. In this measuring chamber, the liquid chocolate mass is brought to solidification, and a device records the temperature pattern in the solidifying chocolate mass in relation to time.... Before chocolate mass is processed from the liquid state and brought to solidification, it has to be heat-treated as is known; that is, it is first heated and thus brought into the liquid state and subsequently cooled, until the fatty fraction in the chocolate mass forms solidification crystals. This process is also known as precrystallization. The properties of the solidified chocolate mass differ according to the composition of the chocolate mass and the heat-treatment process used. For a good gloss, a long shelf life and fine-grained breaking of the final product, it is important that, during heat treatment, fat crystals are formed in a crystal form which is high-melting in temperature terms and that these crystal agglomerates have small dimensions and are distributed homogeneously in the chocolate mass. The degree of heat-treatment or of precrystallization, which is the fraction of solidified fat crystals, is also critical for the production flow. Too low a fraction (inadequate heat-treatment) undoubtedly causes excessively long solidification times during final cooling and can result in a poor gloss and low shelf life. Too high a solidification fraction (excessive heat-treatment) gives rise to an increased viscosity of the chocolate mass to be processed and can result in less contraction during final cooling, a poor gloss and, again, a lower shelf life.... A known apparatus of the type described in the introduction makes it possible to determine crystallization solidification curves. Sampling vessels are used, consisting essentially of a portion of copper tube, on which a small cylindrical container which represents a measuring chamber is formed in one end region. This measuring chamber is filled with liquid chocolate mass. A temperature-measuring sensor is introduced manually into the measuring chamber, that is, it is inserted into the liquid chocolate mass. The other end of the measuring sensor is connected to a recording instrument which, at intervals of time, records the particular temperature of the solidifying chocolate mass. To ensure cooling, the sampling vessel consisting of a copper tube is subjected to cooling at its lower end by being dipped into a vessel containing an ice-water mixture. As a result of the conduction of heat in the copper tube, the liquid chocolate mass in the measuring chamber is also brought to solidification, specifically in a way which can be reproduced over a period of time. A thermocouple can be used, for example, as a temperature-measuring sensor. In the device for recording the temperature pattern, a paper strip is constantly moved sideways, so hat the solidification curves are recorded and thus captured. It is therefore possible, during a production operation, for the heat treatment of the chocolate mass to be processed to be checked repeatedly at intervals of time, in order to ascertain that the heat treatment is being maintained at the desired or necessary level. Correcting measures can then also be taken on the heat-treatment machine accordingly. On the one hand, the known apparatus involves a high outlay, because an attendant is needed to extract the liquid chocolate mass, introduce it into the measuring chamber and carry out the measurement. Furthermore, the measurement is also unreliable since as it is possible for the operation to take place on a completely erroneous basis. Thus, the reference temperature can even deviate from 0.degree. without being noticed. The liquid chocolate mass can experience a change between extraction at the checking point and introduction into the measuring chamber. Due to the possibility of these events, it is difficult to maintain reproducible conditions here. Moreover, the liquid chocolate mass can be extracted only at an open location on a heat-treatment machine or another processing station, and not in a closed pipeline or at other points, where access is difficult. Finally, the sampling vessels have to be cleaned again after the chocolate mass has solidified. For all these reasons, the intervals of time at which such monitoring checks are carried out are often very long.

Web site: http://www.delphion.com/details?pn=US04889434__

- **Apparatus for filling edible rod-shaped hollow bodies with chocolate**

Inventor(s): Yamaguchi; Mitsuo (Sakado, JP), Ohgo; Kenjiro (Sakado, JP), Nagasawa; Makoto (Sakado, JP)

Assignee(s): Meiji Seika Kaisha, Ltd. (Tokyo, JP)

Patent Number: 5,469,780

Date filed: September 27, 1994

Abstract: Disclosed is an apparatus for filling edible, rod-shaped hollow bodies with chocolate comprising a feeding unit (1) for conveying hollow bodies (A), a transport roller (2) positioned close to the feeding unit, a first transfer roller (5) positioned close to the transport roller, a chocolate filling roller (8) positioned close to the first transport roller, a second transfer roller (13) positioned close to the chocolate filling roller, and a discharging unit (14) positioned close to the second transfer roller for receiving and conveying hollow bodies filled with chocolate from the chocolate filling roller via the second transfer roller. The apparatus assures the continuous flow of hollow bodies to the chocolate filling station without any fear of breaking fragile hollow bodies, thereby permitting mass production of chocolate corn cakes, each filled with an exact amount of chocolate.

Excerpt(s): The present invention relates to an apparatus for filling edible, rod-shaped hollow bodies with chocolate. Such edible, rod-shaped hollow bodies are prepared by baking or heating and expanding grain.... An apparatus for making cream cakes or cream puffs functions to fill hollow pieces of light pastry with cream or jam one after another, as disclosed in Japanese Patent 56-64753(A) (Cream Filler). It uses a conveyer equipped with a cream filler, which conveyer can be changed for making a different kind of cream cake or cream puff.... Also, an apparatus for inserting rods into edible rod-shaped bodies, such as sausages is disclosed in Japanese Utility Model 5-14795(Y) (Rod-Inserting Apparatus).

Web site: http://www.delphion.com/details?pn=US05469780__

- **Apparatus for forming an interior chocolate layer on an ice-cream cone**

Inventor(s): Vos; Neale (1599 Castleton Ave., Staten Island, NY 10302)

Assignee(s): none reported

Patent Number: 5,102,672

Date filed: November 28, 1990

Abstract: An apparatus for forming a layer of chocolate on the interior surface of an ice-cream having a cone-shaped mold that is interiorly-cooled by ice-water provided thereto from a bucket, or other source, of ice-water. For forming an interior chocolate coating, liquid chocolate is placed into the interior of the cone, and the cone is then placed onto the cold mold, and centered thereon by the upper end portion of the mold. The cone is allowed to remain there for a short while, while the cold mold-surface solidifies the liquid chocolate, to thereby form the interior layer of chocolate. A stripping device may, if desired, be employed for aiding in the removal of the thus-coated cone from the mold. In the preferred embodiment, the mold is secured directly to the ice-bucket.

Excerpt(s): The present invention is directed to an apparatus by which a layer of chocolate may be coated onto the interior surface of an ice-cream cone. It is known to apply a coating of chocolate to the interior surface of an ice-cream cone, but such has hitherto been done without the aid of any device or apparatus, making it difficult, time-consuming, and haphazard, in that chocolate-coated cones may differ markedly from each other. These drawbacks not only cause poor quality control, but have also made it difficult to provide for the production of such chocolate-coated cones in large quantities, such as would be required at commercial establishments, such as ice-cream shops, parlors, stores, and the like.... The prior art has also consisted of a conically-shaped mold over which an ice-cream cone is laid, which mold is hollow and cooled by refrigerator coils provided in the hollow interior of the mold, so that liquid chocolate spread on the interior of the ice-cream cone may be solidified when the cone is placed over the mold. This type of apparatus requires costly and difficult-to-maintain refrigeration-equipment, and has not been able to consistently and effectively cool the mold in order to solidify the liquid chocolate on the interior surface of the ice-cream cone. Owing to the relatively small size of the mold necessary for receiving a cone thereover, effective cooling of the mold via refrigeration and the tubing associated therewith has not proven practicable nor effective.... It is the primary objective of the present invention to provide an apparatus for coating the interior surfaces of ice-cream cones.

Web site: http://www.delphion.com/details?pn=US05102672__

- **Apparatus for making chocolate-coated ice cream cookie sandwiches**

  Inventor(s): Jones; John F. (140 Summit Rd., Prospect, CT 06712)

  Assignee(s): none reported

  Patent Number: 4,644,901

  Date filed: September 18, 1985

  Abstract: A low labor, highly efficient process and system for manufacturing chocolate coated ice cream cookie sandwiches is achieved by incorporating conveyor means for transporting the ice cream cookie sandwich through the various stages of its manufacture along with uniquely constructed ice cream brick slicing machines and a unique chocolate coating machine. In addition, a pass-through freezer is preferably employed prior to the chocolate coating, in order to assure a high quality, tasty product. The ice cream slicing machine of the present invention employed in the process and manufacturing system of this invention is constructed for receiving a plurality of ice cream bricks and cutting each brick into a plurality of slices in an efficient, automatic, integrated operational procedure and presenting each ice cream slice to a holding zone for placement on a cookie moving along the conveyor means. In addition, the chocolate coating machine of the present invention incorporated into the process and manufacturing system of this invention incorporates a plurality of clamp means controllably driven about the coating machine and positioned for receiving the ice cream cookie sandwich and automatically submerging the sandwich in a chocolate bath and automatically releasing the chocolate-coated ice cream cookie sandwich when the chocolate coating has completely cooled and dried.

Excerpt(s): This invention relates to a process and to machines for making ice cream cookie sandwiches and, more particularly, to the process and machines employed in making chocolate-coated ice cream cookie sandwiches.... Although ice cream sandwiches and ice cream cookie sandwiches have existed for many years and have been manufactured using a variety of alternate methods, no prior art system has been developed which is capable of employing ice cream bricks by cutting the bricks into a plurality of smaller slices, and then assembling the slices between two cookies in an efficient manner wherein labor costs are maintained at a minimum.... Furthermore, no prior art apparatus or process is capable of providing chocolate-coated ice cream cookie sandwiches, wherein the chocolate coating is achieved efficiently, with all used chocolate being recycled. In addition, prior art systems typically require a high degree of handling, thereby reducing production efficiency and causing increased production costs.

Web site: http://www.delphion.com/details?pn=US04644901__

- **Apparatus for mixing and refining a chocolate mass**

Inventor(s): Muntener; Kurt (Bad Salzuflen, DE)

Assignee(s): Richard Frisse GmbH (Bad Salzuflen, DE)

Patent Number: 6,129,008

Date filed: January 3, 2000

Abstract: The present invention is directed to making the mixing and refining of chocolate masses more cost effective by increasing the flow of energy through the material to be treated.

Excerpt(s): In general, conching machines are used for mixing and refining a chocolate mass. Such conching machines comprise typically shearing tools extending mainly in radial direction from a rotor arranged in a partially cylindrical trough. These shearing tools have a surface inclined to the trough wall and end often in a relative sharp edge. In this way, they may act in a double manner, i.e. either by shearing chocolate mass off the trough walls when running in one direction, or by providing a rheological shearing effect onto individual layers of the chocolate mass when running in the other direction where the mass is caught in the gap between the trough walls and the converging surface of the shearing tools.... The expenditure for manufacturing such conching machines is considerable, and so are they in operation. For the individual chocolate mass remains in such a conching machine for a long period while mechanical energy is introduced into the mass to bring it from a more or less dry condition to a pasty condition and to make it eventually liquid.... Therefore, attempts have been made to shorten the conching time and/or to replace conching by other processes, or, at least, to simplify the conching process. An increase of introduced energy to shorten the process is, however, not possible to an unlimited extent, because any mechanical energy introduced into the mass converts itself into heat energy, thus heating up the mass. In doing this, there are certain limits not to be exceeded. Heretofore, conching machines were surrounded by an outer tempering or cooling jacket (at the beginning of operation, a conching machine has often to be first to be heated by means of this jacket to soften the chocolate mass. Thus, "tempering" means both heating and cooling)). This jacket provided for heat dissipation during operation, but had, of course, also some limits.

Web site: http://www.delphion.com/details?pn=US06129008__

- **Apparatus for molding chocolate**

  Inventor(s): Zanetos; Tom (Columbus, OH), Reeder; Paul E. (Columbus, OH)

  Assignee(s): Anthony-Thomas Candy Company (Columbus, OH)

  Patent Number: 4,950,145

  Date filed: June 15, 1989

  Abstract: Chocolate mold filling apparatus having chocolate molds having different number of cavity, cavity volume, cavity fill opening height, and cavity fill opening spacing characteristics. Each mold further has a base flange which incorporates a process code keyed to the mold different characteristics. A sensor detects the base flange process codes and controls a connected conveyor, chocolate metering pump, and chocolate mold fill tube.

  Excerpt(s): The present invention relates generally to molding chocolate, and particularly concerns mold filling apparatus useful to fill tempered chocolate into successive molds having different mold size, mold cavity spacing, and mold cavity chocolate quantity characteristics on a continuous production basis.... Chocolate mold filling apparatus may generally be classified into two types on the basis of production quantity and product variety requirements. A common general-purpose type of chocolate mold filling apparatus selectively and repeatedly pumps an individually-metered adjustable quantity of tempered chocolate from a storage tank to a fill nozzle and into a hand-moved chocolate mold aligned with the fill nozzle. No attempts are made to automatically adjust fill tube heights or fill quantities or to mechanically control mold lateral or longitudinal movements. Hence, such general-purpose mold filling apparatus is well-suited only to a relatively small or hand-production run even though a variety of different chocolate mold sizes can be accommodated.... The common special-purpose type of mold filling apparatus, on the other hand, generally is designed and operated to produce only a single product in quantity and cannot readily accommodate intermediate to large production runs involving different mold sizes and mold cavity spacings.

  Web site: http://www.delphion.com/details?pn=US04950145__

- **Apparatus for molding chocolate bars**

  Inventor(s): Friedwald; Franklin (3781 Mahlon Brower Dr., Oceanside, NY 11572)

  Assignee(s): none reported

  Patent Number: 4,954,069

  Date filed: February 15, 1989

  Abstract: In a machine for moulded chocolate bars of the type having a pair of chains, a plurality of carriers attached to the chains and separate moulds mounted in the carriers; the present invention combines mould and carrier into one piece having a mould and sheath slots to directly connect the mould to pins connected to the chains on machines designed for separate carriers and moulds.

Excerpt(s): This invention relates to machines for moulding candy bars, for instance chocolate bars, and more particularly, for means to combine the mould and carrier in a chain type moulding machine, originally designed for separate carriers and moulds. The device includes a unitary lightweight plastic piece which incorporates the functions of the mould and the carrier. In particular, a fastening means is provided to accommodate pins for supporting the device, which pins extend integrally from the supporting chain into sheaths which form part of the unitary mould/carrier piece.... Machines were generally of the type having a pair of chains carrying carriers. The moulds were placed inside the carriers. Since the carrier pieces were of metal they constituted a very heavy weight since there were very many carriers on a machine. In addition, other dual mould/carrier devices are disclosed in Steels, U.S. Pat. No. 4,229,484, German Patents Nos. 2,517,660 and 2,537,955.... The present invention combines the carrier and the mould in one piece as a lightweight unitary plastic piece for use with existing machines designed to take separate carriers and moulds. In the existing machines the carriers are supported by pins extending from supporting chains.

Web site: http://www.delphion.com/details?pn=US04954069__

- **Apparatus for processing a cocoa butter-containing or similar fat-containing mass, particularly a chocolate mass**

Inventor(s): Koch; Peter (Pinneberg, DE)

Assignee(s): Hosokawa Kreuter GmbH (Hamburg, DE)

Patent Number: 5,947,014

Date filed: October 27, 1998

Abstract: An apparatus for continuously processing a cocoa-butter containing or similar fat-containing mass, particularly a chocolate mass, includes an outer stationary cooling cylinder, wherein the mass to be processed is pumped through the interior of the stationary cooling cylinder from one end face thereof into the area of the other end face. The apparatus further includes a driven agitating element in the interior of the cooling cylinder. A driven inner cylinder having a smaller diameter than the cooling cylinder is arranged concentrically in the cooling cylinder. The cooling cylinder and the inner cylinder form an annular interior in which a number of agitating rollers forming the agitating element are arranged. The axes of the agitating rollers extend parallel to the axis of the cylinders. The axes of the agitating rollers are located on a common circle arranged concentrically to the cylinders. The agitating rollers are driven by the cylinder.

Excerpt(s): The present invention relates to an apparatus for continuously processing a cocoa-butter containing or similar fat-containing mass, particularly a chocolate mass. The apparatus includes an outer stationary cooling cylinder, wherein the mass to be processed is pumped through the interior of the stationary cooling cylinder from one end face thereof into the area of the other end face. The apparatus further includes a driven agitating element in the interior of the cooling cylinder.... In an apparatus of the above-described type which is known in the art, three cylinders are used which are connected in series one behind the other. A driven screw forming the agitating element is arranged in each cylinder. The cylinders form cooling or conditioning zones. The mass to be processed may deposit at the screws, wherein this deposited mass then no longer participates or only participates to a limited extent in the actual processing procedure. The screw also influences the conveyance of the mass through the cylinder, wherein the degree of conveyance is determined by the pitch of the screw. This is not always desirable because this limits the flexibility. Moreover, the apparatus is complicated because several cylinders must be connected one behind the other in series in order to be able to adjust the appropriate processing parameters for each cooling or conditioning stage.... Therefore, it is the primary object of the present invention to provide an apparatus of the above-described type in which a build-up of the mass in the interior or at the agitating element is prevented by contacting all surfaces where possible by other surfaces and, thus, cleaning the surfaces by means of these other surfaces. In addition, all surfaces, even those of the agitating element, are to be utilized for the heat transfer.

Web site: http://www.delphion.com/details?pn=US05947014__

- **Apparatus for the production of shells of fat-containing chocolate-like masses under pressure build-up**

Inventor(s): Aasted; Lars (Charlottenlund, DK)

Assignee(s): Aasted-Mikroverk APS (DK)

Patent Number: 6,497,568

Date filed: October 29, 1999

Abstract: Systems and methods for producing chocolate shells by immersing a core into a liquid filled mold cavity. The temperature of the core member is controlled. A mold cavity closure with shell rim molding surfaces extends peripherally around the core member and, together with outer surfaces of the core and inner surfaces of the mold cavity, the molding surfaces determine the full geometry of the chocolate shell. The cavity closure is axially movable in relation to the core member and has unobstructed travel in relation to the core member, when the mold cavity closure is engaged with the mold. The device includes a load for pressing the core member in direction against the mold cavity to achieve pressure build up in the mass.

Excerpt(s): The present invention concerns a method for the production of fat-containing, chocolate-like masses, in particular for chocolate articles, by which an amount of liquid mass is deposited into a mould cavity, whereafter an associated core member is immersed into the mass, the temperature of which core member is being controlled.... Methods of the above mentioned types as well as associated apparatus are to-day well-known within the prior art, and are being used extensively by the chocolate making industry.... Generally within the present field, chocolate-like masses are suspensions of non-fat particles, such as sugar, milk powders and cocoa solids in a liquid fat phase. The fat phase in most cases comprises an extent of the genuin cocoa butter of until around 30%, but may comprise substitutes as well. Such substitutes may be in the form of other types of fat-containing oils. Chocolate-like masses where the cocoa butter has been replaced wholly or partly by other fats, are often named commercially as compound chocolate, in which the cocoa butter has been replaced by palm-kernel oil, are corresponding oils.

Web site: http://www.delphion.com/details?pn=US06497568__

- **Apparatus for the production of shells of fat-containing, chocolate masses**

Inventor(s): Aasted; Lars (Charlottenlund, DK)

Assignee(s): Aasted-Mikroverk APS (DK)

Patent Number: 6,508,642

Date filed: October 29, 1999

Abstract: A system for the producing of shells of fat-containing, chocolate-like masses, which includes more than one cavity to receive the masses and more than one core member to be immersed in the mass-containing cavity. The core members are independently suspended from a holding device. Further, a mold cavity closure extends peripherally around the core members, and the closure includes shell rim molding surfaces which cooperate with the outer surfaces of the cores and the inner surfaces of the mold cavities to determine completely the geometry of the molded shells in the closed position. The closure is axially movable relative to the core members.

Excerpt(s): The present invention concerns a system for the production of fat-containing, chocolate-like masses, in particular for chocolate articles, by which an amount of liquid mass is deposited into more than one mould cavity, whereafter more than one core member is immersed into the mass forming the shells.... Systems for moulding of shells of fat-containing, chocolate-like masses through immersion of a core member into the liquid mass of an associated cavity and thereby bringing the mass into the desired shape are today well-known within the prior art, and are being used extensively by the chocolate making industry.... Generally within the present field, chocolate-like masses are suspensions of non-fat particles, such as sugar, milk powders and cocoa solids in a liquid fat phase. The fat phase in most cases comprises an extent of the genuine cocoa butter of until around 30%, but may comprise substitutes as well. Such substitutes may be in the form of other types of fat-containing oils. Chocolate-like masses where the cocoa butter has been replaced wholly or partly by other fats, are often named commercially as compound chocolate, in which the cocoa butter has been replaced by palm-kernel oil, or corresponding oils. Shells made of 100% fat being cocobutter or compound is also possible.

Web site: http://www.delphion.com/details?pn=US06508642__

- **Begonia plant named `Boston Cherries 'n Chocolate`**

Inventor(s): Booman; James Lawrence (2302 Bautista Ave., Vista, CA 92084)

Assignee(s): none reported

Patent Number: PP11,947

Date filed: August 17, 1999

Abstract: A new and distinct cultivar of Rex Begonia plant named `Boston Cherries 'n Chocolate`, characterized by its uniform growth habit; moderate plant vigor; no requirement for winter dormancy; and interesting and attractive leaf coloration and pattern.

Excerpt(s): The present invention relates to a new and distinct cultivar of Begonia plant, botanically known as Begonia rex hybrid, commercially known as Rex Begonia, and hereinafter referred to by the name `Boston Cherries 'n Chocolate`.... The new Rex Begonia was discovered and selected by the Inventor in a controlled environment in Vista, Calif., in 1995, within a large group of seedling progeny from multiple crossings of unidentified selections of Begonia rex hybrids.... The selection of this plant was based on its uniform growth habit, moderate plant vigor, salt tolerance and attractive foliage coloration and pattern.

Web site: http://www.delphion.com/details?pn=US0PP11947__

- **Chocolate**

Inventor(s): Kida; Haruyasu (Kitasoma-gun, JP), Arai; Masako (Tsukuba-gun, JP), Tashiro; Yoichi (Kitasoma-gun, JP), Baba; Hideki (Sennan-gun, JP)

Assignee(s): Fuji Oil Company, Limited (Osaka-fu, JP)

Patent Number: 5,532,021

Date filed: June 2, 1995

Abstract: Chocolate having excellent hardness and melting properties in the mouth upon eating at a temperature range of freezing or refrigerating is disclosed. The chocolate is subjected to tempering treatment and has a softening point of 15.degree. to 30.degree. C. Its fat ingredient comprises 95 to 40% by weight of fats rich in 2-unsaturated-1,3-disaturated triglycerides (SUS) the main constituent fatty acids of which are palmitic acid (P) and stearic acid (St) with a P/St ratio of at least 1.0 and 5 to 40% by weigh of lauric fats, the relation of P/St ratio of SUS to the fat content in the chocolate being on or in the higher fat content region above line 1 as shown in FIG. 1.

Excerpt(s): The present invention relates to chocolate suitable for cooling at a low temperature range of freezing or refrigerating and eating at the same temperature range.... It is known that chocolate is made from cacao mass, cacao butter, sugar, powdered milk and the like. Cacao butter is mainly composed of POSt, StOSt and POP glycerides wherein P is palmitic acid, O is oleic acid and St is stearic acid. Typical chocolate which is eaten as it is as sweets (hereinafter referred to as "per se chocolate sweets") contain about 32% by weight of cacao butter. The P/St ratio as an average value calculated from total constituent fatty acids of the glycerides of the cacao butter is about 0.7 to 0.8. Other fats (hard butter) are often used as substitutes for all or a part of cacao butter in order to save production cost or to improve physical properties of chocolate.... In addition to use of chocolate as solid per se chocolate sweets such as bar chocolate, tablet chocolate and the like for tasting its own flavors, tastes and physical mouthfeel, chocolate is used as raw materials of confectionery in combination with other foods, more particularly, chocolate is used as, for example, coating materials, enrobers, filling materials and decorations of iced and baked confectionery. In general, excellent flavor, taste and physical mouthfeel are severely required in the case of the former use, i.e. in the case that chocolate is used as solid per se chocolate sweets.

Web site: http://www.delphion.com/details?pn=US05532021__

- **Chocolate and chocolate additive**

Inventor(s): Koyano; Tetsuo (Kawasaki, JP), Sagi; Nobuo (Sakai, JP), Izumi; Tsugio (Sennan, JP), Fujita; Setsuya (Yokohama, JP), Murata; Tadahiko (Yokohama, JP), Hachiya; Iwao (Yokohama, JP), Mori; Hiroyuki (Sakai, JP)

Assignee(s): Meiji Seika Kaisha, Ltd. (Tokyo, JP), Fuji Oil Company, Limited (Osaka, JP)

Patent Number: 4,877,636

Date filed: October 28, 1987

Abstract: A chocolate additive for preventing fat blooming and useful for omitting or simplifying the tempering operations comprising powder particles composed of as the main component a 2-unsaturated-1,3-disaturated glyceride constituent fatty acids of which are unsaturated fatty acids having at least 18 carbon atoms and saturated fatty acids having 20 to 24 carbon atoms and a chocolate containing the additive.

Excerpt(s): The present invention relates to a chocolate additive. Particularly, the additive of the present invention is suitable for the production of chocolate of such quality that fat bloom is prevented even after standing at a temperature such as about the body temperature at which shape retention is lost for a certain period, and is useful for omitting or simplifying the tempering operation in chocolate production. The present invention also relates to chocolate using the additive of the present invention and a process for producing the same.... The term "chocolate" used herein is not limited to specific kinds of chocolate such as those prescribed by laws and regulations, and means any kind of chocolate including chocolate and other processed food of fats and oils using a so-called cacao butter substitute or an equivalent thereof.... In general, chocolate is produced by appropriately mixing cacao mass, cocoa, cacao butter, a cacao butter substitute, a sweetener, milk powder and the like, and subjecting the resulting chocolate mix to rolling, conching and tempering. In chocolate thus obtained, there is a problem that blooming is often caused during storage, which lowers the commercial value thereof. Blooming is divided into fat blooming caused by unstable crystals of fats and oils, and sugar blooming caused by recrystallization of sugar. Particularly, the former fat blooming is frequently caused.

Web site: http://www.delphion.com/details?pn=US04877636__

- **Chocolate and chocolate-utilizing food**

Inventor(s): Yamaguchi; Kotaro (Sennan, JP), Nishimoto; Tsugio (Naga, JP), Ebihara; Yoshitaka (Sakai, JP), Matsunami; Hidenobu (Sennan, JP), Fujita; Shohei (Miyazaki, JP), Kakurai; Aki (Makabe, JP)

Assignee(s): Fuji Oil Company, Limited (Osaka, JP)

Patent Number: 5,271,950

Date filed: March 4, 1992

Abstract: There is disclosed a chocolate containing as its oil ingredients 10-85 wt % of di-saturated mono-unsaturated glycerides (S.sub.2 U) and 15-90 wt % of di-unsaturated mono-saturated glycerides (SU.sub.2) plus tri-unsaturated glycerides (U.sub.3), at least 35 wt % of the di-saturated mono-unsaturated glycerides (S.sub.2 U) being di-saturated mono-linoleate (S.sub.2 L). Chocolate-utilizing food containing this chocolate such as in frozen desserts and the like are also disclosed.

Excerpt(s): The present invention relates to a chocolate containing a relatively large amount of liquid fats More particularly, it relates not only to a chocolate which has excellent flexibility in molding, such as flexing characteristics, but also to a chocolate for use in frozen desserts. It should be noted that the term "chocolate" used herein has a broad meaning which is not limited by a rule (e.g., "Fair Rule for Designation of Chocolates" in Japan) or a legal provision but includes chocolates or fat-fabricated food using, what is called, a cacao butter substitute. Moreover, the term "fat" used herein has the same meaning as that of "fats and oils", including, what is called, fatty oils that are in the liquid state at room temperature.... Chocolates which have been most commonly seen on the market are required to have snap characteristics as a matter of importance. Such chocolates usually contain only a small amount of low-melting glyceride components, such as di-unsaturated mono-saturated glycerides (SU.sub.2) and tri-unsaturated glycerides (U.sub.3), and they are composed mainly of di-saturated mono-unsaturated glycerides (S.sub.2 U).... On the other hand, there has been known the use of particular chocolates which are required to have moldability rather than snap characteristics as a matter of importance. Typical examples of such chocolates include, what is called, plastic chocolates which can be obtained by blending ordinary chocolates with water-containing materials, such as liquid sugar, and they have been molded into a shape of man, animal or houses for decoration of cakes. However, chocolates using liquid sugar have undesired flavor and also an unfavorable mouth feel. Moreover, such chocolates have difficulty in that water contained therein is evaporated with time and discoloration occurs therewith, whereby blooms appear on their surface and they have a dry and crumbly mouth feel. For this reason, with regard to the conventional plastic chocolates, importance has been attached to the decorating characteristics on their shape rather than the mouth feel thereof. Moreover, the conventional plastic chocolates, although they have high flexibility in molding similarly to the case of clay, have difficulty in handling; for example, they are prone to adhere to fingers and the wall of a vessel.

Web site: http://www.delphion.com/details?pn=US05271950__

- **Chocolate and wafer bar**

Inventor(s): Ferrero; Pietro (Bruxelles, BE)

Assignee(s): Ferrero S.p.A. (IT)

Patent Number: 4,963,379

Date filed: June 12, 1989

Abstract: A chocolate bar is disclosed which comprises a chocolate base, at least one first wafer sheet placed on the chocolate base and having an interconnecting web and a plurality of hollow projections extending from the wafer sheet web on the side opposite the chocolate base. The chocolate bar further includes an anhydrous creamy filling housed in the cavities of the projections and a coating of chocolate deposited on the outer surface of the wafer sheet.

Excerpt(s): The present invention relates to a chocolate bar of the type comprising a base or matrix of chocolate including at least one second food product which contributes to or complements the organoleptic properties of the chocolate.... Chocolate bars including nuts dispersed in the chocolate matrix are known. From the point of view of their appearance, these nut chocolate bars are characterized by the fact that the nuts project partially from at least one surface of the bar and the projecting parts are usually covered by a thin layer of the chocolate constituting the matrix.... If any portion of the projecting surfaces of the nuts is exposed directly to the air as a result of any production defects, there is the problem that the nuts become rancid. There is thus a high risk that the product will age rapidly.

Web site: http://www.delphion.com/details?pn=US04963379__

- **Chocolate articles**

  Inventor(s): Ahlschwede; Wolfgang (Loerrach, DE)

  Assignee(s): Innogram AG (Binningen/Basel, CH), Futurplan AG (Vaduz, LI)

  Patent Number: 5,985,341

  Date filed: October 13, 1998

  Abstract: Chocolate articles, especially a chocolate sweet, with an improved, new kind of taste sensation are described. For this purpose, the chocolate article contains a first filling and a second filling capable of reacting with one another and separated by a barrier which is adapted to be destroyed when the chocolate article is eaten.

  Excerpt(s): The present invention relates to chocolate articles, especially to a chocolate sweet, with two fillings.... Chocolate sweets are known in a great variety of forms and kinds of taste. It is also known to provide chocolate sweets with two fillings, e.g. nougat and marzipan. On eating, the consumer will however, perceive and register the two kinds of taste separately.... It is the object of the present invention to provide chocolate articles, especially a chocolate sweet, giving rise to a new taste sensation and a new eating effect.

  Web site: http://www.delphion.com/details?pn=US05985341__

- **Chocolate beverage and process for the preparation thereof**

  Inventor(s): Caly; William (Dublin, OH), Gullo; Richard Derek (Marysville, OH), Palag; Soledad N. (Hillard, OH), Rosse; Marcel (Sauges, CH)

  Assignee(s): Nestec S.A. (Vevey, CH)

  Patent Number: 5,894,031

  Date filed: October 3, 1996

  Abstract: A beverage mix comprising at least about 40% by weight based on the total weight of the beverage mix of chocolate or compound confectionery pieces whose thickness is from about 0.25 to 0.75 mm together with a powdered cocoa mix or powdered creamer.

  Excerpt(s): The present invention relates to a chocolate beverage mix and more particularly to a hot chocolate beverage mix containing real chocolate or compound confectionery.... Typically, hot cocoa beverage mixes are sold as powders which are mixed into hot water or milk to give the beverage for consumption. The main ingredient of the powder is sugar and, when mixed into hot water or milk, most of the powder is water soluble and dissolves while the remainder of the powder forms a suspension to provide flavour and texture.... b) the appearance of visible oil on the top.

  Web site: http://www.delphion.com/details?pn=US05894031__

- **Chocolate candy imprinting process**

    Inventor(s): Przelomski; Cheryl L. (Wilmington, DE), Cowan; Dennis R. (Middletown, DE)

    Assignee(s): The Planning Factory, Inc. (Wilmington, DE)

    Patent Number: 5,407,691

    Date filed: September 16, 1992

    Abstract: A method for making candy in which a high-resolution image of edible material is imprinted on another edible material, both of which are, in the preferred embodiment, chocolate. The invention includes steps of measuring heated chocolate into a mold, and allowing it to cool to a proper temperature. A screen mesh is laid over partially cooled chocolate pieces, and another chocolate, preferably of a different color than the chocolate pieces, is applied through the mesh. By using a proper combination of materials and conditions, a highly pleasing image is formed, supporting the attractiveness of the resulting candy, especially as a novelty item or souvenir.

    Excerpt(s): The present invention relates to processes for making candy. More specifically, the invention relates to processes for making candy in which a decorative design made of chocolate is imprinted on a piece of candy.... Various methods of applying images are known in the art. Further, some of these methods have been applied in the food preparation field.... For example, U.S. Pat. No. 5,017,394 (McPherson et al.) shows a system for silk screening edible images on a backing material and transferring the image to cake or the like. U.S. Pat. No. 4,946,696 (Nendl et al.) provides a system for applying an image pattern to the surface of a chocolate product. The image of cocoa butter and other ingredients is screened onto a backing material which forms one of the surfaces on which a chocolate body is formed. U.S. Pat. No. 4,369,200 (Iwao et al.) shows a system for marking chocolate or the like by molding and providing a stencil or plate with slits and holes through which the marking material is applied. These patents are incorporated herein by reference as if reproduced in full below.

    Web site: http://www.delphion.com/details?pn=US05407691__

- **Chocolate coated beverage mixes**

    Inventor(s): Camp; William F. (Fulton, NY), Fischbach; Eugene R. (Fulton, NY)

    Assignee(s): Nestec S.A. (Vevey, CH)

    Patent Number: 4,980,181

    Date filed: January 11, 1989

    Abstract: A composition for preparation of a beverage in which agglomerates of a beverage base are coated with chocolate.

    Excerpt(s): The present invention relates to beverage mixes, more particularly to beverage mixes in which beverage base agglomerates are coated with a thin layer of a fat-based confectionery coating.... There is a desire for beverage mixes, which are to be mixed with hot milk or water for consumption, which contain real chocolate.... Beverage mixes are known in which a small amount of chocolate powder is mixed with a beverage powder such as cocoa, but these products suffer from the disadvantages that the presence of chocolate is not self-evident before dissolution or if larger pieces of chocolate are used, the melting and distribution of chocolate throughout the drink is not as rapid as may be desired.

Web site: http://www.delphion.com/details?pn=US04980181__

- **Chocolate coating containing no tropical oils**

Inventor(s): Meidenbauer; Arlen R. (New Berlin, WI)

Assignee(s): Eskimo Pie Corporation (Richmond, VA)

Patent Number: 5,215,780

Date filed: July 10, 1990

Abstract: A chocolate coating for frozen desserts or the like containing no tropical oils but including a mixture of first and second oils having a different degree of hydrogenation and different melting temperatures and other compatible ingredients.

Excerpt(s): This invention relates generally to a chocolate coating for a dairy dessert and more particularly, to a novel chocolate coating low in saturated fats for use in conjunction with a frozen dairy dessert such as an ice cream bar, cone, or the like.... Consumers have become increasingly concerned about the saturated fat content of the foods which they eat and the effect of such foods on their health and general well-being. Saturated fat has been shown to increase levels of cholesterol in the blood and has been linked to heart disease. Prudent consumers thus consciously seek foods having low saturated fat content.... Chocolate coatings for dairy desserts traditionally have been manufactured with tropical oils, particularly coconut oil which is high in saturated fat. Coconut oil has been preferred because of its reasonable cost, its compatibility with chocolate liquors and its neutral flavor which lets the chocolate flavor come through on the finished product. It has a good shelf life and does not have a waxy taste. Coconut oil is also beneficial to the production process since it dries quickly on the frozen dessert and is very compatible with automatic dipping machines used in the manufacturing process.

Web site: http://www.delphion.com/details?pn=US05215780__

- **Chocolate component-containing food and method for preparing same**

Inventor(s): Kawabata; Yasushi (Ibaraki, JP), Hoshino; Terue (Tsuchiura, JP), Kobayashi; Makoto (Ibaraki, JP)

Assignee(s): Fuji Oil Co., Ltd. (Osaka, JP)

Patent Number: 5,460,847

Date filed: July 15, 1994

Abstract: A chocolate component containing food, and a method for preparing the same, characterized as an oil-in-water emulsion and a non-fluidized state at 5.degree. C. containing 5-50 wt % of fat-free cacao, 10-44 wt % of oils, fats, or combination thereof, 0.5-20 wt % of non-fat milk solid, 10-50 wt % water and 0.05-1 wt % of polyglycerol fatty acid ester having an HLB value of not less than 8 as an emulsifier, and having an emulsion particle diameter in accordance with a laser diffraction particle size distribution measuring device of less than 7.mu.m in median diameter, and said food being in a non-fluidized state at 5.degree. C. This food does not experience oil separation even if repeatedly melted, and has good workability.

Excerpt(s): The present invention relates to a chocolate component containing food, more particularly, a chocolate component containing food that is in a non-fluidized state at 5.degree. C., is considered a "ganache", and from which oil does not separate even if melted repeatedly.... A "ganache", which is prepared by mixing chocolate and cream, is a material for confectionery, which is used, for example, on a cake, in the form of flowers, or for sandwiching between cake dough. However, a ganache with good physical properties has not been obtained because conventional ganaches are unstable in the emulsified state, separate when used, and become difficult to apply because of increasing viscosity, and in particular, when they are solidified by cooling and then heated oil separates therefrom.... Heretofore, many kinds of oil-in-water type processed chocolate foods have been disclosed. For example, JP.A.62-163658 discloses a processed chocolate food that is improved in the emulsified state. It uses sucrose fatty acid ester and lecithin as an emulsifier. Also, in JP.A.2-171154 and 3-139241, a sucrose fatty acid ester is utilized as an emulsifier. However, in these references, a sufficient result is not obtained. For example, when using sucrose fatty acid ester and lecithin as an emulsifier, viscosity increases in a system that contains large amount of cacao solid contents containing milk solid.

Web site: http://www.delphion.com/details?pn=US05460847__

- **Chocolate composition**

  Inventor(s): Gonze; Michel Henri Andre (Brussels, BE), Van Der Schueren; Freddy Maurits Luc (Aalst, BE)

  Assignee(s): Cerestar Holding B.V. (Sas van Gent, NL)

  Patent Number: 6,143,345

  Date filed: February 8, 1996

  Abstract: The present invention discloses a chocolate composition. The composition is characterised in that the normal sugar is replaced with a mixture of sugar alcohols. The mixture contains erythritol and maltitol in such a ratio that the cooling effect of erythritol is considerably reduced.

  Excerpt(s): The present invention discloses a chocolate composition. The present invention also discloses a method for producing a chocolate with the said composition. The composition of the present invention comprises both erythritol and maltitol. Chocolates prepared using this composition have a mouthfeel which corresponds to the mouthfeel of a chocolate containing conventional sugars. The chocolates prepared show a considerable calorie reduction and the `cooling effect` of erythritol is masked by the presence of maltitol.... European patent application EP 0 498 515 describes a process for the production of chocolate. The application discloses that with the use of erythritol or maltitol as sweeteners the conching step used in the production of chocolates is carried out in the form of a dry conching step moreover, this step can be carried out at temperatures well above the normal temperature of 65.degree. C. and suitably for a period of 6 to 16 hours. It is disclosed that the dry conching step can be used with both erythritol and maltitol.... The use of erythritol or maltitol as the sweetener instead of sucrose in the chocolate results in a product of similar appearance and organoleptic properties to an equivalent sucrose based chocolate. It is further shown in the application that the amount of cocoa butter can be reduced by 2 to 15% by weight there is therefore a considerable reduction in the amount of fat (calories).

  Web site: http://www.delphion.com/details?pn=US06143345__

- **Chocolate composition for the preparation of heat-resistant chocolate articles and process for its preparation**

  Inventor(s): Giddey; Claude (Geneva, CH), Dove; Georges (Carouge, CH)

  Assignee(s): Battelle Memorial Institute (Carouge, CH)

  Patent Number: 4,446,166

  Date filed: March 17, 1983

  Abstract: A chocolate composition for use in the preparation of a heat-resistant chocolate article comprising a chocolate mass containing cocoa butter, sugar, milk solids and cocoa solids and, dispersed throughout the mass, from 2 to 10% by weight of the composition of a water-in-fat emulsion, at least a portion of the fat being in solid form.

  Excerpt(s): The present invention concerns the field of foodstuff articles, especially of chocolate which resists, without softening, summer temperatures or the heat of tropical countries. Such a chocolate is often called "tropicalized" chocolate.... An object of the present invention therefore is to provide a chocolate composition for use in the preparation of tropicalized chocolate articles and a method for its manufacture.... Ordinary chocolate is composed of fats or fatty substances (cocoa-butter) in which there are dispersed non fat products such as cocoa components (cellulosic substances, flavors, theobromine, etc..), sugars, proteins (that of milk, for instance). Besides, there can be present in chocolate also various ingredients (fruits, peeled almonds, hazelnuts, special aromas, etc..). Thus, the main phase of chocolate is constituted by fat bodies and its melting temperature is generally not high. This phase essentially comprises cocoa-butter (a mixture of stearyl, oleyl, palmityl and linoleyl glycerides)and it starts softening at 28.degree. C. with consequent loss of strength of the whole mass of chocolate. This mass does not neatly "break", anymore and it tends to flow and sticks annoyingly to the wrapper. Furthermore, after cooling, there can form, on the surface of the chocolate growths of crystallized cocoa butter (blooming) which looks like mold.

  Web site: http://www.delphion.com/details?pn=US04446166__

- **Chocolate compositions**

  Inventor(s): Cain; Frederick W. (Voorburg, NL), Hughes; Adrian D. ('s-Gravenhage, NL), Talbot; Geoffrey (Kempston, GB3)

  Assignee(s): Van Den Bergh Foods Co., division of Conopco Inc. (Lisle, IL)

  Patent Number: 5,324,533

  Date filed: July 1, 1992

  Abstract: Incorporation of at least 0.5 wt. % of a hardstock rich in ($H_2 M + HM_2$)-fat into chocolate compositions results in chocolates that display improved bloom characteristics. H=saturated fatty acid with.gtoreq.C_{16}; M=saturated fatty acid with C_8-C_{14}, in particular C_{12}-C_{14}.

  Excerpt(s): Chocolate compositions containing such conventional ingredients as cocoa powder, cocoa butter, cocoa butter equivalents, sugar, emulsifier need to be tempered because of the presence of polymorphic fats such as POP, POSt and/or StOSt (P=palmitic acid, St=stearic acid and O= oleic acid). Still, it was very difficult to avoid bloom formation, i.e. a polymorphic transformation of the crystal lattice. Therefore, many attempts have been made to find additives that could prevent bloom formation in chocolate compositions. Examples of such additives are butterfat, fully hardened, higherucic rapeseed and BOB (B=behenic, O= oleic).... However, very often the results obtainable with these additives are not satisfactory. Therefore, we have conducted a study in order to find out whether it was possible to find a new, more effective additive.... From U.S. Pat. No. 2,979,407 stabilizing ingredients for solid chocolate materials or chocolate-coated products are known that are included in the chocolate in amounts of 0.5-5 wt. %. The stabilizing ingredients consist of triglycerides of lauric, myristic and palmitic acid, preferably in molar ratios of 2.0:1.2:2.0. Minor amounts of other fatty acids do not change the basic character of the ingredients. The ingredients are used to stabilize the colour of chocolate upon storage. Because of the very strict requirements set to the fatty acid components of the triglycerides that may be used, these products have never been applied commercially.

Web site: http://www.delphion.com/details?pn=US05324533__

- **Chocolate compositions and utilization thereof**

  Inventor(s): Kawabata; Yasushi (Izumisano, JP), Morikawa; Kazutoshi (Ibaraki, JP), Nakajima; Satoko (Izumisano, JP), Shiota; Fumiko (Izumisano, JP), Kurooka; Akira (Izumisano, JP), Yamawaki; Yoshio (Ibaraki, JP), Umeno; Koji (Ibaraki, JP), Kobayashi; Makoto (Ibaraki, JP)

  Assignee(s): Fuji Oil Co., Ltd. (Osaka, JP)

  Patent Number: 6,537,602

  Date filed: June 2, 2000

  Abstract: The present invention provides a ganache-type chocolate composition outstanding in inclusion (mechanical) fitness when contained in confectionery dough, and moreover having good baking tolerance. The chocolate composition includes 1 to 30 wt. % non-fat cacao part, 10 to 50 wt. % fats/oils, 4 to 40 wt. % moisture and by anhydride conversion, 0.2 to 10 wt. % heat-coagulating proteins, and is in non-liquid at 5.degree. C. Chocolate confectionery may be easily manufactured by including or coating this chocolate composition in/on other confectionery dough. Moreover, separately baking the chocolate composition itself can provide chocolate confectionery having new tastes/textures.

  Excerpt(s): The present invention relates to chocolate compositions; in particular it relates to oil-in-water type water-containing chocolate compositions referred to as ganache-type, and to uses thereof.... Oil-in-water type water-containing chocolate compositions (which in general are called "ganaches"), manufactured by mixing chocolate foodstuff with moisture in for example creams, are used as high-grade confectionery materials. Ganaches may be used for napping cakes (i.e., coating onto cake surfaces with a spatula), for flower-making using confectionery tools, or they may be sandwiched between tortes.... Nevertheless, problems with conventional ganaches have been pointed out, such as the following.

  Web site: http://www.delphion.com/details?pn=US06537602__

- **Chocolate compositions of increased viscosity and method for preparing such compositions**

Inventor(s): Finkel; Gilbert (Morristown, NJ)

Assignee(s): Food-Tek, Inc. (Morris Plains, NJ)

Patent Number: 4,980,192

Date filed: March 14, 1989

Abstract: The addition of polyol, such as glycerine or sorbitol, to a system containing a low melting point fat or oil greatly increases the viscosity of the fat or oil thereby immobilizing it even at temperatures which are well above its normal melting point. When a polyol is added to chocolate, the resulting product does not stick to wrappers or fingers even at elevated temperatures where the cocoa butter in the chocolate would normally flow.

Excerpt(s): The present invention relates to a method of increasing the viscosity of a fat or oil and to the product produced by that method. More particularly, this invention is directed to a technique for immobilizing the normally flowable fats or oils in systems containing these materials so that they remain substantially non-flowable even at temperatures which are above their normal melting point.... Fats and oils are widely used in food, cosmetic and pharmaceutical products. Unfortunately, many naturally occurring oils and some fats have very low melting (flow) points and, therefore, impart an undesired physical characteristic to products which contain them. The separation of peanut oil in peanut butter is one typical example of the problem. Another example is the tendency of natural chocolate products containing cocoa butter to stick to product wrappers or to fingers, particularly during the summer months. The separation of butter from dough in the preparation of dough for pastry products, such as croissants or danish pastry, and the surface greasiness of such products is yet another example of an adverse product characteristic resulting from the low melting and flow point of a fat-containing product.... Oils and fats can be immobilized by hydrogenation but this approach is expensive and leads to physiological properties which may be undesirable in food products. Hard fats may be substituted for oils or lower melting point fats, but this substitution often changes the texture or other eating characteristics of the product. Immobilization of fats may also be achieved by the use of stabilizers. However, such additivies are often expensive and may be comprised of undesirable synthetic materials. Moreover, there is a consumer trend away from food products which contain unnatural additivies. In addition, in the case of some products, such as chocolate, the addition of a stabilizer may constitute a material departure from the standard of identity for "chocolate", thereby depriving a manufacturer of the ability to call a particular product a "chocolate" product.

Web site: http://www.delphion.com/details?pn=US04980192__

- **Chocolate conching**

Inventor(s): Capodieci; Roberto A. (Glen Ellyn, IL)

Assignee(s): Mars, Incorporated (McLean, VA)

Patent Number: 5,332,588

Date filed: March 1, 1993

Abstract: A process and a system for combining and physically working chocolate-making ingredients are provided. A variable frequency drive controls the motor of a conching device to increase the efficiency by which energy is imparted to chocolate ingredients during conching. This automatic variable speed approach permits the power to be maintained at a relatively constant and maximum rate, with the speed being determined by the consistency of the ingredients themselves. Feedback associated with the automatic speed variation can be used in order to reduce conching times and vary the quantity of certain ingredients and the timing of and location of their introduction. By the invention, it is possible to standardize the chocolate product during the conching operation and thereby avoid a post-conching standardization procedure with respect to characteristics such as viscosity and fat content.

Excerpt(s): The present invention generally relates to the production of chocolate by an improved process and system. More particularly, the invention relates to chocolate production that includes imparting a substantially constant power level to the chocolate refinings being conched. Included is an arrangement for varying the drive speed of the conching equipment in response to the changing consistency of the intermediate chocolate product being conched. The invention enhances chocolate production efficiency by making additional energy available in order to achieve one or more advantages, especially reduction in processing times and optimization of the addition of costly ingredients such as cocoa butter.... Chocolate is a mixture of finely milled solids, chocolate liquor, sugar, milk crumb or powder, all suspended or well dispersed in cocoa butter and/or substitute fat, which at normal processing temperatures is the liquid carrying medium. Raw materials such as chocolate liquor, sugar, water and milk are processed into chocolate through a series of processed steps including, for example, crumb making, paste mixing, refining, conching and standardizing. Usually, an emulsifier or an emulsifying system is added during conching.... During conching, chemical and physical processes take place. These include the development of the full desirable chocolate flavor and the conversion of the powdery, crumbly refined product into the chocolate. Conching imparts shearing stresses and kneading action which serve both to liquify the masse and to positively influence and accelerate the flavor development processes. Important physical tasks of conching are to disperse, to dehumidify or remove moisture, to remove unwanted volatile flavors, to break up solid particle agglomerates, to round particle edges and to homogenize. Viscosity is lowered, and flowability and texture are improved.

Web site: http://www.delphion.com/details?pn=US05332588__

- **Chocolate conching**

  Inventor(s): Capodieci; Roberto A. (Glen Ellyn, IL)

  Assignee(s): Mars, Incorporated (McLean, VA)

  Patent Number: 5,460,840

  Date filed: July 12, 1994

  Abstract: A process and a system for combining and physically working chocolate-making ingredients are provided. A variable frequency drive controls the motor of a conching device to increase the efficiency by which energy is imparted to chocolate ingredients during conching. This automatic variable speed approach permits the power to be maintained at a relatively constant and maximum rate, with the speed being determined by the consistency of the ingredients themselves. Feedback associated with the automatic speed variation can be used in order to reduce conching times and vary the quantity of certain ingredients and the timing of and location of their introduction. By the invention, it is possible to standardize the chocolate product during the conching operation and thereby avoid a post-conching standardization procedure with respect to characteristics such as viscosity and fat content.

Excerpt(s): The present invention generally relates to the production of chocolate by an improved process and system. More particularly, the invention relates to chocolate production that includes imparting a substantially constant power level to the chocolate refinings being conched. Included is an arrangement for varying the drive speed of the conching equipment in response to the changing consistency of the intermediate chocolate product being conched. The invention enhances chocolate production efficiency by making additional energy available in order to achieve one or more advantages, especially reduction in processing times and optimization of the addition of costly ingredients such as cocoa butter.... Chocolate is a mixture of finely milled solids, chocolate liquor, sugar, milk crumb or powder, all suspended or well dispersed in cocoa butter and/or substitute fat, which at normal processing temperatures is the liquid carrying medium. Raw materials such as chocolate liquor, sugar, water and milk are processed into chocolate through a series of processed steps including, for example, crumb making, paste mixing, refining, conching and standardizing. Usually, an emulsifier or an emulsifying system is added during conching.... During conching, chemical and physical processes take place. These include the development of the full desirable chocolate flavor and the conversion of the powdery, crumbly refined product into the chocolate. Conching imparts shearing stresses and kneading action which serve both to liquify the masse and to positively influence and accelerate the flavor development processes. Important physical tasks of conching are to disperse, to dehumidify or remove moisture, to remove unwanted volatile flavors, to break up solid particle agglomerates, to round particle edges and to homogenize. Viscosity is lowered, and flowability and texture are improved.

Web site: http://www.delphion.com/details?pn=US05460840__

- **Chocolate confection**

Inventor(s): Krawczyk; Gregory R. (Princeton Junction, NJ), Selinger; Edward (Langhorne, PA), McGinley; Emanuel J. (Morrisville, PA)

Assignee(s): FMC Corporation (Philadelphia, PA)

Patent Number: 5,505,982

Date filed: January 27, 1995

Abstract: A chocolate that contains a composite of surfactant/cellulose. The composite is made by the process of coprocessing the cellulose with a surfactant. The composite can be used as a bulking agent or functional formulary aid in low-moisture or in fat phase compositions.

Excerpt(s): This invention relates to new functional bulking and texturizing materials used as an ingredient in chocolate. More particularly, the invention relates to an improved chocolate containing a particulate coprocessed cellulose.... In this era of calorie consciousness in which many consumers are interested in reducing their calorie intake, particularly their fat intake, without reducing their food consumption, there is a need for reduced calorie food ingredients that provide bulk, but few, if any, calories. These bulking aids can be incorporated into specific foods to replace or otherwise reduce the amount of fat and/or other calorie source that would normally have been present in the food. Typically, although not always, these bulking aids preserve the texture of the food and the mouthfeel of the food and preferably enhance either the functionality of other food ingredients or the efficiency of the process of forming the foods.... Cellulose is one such material that has historically served as a functional formulary aid in a wide range of food applications. The use of cellulose as a non-nutritive bulking agent in food systems, especially in nonaqueous food systems, is limited by several characteristics of cellulose. These include an inherent chalky or other disagreeable taste, especially at high use levels; difficulty in forming a dispersion, which adversely affects its mouth feel; and an adverse affect on texture or consistency.

Web site: http://www.delphion.com/details?pn=US05505982_

- **Chocolate confection containing carbonated hard candy crystals dispersed therein**

  Inventor(s): Mangano; Santi F. (Perugia, IT)

  Assignee(s): I.B.P. Industrie Buitoni Perugina S.p.A. (Perugia, IT)

  Patent Number: 4,287,216

  Date filed: December 31, 1979

  Abstract: A confectionery product comprising at least two components, the first component being chocolate, and the second component being a certain amount of candied popping crystals, said two components having both a moisture content between about 0.1 and 5.0%; the product is manufactured substantially with moisture proof material.

  Excerpt(s): This invention concerns a confectionery product which comprises at least two components, the first component being chocolate, a surrogate thereof or the like, and the second component being a certain amount of candied popping crystals; such a product may be in the form of chocolate, a surrogate thereof or the like, containing said crystals scattered in its mass.... Chocolate is a known confectionery product manufactured with the following raw materials: sugar, cocoa, cocoa butter, milk, nuts and aromas; the term surrogate here is to be intended as describing a confectionery product having a structure, consistency, color and taste, all of which recall those of chocolate; the term "and the like" is to be intended here as describing confectionery products not containing cocoa and having a structure and consistency which recall those of surrogate and chocolate.... Chocolate or surrogate or like confectionery products are all suitable for use in manufacturing this new confectionery product, although they must nevertheless be obtained, as will be explained further on, through an accurate technological process. In the following description, the component known as chocolate, surrogate or like confectionery product will be referred to simply as "chocolate or the like".

  Web site: http://www.delphion.com/details?pn=US04287216_

- **Chocolate confectionery and hard fat emulsion contained therein**

  Inventor(s): Padley; Frederick B. (Bedford, GB3), Talbot; Geoffrey (Kempston, GB3)

  Assignee(s): Van den Bergh Foods Co., division of Conopco, Inc. (Lisle, IL)

  Patent Number: 5,104,680

  Date filed: May 10, 1990

Abstract: Compositions, suitable for chocolate filling, comprising a water in hard fat emulsion, wherein the particle size of the dispersed water phase is at most 50.mu.m, are obtained by a process in which a melt of the hard fat is dispersed in an aqueous phase, after which a phase inversion is effected and the water in hard fat emulsion is obtained.

Excerpt(s): This invention relates to chocolate confectionery compositions and in particular to chocolate fillings containing fat compositions.... Chocolate confectionery includes much of the sugar confectionery covered in chocolate, for example chocolate fillings. Chocolate confectionery containing fat compositions frequently include aqueous components including water-soluble flavouring agents in addition to sugar. The latter is present not only for its sweetening effect but also to provide adequate microbiological stability. The increasing emphasis on healthier eating provides a demand for chocolate confectionery with a lower calorific content. The present invention provides chocolate confectionery suitable for chocolate fillings meeting this demand. The present invention therefore provides confectionery compositions suitable for chocolate fillings comprising hard fat in which an aqueous phase is dispersed having a droplet size not exceeding 50 microns, preferably 35 microns or less and more preferably not exceeding 10 microns, and preferably including flavouring agents and sugar.... The hard fat emulsions of the compositions of the present invention exhibit a hardness or C-value of at least 1600 at 20.degree. C. Hardness determined by C-values are measured in accordance with the method described by Haighton et al, JAOCS, 36, 345 (1959) using a cone angle at 40.degree. with a weight of 240 grams. The water-in-fat emulsion comprising the invention may be prepared in a manner conventional for margarine and other plastified water-in-fat emulsion products, as for example by churning or by processing in scraped-surface heat exchanger units for example Votator units, in which an emulsion of fully melted fat and aqueous phase is chilled and worked to provide a matrix of fat crystals in which the aqueous phase is dispersed, an emulsifier suitable for the purpose being present in the composition. Water-soluble ingredients are preferably dissolved or dispersed in the aqueous phase before the emulsion is prepared. Preferably the initial emulsion of liquefied fat and aqueous phase is in the form of a cream i.e. a dispersion of liquid fat in the aqueous phase, conditions being selected during the chilling and working stages of the process to effect inversion of the composition to a water-in-fat dispersed product. By appropriate choice of emulsifier, the product retains an inherent propensity to revert by phase inversion at body temperature, providing a continuous aqueous phase affording more immediate response to the flavour components in the aqueous phase when the product is consumed.

Web site: http://www.delphion.com/details?pn=US05104680__

- **Chocolate containing spray dried glucose**

  Inventor(s): Van Der Schueren; Freddy Maurits Luc (Aalst, BE), Solner; Mari Cornelis Willem (Reeuwijk, NL)

  Assignee(s): Cerestar Holding B.V. (LA Sas van Gent, NL)

  Patent Number: 5,976,605

  Date filed: September 26, 1997

Abstract: The present invention describes the use of spray dried glucose as sweetening agent in chocolate compositions. The spay dried glucose is used to replace between 5 and 100% of the normal sweetening agent which is sucrose. The spray dried glucose is used in dark, milk and white chocolate. This replacement leads to product having lower viscosity and which is therefore easier to handle.

Excerpt(s): The present invention discloses a chocolate composition containing spray dried glucose and chocolates obtained therewith. The invention also describes a method for obtaining chocolates containing the said spray dried glucose.... The conventional chocolate composition contains sucrose as a sweetener. The essential components of chocolate are cocoa nib, i.e. the roasted cocoa bean with shell and germ removed, sugar and cocoa butter. Cocoa nib is approximately 55% cocoa butter, the balance being proteins, carbohydrates, tannins, acids etc. The cocoa butter content of the chocolate controls its setting characteristics and largely governs its cost. Different types of chocolate are obtained by varying the ratio of cocoa nib to sugar. The amount of cocoa butter varies according to its application; bitter sweet chocolate has a ratio of nib to sugar of 2:1 while sweet chocolate has a ratio of 1:2.... Nowadays there is a strong interest in reducing the amount of calories contained in chocolate. Two approaches are taken, a reduction of the amount of butter (fat) and/or a reduction of the amount of sugar. The amount of sugar calories is reduced by replacing sucrose with polyols such as maltitol, lactitol, sorbitol, xylitol and erythritol. This replacement often has a double advantage in that not only there is a calorie reduction but also some of the polyols are non-cariogenic.

Web site: http://www.delphion.com/details?pn=US05976605__

- **Chocolate enrobed wafer products and method for preparing the same**

  Inventor(s): Finkel; Gilbert (Parsippany, NJ)

  Assignee(s): Food-Tek, Inc. (Morris Plains, NJ)

  Patent Number: 4,812,318

  Date filed: May 12, 1987

  Abstract: A liquid polyol is added to a flowable chocolate mixture after it has been tempered to increase the viscosity thereof. Utilizing concentric nozzles, the chocolate is simultaneously extruded around a non-aqueous stabilized batter material thus producing an outer cylinder of stabilized chocolate and an inner core of stabilized batter. The co-extruded entity is then cooked briefly in a microwave oven in order to set the batter into a stiff wafer-like material while leaving the outer chocolate coating essentially unchanged.

  Excerpt(s): The present invention relates to a method of increasing the viscosity of a fat or oil and to the product produced by that method. More particularly, this invention is directed to a technique for immobilizing the normally flowable fats or oils in systems containing these materials so that they remain substantially non-flowable even at temperatures which are above their normal melting point.... Fats and oils are widely used in food, cosmetic and pharmaceutical products. Unfortunately, many naturally occurring oils and some fats have very low melting (flow) points and, therefore, impart an undesired physical characteristic to products which contain them. The separation of peanut oil in peanut butter is one typical example of the problem. Another example is the tendency of natural chocolate products containing cocoa butter to stick to product wrappers or to fingers, particularly during the summer months. The separation of butter from dough in the preparation of dough for pastry products, such as croissants or danish pastry, and the surface greasiness of such products is yet another example of an adverse product characteristic resulting from the low melting and flow point of a fat-containing product.... Oils and fats can be immobilized by hydrogenation but this approach is expensive and leads to physiological properties which may be undesirable in food products. Hard fats may be substituted for oils or lower melting point fats, but this substitution often changes the texture or other eating characteristics of the product. Immobilization of fats may also be achieved by the use of stabilizers. However, such additivies are often expensive and may be comprised of undesirable synthetic materials. Moreover, there is a consumer trend away from food products which contain unnatural additivies. In addition, in the case of some products, such as chocolate, the addition of a stabilizer may constitute a material departure from the standard of identity for "chocolate", thereby depriving a manufacturer of the ability to call a particular product a "chocolate" product.

Web site: http://www.delphion.com/details?pn=US04812318__

- **Chocolate feeding device for chocolate refiners**

  Inventor(s): Ripani; Sergio (Milan, IT), Serafini; Giulio (Milan, IT)

  Assignee(s): Carle & Montanari S.p.A. (Milan, IT)

  Patent Number: 4,688,177

  Date filed: May 6, 1985

  Abstract: A chocolate feeding device for chocolate refiners which has a chocolate feeding conveyor provided with movable pick-up blades feeding the chocolate to several points in an adjacent refiner feeding hopper which cooperates with an electric cell, the output of which is representative of the chocolate quantity in said feeding hopper. The feeding hopper is provided with an oscillable shield-like bottom wall the movements of which are controlled by a pneumatic cylinder/piston unit connected to it and controlled in turn by an actuator having a circuit controlled by an oscillable front wall of a chocolate-receiving chamber of the chocolate refiner.

  Excerpt(s): This invention relates to a chocolate feeding and control system for chocolate refiners.... As is known in the art, chocolate refiners have the function of "rolling" the chocolate paste being fed in in order to impart to it a desired fineness. This is selected according to the intended final use of the chocolate in a variety of different products. Measuring the fineness of the chocolate film being delivered by the refiners presents considerable difficulties and is generally carried out in an empirical fashion.... Italian Patent Application No. 20 718 A/83 (U.S. Pat. No. 4,519,304) by this Applicant discloses a device for adjusting and monitoring the thickness of the film being delivered by refiners, which enables the achievement of fineness grades which are required and preset. With that device, it is possible to directly adjust a refiner so as to maintain set fineness values.

  Web site: http://www.delphion.com/details?pn=US04688177__

- **Chocolate flavored hard candy**

  Inventor(s): Carpenter; John R. (Hershey, PA), Gutshall-Zakis; Ann L. (Harrisburg, PA), Ejike; Ofomata E. (Palmyra, PA), Heim; R. Mark (Haarrisburg, PA)

  Assignee(s): Hershey Foods Corporation (Hershey, PA)

  Patent Number: 5,637,344

  Date filed: October 20, 1995

  Abstract: The present invention relates to an amorphous crystalline chocolate flavored hard candy confection utilizing air-jet milled cocoa powder in which the particles thereof are less than about 15 microns in size and generally have rounded edges to achieve a desirable smooth texture and to the process of preparing the same.

Excerpt(s): The present invention is directed to a method of preparing chocolate flavored amorphous hard candy utilizing air-jet milled cocoa powder and the product prepared thereby.... Hard candy confections are very popular in the United States. They are amorphous confections having a relatively smooth and glassy surface. They appear in various shapes and sizes and come in various flavors, such as fruit, mint, butterscotch, peppermint, and the like. Although chocolate is a very popular flavor in other types of confections, it is surprising that chocolate flavored hard candy makes up only a small percentage of the hard candy market. An example of a hard candy chocolate product was sold in Japan and named BLACK and WHITE. It was manufactured by Kanro and was sold as part of a pair of products. The BLACK hard candy contained a chocolate flavored hard candy center, and the surface thereof was dusted with cocoa powder, while in the product called "WHITE", the candy contained a hard candy center and the surface was dusted with milk powder. The "BLACK" product had a rough, coarse, sandy surface--characteristics which are not acceptable for hard candy.... Thus, the present inventors sought to make a chocolate flavored hard candy which exhibits mouthfeel, texture and organoleptic characteristics typical of hard candy. First, they used commercial cocoa powder to make the hard candy.

Web site: http://www.delphion.com/details?pn=US05637344__

- **Chocolate for use in producing rolled chocolate**

Inventor(s): Yamaguchi; Kotaro (Sennan, JP), Nishimoto; Tsugio (Naga, JP), Ebihara; Yoshitaka (Sakai, JP), Matsunami; Hidenobu (Senna, JP)

Assignee(s): Fuji Oil Company, Limited (Osaka, JP)

Patent Number: 5,286,515

Date filed: March 4, 1992

Abstract: There is disclosed a chocolate containing disaturated monolinoleate and non-tempering type hard butter as its oil ingredients. A process for producing a rolled chocolate by rolling-up a chocolate containing disaturated monolinoleate and non-tempering type hard butter as its oil ingredients is also disclosed.

Excerpt(s): The present invention relates to a chocolate, in particular, a chocolate which is suitable for rolling-up, and to a rolled chocolate. The term "chocolate" used herein is not limited to specific kinds of chocolate such as those prescribed by agreements, e.g., "Fair Agreements on Indication of Chocolates" as well as laws and regulations, and it is intended that other chocolates and other processed food of fats and oils using a so-called cacao butter substitute are also included.... A rolled chocolate used for decorating cakes and the like has been produced by manually scraping a plate-like chocolate with a spoon or the like. However, since this requires skill, and it is difficult to obtain uniform products, the mass production thereof by a machine has been recently employed (JP-A 59-66842, JP-A 63-263048, etc.). In such a mechanical treatment, there is a rolling-up step such as peeling off a chocolate spread on a belt with a scraper or shaving it off therefrom with a cutting blade. Since extremely severe temperature control is required in such a rolling-up step and the shape and size become uneven in many cases even in such a highly mechanized step, the yield in the rolling-up step is usually from 50 to 70%. Further, a cylindrical inner surface of the rolled chocolate thus produced tends to become whitish and this is undesirable from the viewpoint of appearance.... One object of the present invention is to provide a chocolate which is suitable for the production of a rolled chocolate.

Web site: http://www.delphion.com/details?pn=US05286515__

- **Chocolate having defined hard fat**

  Inventor(s): Padley; Frederick B. (Welwyn Garden City, GB2), Paulussen; Cornelis N. (Uitgeest, NL), Soeters; Cornelis (Rotterdam, NL), Tresser; David (London, GB2)

  Assignee(s): Lever Brothers Company (New York, NY)

  Patent Number: 4,276,322

  Date filed: May 11, 1977

  Abstract: Chocolate is provided containing a hard fat comprising a mixture of a natural, high POP/POS/SOS-fat and a narrowly defined SOS/POS-fat. The hard fat lies within an area defined in FIG. 18, 19 or 20; in the absence of the SOS/POS-fat, the hard fat lies outside the area. Particular mixtures are also claimed for use as hard fats. Palm mid-fraction is a preferred natural, high POP/POS/SOS-fat.

  Excerpt(s): Reference is made to our copending application Ser. No. 751,309 which is a continuation of Ser. No. 417,865 which was itself a continuation of Ser. No. 240,265. Both Ser. No. 417,865 and 240,265 are now abandoned.... The invention relates to fats, particularly to hard fats, often called hard butters.... Hard fats are specially important in confectionery, bakery and pharmaceutical products. Such fats have the special property that at room temperature they are hard but melt quickly at body temperature, e.g. in the mouth. The most important example of a hard fat is cocoabutter. Because of its very special properties, although also because of long association, cocoabutter can command high prices. There has been a long-standing need for fats that can act as replacers, for example, for cocoa-butter. As more fully explained below, fats have been developed that partly meet this need. But all these fats suffer from one or more disadvantages.

  Web site: http://www.delphion.com/details?pn=US04276322__

- **Chocolate heat-resistance by particulate polyol gel addition**

  Inventor(s): Mandralis; Zenon I. (Dublin, OH), Weitzenecker; Don P. (Urbana Pike, OH)

  Assignee(s): Nestec S.A (Vevey, CH)

  Patent Number: 5,523,110

  Date filed: June 23, 1994

  Abstract: Chocolate-based confectionery products having improved heat-resistance are prepared by mixing a polyol gel in particulate form with a flowable chocolate or a flowable mixture of ingredients for preparing a chocolate or chocolate-type composition in an amount to obtain a product having, based upon the product weight, a polyol content of from 0.2% to 60% by weight.

  Excerpt(s): The present invention relates to improving the heat resistance of chocolate or chocolate-type products so that they have a reduced tendency to deform or melt at elevated temperatures or to stick to the packaging material.... Chocolate products are usually thorough mixtures of liquid cocoa, cocoa butter, sugar, lecithin and possibly milk and flavouring substances. They therefore contain fatty substances which soften and melt between 30.degree. and 35.degree. C.... When articles which consist entirely or partly of these products are exposed to temperatures lying above the melting point of the aforesaid fatty substances, (i.e., temperatures occurring during the summer season or in tropical countries), they tend to lose their original shape and appearance, and become soft and unpleasant to handle. If they are wrapped, the surface of the article may adhere to the wrapper and may produce unsightly fat staining.

Web site: http://www.delphion.com/details?pn=US05523110__

- **Chocolate plant**

  Inventor(s): Bindler; Uwe (Bergneustadt, DE)

  Assignee(s): Gebr, Bindler Maschinenfabrik GmbH & Co. KG (Bergneustadt, DE)

  Patent Number: 6,135,016

  Date filed: February 26, 1999

  Abstract: A plant for producing foodstuffs is particularly suited for use as a chocolate plant, and permits facilitated tailoring thereof for a particular production purpose by including at least two sections, at least a portion of which are mechanically independent of one another. The foodstuffs are advantageously processable and/or conveyable in product carriers, and optionally delivered from one section to another by transfer devices located therebetween. Optionally, intermediate storage devices may also be provided between the portion of the sections which are mechanically independent of one another.

  Excerpt(s): The invention relates to a plant for producing foodstuffs, in particular a chocolate plant, comprising at least two sections, with the foodstuffs in the sections preferably being processable and/or conveyable in product carriers.... The chocolate plants known from the state of the art are always built as entire plants comprising various sections, e.g. mold changing sections, warming-up sections, refrigeration sections and mold release sections. The known plants are tailor-made for a particular purpose, e.g. for producing Advent calendars, for producing chocolate bars or similar products. As a rule, reconfiguring the known plant from a plant for producing Advent calendars to a plant for producing chocolate bars is expensive, and sometimes even impossible. However, due to their special design, the known chocolate plants achieve high rates of throughput when producing those products for which a particular plant is tailor-made.... Based on the above-mentioned problems, it is the object of the invention to provide a plant for producing foodstuffs, in particular a chocolate plant, which ensures flexible production of usually small batches of various products.

  Web site: http://www.delphion.com/details?pn=US06135016__

- **Chocolate product containing dipeptide-cocoa butter composition**

  Inventor(s): Frost; John R. (Tarrytown, NY), Sarich; Nancy J. (Putnam Valley, NY), Schenz; Timothy W. (Haworth, NJ), Glatz; Alfred C. (Summit, NJ)

  Assignee(s): General Foods Corporation (White Plains, NY)

  Patent Number: 4,701,337

  Date filed: September 30, 1985

Abstract: A composition which modifies the physical characteristics of a lipid is disclosed. This composition comprises a hydrated, crystalline dipeptide sweetener and a lipid and can be used to produce a non-waxy, no melt chocolate by utilizing cocoa butter as the lipid source.

Excerpt(s): The present invention relates to a dipeptide-cocoa butter composition. More particularly the present invention is concerned with a chocolate product containing a dipeptide-cocoa butter composition.... Dipeptide sweeteners such as.alpha.-L-aspartyl-L-phenylalanime-methyl ester (aspartame or APM) disclosed by Schlatter in U.S. Pat. No. 3,492,131; the L-aspartyl-D-alaninamides and L-aspartyl-D-serinamided disclosed in U.S. Pat. No. 4,373,430; and L.alpha.-aspartyl-L-tyrosine disclosed n U.S. Pat. No. 4,017,422 are generally known as low-calorie sweetening agents which have the quality of possessing a clear initial taste without an unpleasant bitter aftertaste. Nonetheless, heat and enzymes readily degrade aspartame in an aqueous environment causing aspartame to be far less stable then other well-known sweeteners such as sugars, polyols and synthetic chemical sweeteners such as cyclamate and saccharin. Because of this stability, food processors need a means of preserving dipeptide sweeteners throughout standard food processing procedures.... Unlike dipeptide sweeteners, lipids, even in an aqueous environment, can withstand considerable heat. Nonetheless, the physical structure of a lipid--its double bonds, the location of its double bonds, and the stereochemistry of its double bonds--normally determines the lipids other properties. However, food processors typically desire a mix of properties not available with any one particular lipid, for example, a flaky pie crust requires a hard fat, but nutritionally, polyunsaturated oils are preferred. Consequently, food processors desire a method for modifying lipid properties.

Web site: http://www.delphion.com/details?pn=US04701337__

- **Chocolate products with increased protein content and process for the production of such type products**

  Inventor(s): Vajda; Gabor (Budapest, HU), Ravasz; Laszlo (Budapest, HU), Karacsonyi; Bela (Budapest, HU), Tabajdi; Gabor (Budapest, HU)

  Assignee(s): Kozponti Valto- es Hitelbank RT. Innovacios Alap (Budapest, HU)

  Patent Number: 4,493,853

  Date filed: January 31, 1983

  Abstract: A chocolate product with increased protein content and having decreased carbohydrate content is disclosed. The product comprises substantially of a processed cheese and chocolate melt made perfectly homogeneous in a weight ratio of 1:1-1,5, being solid or semi-solid at environmental temperature. The carbohydrate content of the chocolate is partially replaced by decomposed milk or cheese protein. This product is manufactured by mixing melted cheese with a chocolate melt at 50.degree. C. or higher temperature by intensive stirring and homogenizing the mass, which is allowed to solidify preferably after it is formed. The formed product can be immersed into chocolate to obtain a chocolate icing on the surface of the product.

  Excerpt(s): This invention relates to chocolate products with increased protein content and to a process for the manufacturing of such type chocolate products to increase the assortment of products of the sweet industry.... It is well-known, that among the products of the sweet industry, chocolates and products containing purely chocolate, are the most favourable. Depending on the kind of the chocolate it contains 40-60 weight

% carbohydrate whereas the carbohydrate content of the products of the sweet industry with chocolate-content or chocolate icing is still even greater as mentioned. Chocolates contain in addition to carbohydrate alkaloids as well e.g. theobromine, tannin-derivatives cocoared and catechine, further mineral substances, which are physiologically useful and easily digestible.... Many experiments were made to increase the protein and to reduce the carbohydrate content of chocolates maintaining at the same time their deliciousness. These experiments, however, failed and therefore the proportion of the protein could not be increased at the expense of the carbohydrate. Chocolates form a heterogenous, polydisperse system, which contains sugar dispersed in cocoa-butter, cocoa-starch and other solid components, e.g. mineral substances. The cocoa-butter--as dispersing medium--is solid at room-temperature. The viscosity of the dispersing medium depends on the proportion of the cocoa-butter at a given temperature, as well as on the quantity of additives which reduce the viscosity of the product. Chocolate has a lypophobic character and cannot absorb more than 2-3 weight % of water, The homogeneity of the chocolate mass is destroyed, if it contains more than 5 weight % of water. Under influence of the water the sugar content of the chocolate dissolves and the formed sugar syrup is not able to redisperse in the dispersing medium, which is the cocoa-butter. Consequently small water- and fat droplets form within the originally homogeneous chocolate mass at 32.degree. C. The unhomogeneous chocolate mass cannot be processed further and it becomes lumpy. This is the reason why chocolates could be enriched, or mixed respectively, with anhydrous substances or substances only containing very small water e.g. dried milk, roasted and milled seeds. This is the method which is suitable to produce milk-chocolate, and whole-nut-chocolate. If chocolate is mixed with substances having great water content, than this water content should be eliminated by heating during the refining process. If the water content of the chocolate is greater than the usual amount, the substance becomes lumpy and tastes gritty.

Web site: http://www.delphion.com/details?pn=US04493853__

- **Chocolate products with sucrose fatty acid polyester fat substitutes**

  Inventor(s): Miller; Mark S. (Arlington Heights, IL), Surber; Kevin J. (Lombard, IL)

  Assignee(s): Kraft Foods, Inc. (Northfield, IL)

  Patent Number: 5,518,754

  Date filed: August 19, 1994

  Abstract: Low-fat or reduced-fat chocolate products containing sucrose fatty acid polyesters are provided which have texture and mouthfeel properties similar to conventional chocolate products. These chocolate products are prepared using a sucrose fatty acid polyester or a blend of sucrose fatty acid polyesters in place of the conventional cocoa butter constituent. The sucrose fatty acid polyesters used do not necessarily mimic the theological and thermal properties of cocoa butter. Rather, the desired texture and mouthfeel properties of the chocolate products of this invention are obtained by incorporating a hydrogenated or hardened oil (i.e., a hardstock triglyceride) and an emulsifier selected from the group consisting of lactylated glycerides, sorbitan esters, acetylated glycerides, polysorbate esters, and polyglycerol esters, along with the one or more sucrose fatty acid polyesters, into conventional chocolate formulations containing essentially no cocoa butter or substantially reduced levels of cocoa butter. In one especially preferred embodiment, two sucrose fatty acid polyesters of different firmness and having high levels of sucrose fatty acid octaesters are employed. The improved chocolate products have similar texture and mouthfeel properties of conventional chocolate with significantly fewer calories and lower fat content. Moreover, the texture and mouthfeel properties can be varied for various uses by varying the relative proportions of the sucrose fatty acid polyesters and the hardened oil.

Excerpt(s): The invention generally relates to the field of chocolate products, especially low-fat or reduced-fat chocolate products. More specifically, this invention relates to low-fat or reduced-fat chocolate products having texture and mouthfeel similar to conventional chocolate products. The chocolate products of this invention are prepared using a sucrose fatty acid polyester or a blend of sucrose fatty acid polyesters in place of the conventional cocoa butter constituent.... Chocolate is a highly desirable confection product which has unique texture and flavor release properties in the mouth. Many of these desirable properties are generally attributable to the fat component of chocolate--cocoa butter--which has a narrow melting point range just slightly below normal body temperature and a sharp melting curve. Accordingly, the desirable flavor release and organoleptic sensations of chocolate occur rapidly as the chocolate melts in the mouth.... Conventional chocolate products generally contain about 30 to 60 percent sugar, about 10 to 70 percent chocolate liquor (which normally contains about percent cocoa butter), about 20 to 25 percent added cocoa butter, and about 1 percent flavor and other constituents. Typically, such chocolate products contain about 30 to 34 percent total fat in the form of cocoa butter. Unfortunately, therefore, conventional chocolate products are generally high in undesirable saturated fats and calories. Due to the relatively recent interest in reducing calorie and saturated fat intake in the diet, there has been an increased interest in providing reduced-calorie and/or reduced-fat chocolate products. Most of these efforts have attempted to provide a substitute for the cocoa butter component in conventional chocolate products.

Web site: http://www.delphion.com/details?pn=US05518754__

- **Chocolate refining process**

    Inventor(s): Carvallo; Federico de Loyola (Arlington Heights, IL), Hine; William Scott (McMahons Point, AU), Helmreich; Andreas Valentin (Aying, DE)

    Assignee(s): Kraft Foods, Inc. (Northfield, IL)

    Patent Number: 6,238,724

    Date filed: October 19, 1999

    Abstract: An improved chocolate manufacturing and/or refining process is provided. This process allows chocolate refining at a significantly increased throughput rate while maintaining the particle size distribution at the desired level. Thus, the production rates of existing or newly designed chocolate-making processes can be increased significantly. High shear is applied to the chocolate mass during the later stages of refining and before conching. Generally, this high shear is in the range of about 200,000 to about 1,000,000 sec.sup.-1. By significantly increasing the shear rate in the later stages of the refining process, the throughput of refining process, and thus the overall chocolate manufacturing process, can be significantly increased without significantly increasing the particle size of the chocolate mass entering the conching step.

    Excerpt(s): The present invention is directed to an improved chocolate refining process. More particularly, the present invention is directed to a process which allows chocolate refining at a significantly increased throughput rate while maintaining the particle size distribution at the desired level. Thus, using the methods of this invention, the production rates of existing or newly designed chocolate-making processes can be increased significantly. As used herein, the term chocolate means confectionery masses containing cocoa butter and/or other vegetable fats.... The essential components of a conventional chocolate formulation are cocoa "nib" (i.e., the roasted cocoa bean with shell and germ removed), sugar, and cocoa butter in addition to the cocoa butter contained in the nib. Cocoa nib is approximately 50% cocoa butter, the balance being proteins, carbohydrates, tannins, acids, and the like. The cocoa butter content of the chocolate controls its setting characteristics and largely governs its cost. While the ratio of cocoa nib to sugar determines the type of chocolate, the cocoa butter content varies according to the application. Thus, bitter sweet chocolate has a nib to sugar ratio of about 2 to 1 while sweet chocolate has a ratio of about 1 to 2. Molding chocolate may have a fat content of about 25% to 40%, covering chocolate about 33 to 36%, chocolate for hollow goods about 38 to 40%, and chocolate for covering ice cream about 50 to 60%.... The typical preparation of chocolate involves four general operations or steps. In the first operator, the ingredients are mixed together in a process which also involves grinding or rubbing (e.g., on a multiple roll press) to provide a smooth fluid paste of uniform and specific particle size. The ingredients may be added sequentially and/or, in particular the cocoa butter, may be added stepwise to help control the viscosity of the composition. The sugar may also be preground to a smaller particle size to reduce the length of time required in the grinding/rubbing (i.e., refining) of the chocolate mixture. Most chocolate, and certainly all good quality chocolate, is subjected after refining or mixing to the process of "conching" in which the chocolate mixture is subjected to temperature treatment and mechanical working to give the chocolate an improved texture and a fuller and more homogeneous flavor. Other ingredients such as flavors (e.g., vanilla and extra cocoa butter) may be added during this operation, if desired. A frequently added additional ingredient is lecithin or other emulsifiers which improves the flow properties of the chocolate and thereby enables the amount of fat to be reduced. The third operation of the chocolate preparation is called "tempering" in which nuclei are provided in the liquid chocolate composition to facilitate the rapid crystallization of selected stable fat crystals on cooling. The final appearance of the chocolate, its texture and keeping properties depend upon correct tempering conditions. After tempering, the chocolate may finally be cast into molds to set or may be used in an enrobing process to produce the desired chocolate products.

Web site: http://www.delphion.com/details?pn=US06238724__

- **Chocolate shape mold assembly**

  Inventor(s): Zanetos; Tom (Columbus, OH), Zanetos; Joseph C. (Columbus, OH)

  Assignee(s): Anthony-Thomas Candy Company, Inc. (Columbus, OH)

  Patent Number: 5,033,947

  Date filed: May 7, 1990

  Abstract: A mold assembly for forming solid molded chocolate shapes is formed from first and second sheet-like mold halves separably joined by permanent magnets and having base flanges that support the mold assembly in an upright position for filling through an edge fill opening. The base flanges for the mold assembly include binary-coded mold fill information utilized in chocolate shape production apparatus and specific to that particular mold assembly.

Excerpt(s): The present invention relates generally to molding chocolate, and particularly concerns a mold assembly for forming solid molded chocolate shapes.... Chocolate mold filling apparatus may generally be classified into two types on the basis of production quantity and product variety requirements. A common general-purpose type of chocolate mold filling apparatus selectively and repeatedly pumps an individually-metered adjusted quantity of tempered chocolate from a storage tank to a fill nozzle and into a hand-moved chocolate mold aligned with the fill nozzle. No attempts are made to automatically adjust fill tubes heights or fill quantities or to mechanically control mold lateral or longitudinal movements. Hence, such general-purpose mold filling apparatus is well-suited only to a relatively small or hand-production run even though a variety of different chocolate mold sizes can be accommodated.... The common special-purpose type of mold filling apparatus, on the other hand, generally is designed and operated to produce only a single product in quantity and cannot readily accommodate intermediate to large production runs involving different mold sizes and mold cavity spacings.

Web site: http://www.delphion.com/details?pn=US05033947__

- **Chocolate shape retention**

  Inventor(s): Beckett; Stephen T. (York, GB2)

  Assignee(s): Nestec S.A. (Vevey, CH)

  Patent Number: 5,445,843

  Date filed: July 8, 1994

  Abstract: A process for improving the shape retention of chocolate or chocolate type products so that they have a reduced tendency to deform at elevated temperatures which comprises mixing an encapsulated product in particulate form comprising capsules of a polyol enclosed within an edible lipid with a flowable mixture of chocolate type ingredients, the encapsulated product being added in an amount to achieve a polyol content of from 0.2 to 5% by weight based on the total amount of the resultant chocolate.

  Excerpt(s): The present invention relates to a process for improving the shape retention of chocolate or chocolate type products so that they have a reduced tendency to deform or melt at elevated temperatures or to stick to the packaging material.... Chocolate products are usually thorough mixtures of liquid cocoa, cocoa butter, sugar, lecithin and possibly milk and flavouring substances. They therefore contain fatty substances which soften and melt between 30.degree. and 35.degree. C.... When articles which consist entirely or partly of these products are exposed to temperatures lying above the melting point of the aforesaid fatty substances, (i.e. temperatures occurring during the summer season or in tropical countries), they tend to lose their original shape and appearance, and become soft and unpleasant to handle. If they are wrapped, the surface of the article may adhere to the wrapper and may produce unsightly fat staining.

  Web site: http://www.delphion.com/details?pn=US05445843__

- **Chocolate solid wafer and method of manufacture**

Inventor(s): Warkentin; Brian T. (Sunnyvale, CA)

Assignee(s): Shade Foods, Inc. (Belmont, CA)

Patent Number: 3,966,997

Date filed: February 3, 1975

Abstract: A substantially unsweetened homogeneous solid chocolate composition useful as an intermediate in producing chocolate fudge toppings and chocolate variegating sauces for ice cream and method for preparation thereof which composition consists essentially of 25 to 40 weight percent of cocoa determined on a fat-free basis, 30 to 40 weight percent of a mixture of hydrogenated vegetable oil and cocoa butter, 18 to 25 weight percent of starch, 0 to 10 weight percent of low fat milk powder, 0.5 to 2.0 weight percent of lecithin and 0.5 to 3.0 weight percent of salt. Small amounts of flavor imparting materials such as vanillin may be present.

Excerpt(s): Chocolate fudge toppings for ice cream are widely used confections. Currently they are manufactured by separately adding weighed quantities of chocolate liquor, cocoa, salt, vanillin, vegetable oil, stabilizer, emulsifier and milk powder to a measured quantity of corn syrup, sugar and water residing in a kettle. This mixture is agitated and heated in the kettle until an intimate mixture of all of the materials is produced. The resultant intimate mixture is then packed in small bottles for direct consumer use or in large cans for institutional use. Some manufacturers run the mixture produced in the kettle through a homogenizer before packing. This method of manufacture has certain disadvantages. The manufacturer is required to purchase, store, inventory, handle and weigh a large number of ingredients in formulating a kettle batch, errors are common. Unless the product from the kettle is run through a homogenizer before packing the product is frequently gritty due to the presence of large particles of cocoa powder or cocoa solids in the mixture. The product, whether the homogenization step is used or not, is a thin liquid which must be stored in the containers for as long as four to six weeks before it develops the thick creamy character of an acceptable fudge topping. Immediately after packaging, it can be poured from the container as a thin syrup, but after the four to six weeks storage period, it has thickened to the point where it must be spooned from the container and has all of the desired characteristics of a fudge topping.... It would be desirable to simplify the manufacturing procedure for topping producers by reducing the number of ingredients which they must store, inventory and measure and it would be especially desirable to enable them to avoid the four to six weeks storage period required for the product to develop a thick creamy consistency so that it is in a condition suitable for sale to the consumer.... Pursuant to the present invention, a solid chocolate product is produced which can be added to corn syrup, invert sugar and water, heated to elevated temperature for a few minutes to form a fudge topping which can be packaged and immediately sold for consumer use. The fudgy consistency appears promptly after the mixture is cooled and no storage period is required for the product to develop an acceptable fudgy consistency.

Web site: http://www.delphion.com/details?pn=US03966997__

- **Chocolate syrup and method of making same**

Inventor(s): Dow; Douglas (1080 Iroquois, Detroit, MI 48214), Flanagan; Patricia J. (18917 Highlite Dr., S., Mt. Clemens, MI 48043)

Assignee(s): none reported

Patent Number: 4,880,655

Date filed: July 29, 1985

Abstract: A chocolate syrup sweetened by honey which allows the syrup to be kept at room temperature even after opening. An approximate ratio of 8 parts honey to 1 part cocoa by weight is maintained in the formulations. When these are mixed together, water is also added which will vary from between 4 to 25% by weight of the total mixture. A flavoring, in less than 2% by weight of the syrup, can also be mixed into the syrup.

Excerpt(s): The invention concerns a chocolate syrup that can be readily applied to ice cream and mixed with drinks while not requiring refrigeration.... There are a number of commercially available chocolate flavored syrups which are marketed under such trade names as HERSHEY'S and NESTLE'S; however, these all suffer the disadvantage of having to be refrigerated upon opening and further make use of numerous additives. The inconvenience of having to refrigerate the syrups discourages their use as does the increasing recognition of the desire to avoid additives in foods for better health.... Described is a chocolate syrup which can be made from three natural ingredients, with perhaps a flavoring added. The ingredients are: cocoa, honey and water. When these are combined by maintaining an approximate 8 to 1 ratio between the honey and the cocoa with water added varying between 4 and 25% depending on the desired use of the end product, a chocolate syrup will result which not only tastes good but is easily usable and does not need refrigeration.

Web site: http://www.delphion.com/details?pn=US04880655__

- **Chocolate with improved and enriched aroma, and a process of its production**

Inventor(s): Takemori; Toshio (Tokyo, JP), Tsurumi; Toshinobu (Saitama, JP), Ito; Masanori (Saitama, JP), Kamiwaki; Tatsuya (Saitama, JP)

Assignee(s): Lotte Company Limited (Tokyo, JP)

Patent Number: 5,635,183

Date filed: March 30, 1994

Abstract: A raw material cacao for chocolate may be improved and enriched in its aroma, thereby providing a chocolate whose consumption results in increased mental concentration, and which has an improved cacao aroma and reduced sweetness. The chocolate of the invention is produced by using the improved and enriched cacao nibs produced by an alkali-treatment of cacao beans. The process for producing the chocolate using cacao nibs of improved and enriched aroma comprises removing shells and germs from raw or semi-roasted cacao beans to prepare cacao nibs, adding an alkali thereto and stirring for reaction thereof with the alkali, subsequently drying and roasting the same and finally grinding and pulverizing the alkali-treated cacao nibs to prepare a cacao mass to be used for producing the chocolate in the conventional way. The alkali is preferably calcium hydroxide.

Excerpt(s): The invention relates to a chocolate of reduced sweetness and to a process of producing the same, in which the flavor of main raw cacao material for the chocolate is improved to enrich the cacao.... For the purpose of producing a chocolate, there have been neither ideas nor practices for treating the material cacao with alkali. Heretofore, the cacao has been treated with alkali for another purpose, that is merely to improve an aroma, color, dispersibility in water and the like of cocoa powder.... Further, there have been several cases of the alkali-treatment of cacao other than production of cocoa powder. For example, an attempt of treating the cacao with an aqueous solution of weakly alkaline salt for the purpose of sterilization is disclosed in the Japanese Patent Publication No. 291233/1990. An attempt of neutralizing organic acids with ammonia for the purpose of improvement in aroma of cacao beans of low grade is disclosed in the Japanese Patent Publication No. 56975/1986. An attempt of increasing water-dispersibility of chocolate for food materials used in a pudding or jelly is disclosed in the Japanese Patent Publication No. 10094/1986.

Web site: http://www.delphion.com/details?pn=US05635183__

- ## Chocolate yogurt and preparation

Inventor(s): Lee; Thomas D. (Scarsdale, NY), Dell; William J. (Wappinger Falls, NY), Bissonnette; Madeline M. (Mahopac, NY), Barnard; David J. (Des Plaines, IL)

Assignee(s): Kraft Foods, Inc (Northfield, IL)

Patent Number: 6,068,865

Date filed: November 7, 1997

Abstract: A chocolate yogurt containing active cultures and having a diminished acid taste compatible with chocolate and a new product form that enables the enjoyment of the product utilizing only normal channels of distribution are enabled by separately preparing and packaging a yogurt base portion and a chocolate flavoring portion. The yogurt base portion contains active cultures and has a pH of less than about 4.6. The chocolate flavoring portion containing cocoa, nonfat dry milk solids, and a buffering salt. The two portions are packed, preferably, in a two-piece composite package. The two packages are opened and the contents mixed just prior to consumption.

Excerpt(s): The invention relates to chocolate yogurt, and particularly to a chocolate yogurt containing active cultures and having a diminished acid taste compatible with chocolate, a new product form that enables the enjoyment of the product utilizing only normal channels of distribution, and processes for preparing them.... Yogurt has been prepared for centuries in essentially the same way. Simply, pasteurized milk is inoculated with a preferred culture and held at a suitable temperature for long enough (e.g. , 3 to 6 hours) for the active cultures to grow in the milk. A natural consequence of the culturing process is the development of a sour taste due to the production of lactic acid. The acid has several benefits, including providing a clean, fresh taste and aiding preservation. If the yogurt is made with good manufacturing practices and cultured until the pH is less than about 4.6, the product should be stable for several weeks under refrigeration.... However, the acid flavor is incompatible with some flavors such as chocolate. Attempts to reduce the acid flavor by the use of buffering salts is not effective because the salts tend to increase the pH to an extent that preservation cannot be assured. Heating the yogurt to assure stability kills the active cultures, making the product less desirable to many consumers. Also, the buffering tends to add an off flavor, incompatible with both yogurt and chocolate.

Web site: http://www.delphion.com/details?pn=US06068865__

- **Chocolate-coated beverage container and method for making it**

  Inventor(s): Sweesy; Millie (5582 Mossvale Cir., Huntington Beach, CA 92649)

  Assignee(s): none reported

  Patent Number: 6,129,938

  Date filed: March 31, 1999

  Abstract: The subject invention is a chocolate-coated beverage container and method for making it. A pull ribbon is affixed to the container over which a plastic inner sleeve comprised of shrink plastic with a tearable portion is positioned. The inner sleeve is heated to conform to the surface of the container so that the tearable portion is adjacent to the pull ribbon. Then, the container is coated with chocolate, keeping an end of the pull ribbon exposed, and the chocolate coating is cooled until it solidifies. Additionally, a transparent outer sleeve comprised of shrink plastic can be placed over the coated beverage container, and heated to conform to the surface of the chocolate coating.

  Excerpt(s): The invention relates generally to chocolate-coated beverage containers, and more particularly, to chocolate-coated beverage containers in which the chocolate can be removed with ease by the consumer.... Beverage containers can be coated with chocolate to allow for a novel and appealing product in which the chocolate and the beverage in the container can be enjoyed simultaneously and conveniently. Prior methods for coating beverage containers with a layer of chocolate involved wrapping the container with commercially available standard plastic food wrap, by placing the wrap on the container in a spiral and tapering the wrap off at the top. One disadvantage of this method has been that the thin, low-gauge plastic of which the food wrap is composed can stretch and tear as the chocolate coating is removed. This can cause the chocolate coating to spray from the container, creating an untidy and aesthetically unpleasing situation, and making consumption of the chocolate more difficult.... One attempt to rectify this problem has been to use a cylindrically-shaped plastic sleeve, with a serration extending down along the length of the cylinder. This sleeve has no plastic area to cover the base of the container; to seal off the base of the container, a suitably-sized piece of tape is applied. Making such a chocolate-coated beverage container is labor-and time-intensive, and it requires additional sections of plastic, leading to increased cost. Also, the tape sections can sometimes disengage while the container is being dipped in chocolate, leading to delay and possible interference with equipment.

  Web site: http://www.delphion.com/details?pn=US06129938__

- **Chocolate-encapsulated fillings**

  Inventor(s): Cain; Frederick W. (Voorburg, NL), Hughes; Adrian D. ('s-Gravenhage, NL), Talbot; Geoffrey (Kempston, GB3)

  Assignee(s): Van Den Bergh Foods Co., Division of Conopco Inc. (Lisle, IL)

  Patent Number: 5,385,744

  Date filed: July 1, 1992

  Abstract: The presence of a specific (H.sub.2 M+HM.sub.2)-fat, either in the filling or in the coating of encapsulated fillings, results in the retardation of bloom of the chocolate composition. Therefore, the invention is concerned with encapsulated fillings, wherein the coatings display a defined (H.sub.2 M+HM.sub.2)-content. A process of preparing these encapsulated products is also included. Encapsulated products are, e.g., chocolates, pralines, biscuits, cookies, toffees, fried snacks or cakes.

Excerpt(s): Chocolate-encapsulated fillings consisting of at least a filling and a chocolate coating, wherein the filling comprises conventional filling ingredients, such as sugar, skimmed milk powder, salt or emulsifier and at least 35 wt. % of a filling fat, are well-known products. So far, however, these products have displayed a big disadvantage, in particular when the filling is liquid, i.e. fat present in the liquid filling migrates into the coating layer. Because of this migration, blooming of the chocolate occurs.... In order to overcome this problem, a solution was sought in the use of an intermediate layer between the liquid filling and the coating. However, such an extra layer complicates the production process and often has a negative influence on the mouthfeel of the product.... Therefore, we have conducted a study in order to find out whether it is possible to avoid the necessity of such an extra layer while the product properties are as good or even better.

Web site: http://www.delphion.com/details?pn=US05385744__

- **Chocolate-flavored confections and method for manufacturing**

Inventor(s): Moore; Carl O. (Rochester, IL), Dial; James R. (Moweaqua, IL)

Assignee(s): A. E. Staley Manufacturing Co. (Decatur, IL)

Patent Number: 5,258,199

Date filed: August 30, 1991

Abstract: Chocolate-flavored morsels essentially free of fat and a method for their preparation are provided. The morsels are manufactured by first preparing a mixture comprised of a major amount by weight of an aqueous syrup comprised of a crystallizable saccharide, said aqueous syrup being supersaturated with respect to said crystallizable saccharide, a minor amount by weight of defatted cocoa powder, a minor amount by weight of said crystallizable saccharide in crystalline form, and a minor amount by weight of an instant starch having a cold-water solubility of greater than 50 weight percent (and preferably a fat content of less than 0.25 weight percent), the amount of water in said aqueous syrup being insufficient to dissolve a major portion of said minor amount of instant starch. The morsels are then prepared by dividing said mixture into separate portions and forming said portions into discrete morsels in an environment which allows crystallizable saccharide to crystallize from said syrup onto said crystallizable saccharide in crystalline form. The chocolate-flavored morsels can be used in baked goods, particularly in cookies, to provide a chocolate-flavored morsel as a flavoring ingredient without adding fat to the baked good.

Excerpt(s): This invention relates to a method useful in the manufacture of confections having a chocolate flavor and to chocolate-flavored confections useful in the preparation of baked goods.... Processes and recipes for various confections, including chocolate and other confections, are disclosed and discussed by B. W. Minifie, Chocolate, Cocoa and Confectionery: Science and Technology, pp. 28-141, (AVI Publ. Co., Westport, Conn., 1980, 2d ed.). The passage at pages 128 to 141 discusses chocolate coatings, made with partial substitution of a vegetable fat for the cocoa butter, and dietetic chocolates, made by replacing sweeteners with low or non-caloric substitutes or by incorporating ingredients low in fat and carbohydrate, e.g. soy protein or carboxymethyl cellulose....

U.S. Pat. No. 3,184,315 (Wolf) discloses chocolate flavored confections to be used in frozen foods such as ice cream, frozen cake batters and doughs, and the like. It is disclosed that the confection is made from cocoa and sugar and that it has sufficiently low fat and moisture content to avoid being brittle at low temperatures. It is disclosed that when cocoa is employed without added chocolate liquor, a small amount of a fat, e.g. cocoa butter, natural fat or hydrogenated vegetable oil, is added.

Web site: http://www.delphion.com/details?pn=US05258199__

- **Coating machine for the processing of chocolate and similar masses**

  Inventor(s): Sollich; Helmut (Rabenkirchen, DE)

  Assignee(s): Sollich GmbH & Co. KG (Salzuflen, DE)

  Patent Number: 5,437,723

  Date filed: November 19, 1993

  Abstract: A coating machine for the processing of chocolate and similar masses having a frame and a circularly driven grating belt supported thereon for the reception of the articles to be coated. The grating belt is guided by deflectors and has a tensioning device. Coating machine components are arranged below the upper run of the grating belt. The tensioning device has an extended travel enabling the lifting of the grating belt. A plurality of supports are provided to support the lifted grating belt, the supports including carriers on the frame of the coating machine.

  Excerpt(s): The invention relates to a coating machine for the processing of chocolate and similar masses, having a frame and bearing therein a circularly driven grating belt for the reception of the articles to be coated, which is guided by deflectors and has a tensioning device, and with pieces of the coating machine, especially a shaking device, arranged under the upper run of the grating belt. Such a coating machine serves to cover the articles on the grating belt with chocolate, the chocolate flowing in surplus through the coating machine penetrating the grating belt and coming into contact with many parts of the coating machine. It may be a coating machine which has a covering station in which the liquid chocolate reaches the articles in free fall. The coating machine may also have a bottom covering station and/or a blower to blow off any surplus chocolate. Masses other than chocolate, such as fat-containing masses, coating masses and, caramel masses may also be processed with such a coating machine.... When changing the mass in the coating machine, that is when a dark chocolate has been processed and the following articles are to be coated with a light chocolate or even a white coating mass, the problem to remove the previously processed mass and to clean all parts which have been in contact with this mass, so that the new mass, for example a white coating mass, can be used in the coating machine, arises.... It is known that in order to complete such a change of masses the coating machine including the previously processed mass is heated and emptied by removing the previously processed mass using a recovery pump. Then a cleaning mass such as cocoa butter or some other fatty solution is introduced into the coating machine. The coating machine is then put into action without any articles passing through, so that the cleaning mass is continuously recirculated and passes through the machine station. By this the cleaning mass reaches a large fraction of the parts of the coating machine contaminated with the old mass and cleans these more or less completely by melting off the old mass. But not all parts of the coating machine are reached by the cleaning mass, so that the cleaning action is incomplete. The cleaning mass is removed from the coating machine at the end of the cleaning and used in the normal production of chocolate. Afterwards the coating machine can be filled with the new coating mass.

Web site: http://www.delphion.com/details?pn=US05437723__

- **Conched chocolate**

Inventor(s): Capodieci; Roberto A. (Glen Ellyn, IL)

Assignee(s): Mars, Incorporated (McLean, VA)

Patent Number: 5,591,476

Date filed: October 18, 1995

Abstract: A process and a system for combining and physically working chocolate-making ingredients are provided. A variable frequency drive controls the motor of a conching device to increase the efficiency by which energy is imparted to chocolate ingredients during conching. This automatic variable speed approach permits the power to be maintained at a relatively constant and maximum rate, with the speed being determined by the consistency of the ingredients themselves. Feedback associated with the automatic speed variation can be used in order to reduce conching times and vary the quantity of certain ingredients and the timing of and location of their introduction. By the invention, it is possible to standardize the chocolate product during the conching operation and thereby avoid a post-conching standardization procedure with respect to characteristics such as viscosity and fat content.

Excerpt(s): The present invention generally relates to the production of chocolate by an improved process and system. More particularly, the invention relates to chocolate production that includes imparting a substantially constant power level to the chocolate refinings being conched. Included is an arrangement for varying the drive speed of the conching equipment in response to the changing consistency of the intermediate chocolate product being conched. The invention enhances chocolate production efficiency by making additional energy available in order to achieve one or more advantages, especially reduction in processing times and optimization of the addition of costly ingredients such as cocoa butter.... Chocolate is a mixture of finely milled solids, chocolate liquor, sugar, milk crumb or powder, all suspended or well dispersed in cocoa butter and/or substitute fat, which at normal processing temperature is the liquid carrying medium. Raw materials such as chocolate liquor, sugar, water and milk are processed into chocolate through a series of processed steps including, for example, crumb making, paste mixing, refining, conching and standardizing. Usually, an emulsifier or an emulsifying system is added during conching.... During conching, chemical and physical processes take place. These include the development of the full desirable chocolate flavor and the conversion of the powdery, crumbly refined product into the chocolate. Conching imparts shearing stresses and kneading action which serve both to liquify the masse and to positively influence and accelerate the flavor development processes. Important physical tasks of conching are to disperse, to dehumidify or remove moisture, to remove unwanted volatile flavors, to break up solid particle agglomerates, to round particle edges and to homogenize. Viscosity is lowered, and flowability and texture are improved.

Web site: http://www.delphion.com/details?pn=US05591476__

- **Conchless high protein chocolate flavored composition and method of making same**

Inventor(s): de Paolis; Potito U. (131 Groverton Pl., Los Angeles, CA 90024)

Assignee(s): none reported

Patent Number: 4,296,141

Date filed: August 27, 1979

Abstract: The invention is directed to a method of making a conchless chocolate-flavored confectionary coating and composition and to the products resulting therefrom. This is accomplished by the use of 3-40 parts, by weight, of a soya protein isolate as the main emulsifier in combination with: (a) 10-65 parts by weight, edible fats (such as hydrogenated cottonseed or soybean oils); (b) 40-70 parts, by weight, sweeteners, i.e., sugar or sugar substitutes, such as corn flour, tapioca flour, or corn syrup solids; and (c) 2-60 parts, by weight, chocolate flavorings, such as cocoa or carob, plus trace amounts of other flavoring agents. The edible fats (less a hold-back of 40-50%) sugar or sugar substitutes, flavorings and emulsifier are admixed (except for a substantial portion of the fat) to form a paste. The paste is extruded, between a series of stainless steel paired rollers to form a smooth, homogeneous but very viscous, paste of the order of 45-60 McMichael viscosity. Blended into the resulting extruded viscous paste are the balance of the fats to form a liquified blend. The liquified blend is then heated to between about 110.degree. F.-140.degree. F. for about 10-30 minutes under agitation, and then passed through an extruder, cooled, cut into chips, and packaged, for later use by manufacturers as a confectionary coating, or directly admixed with fruits, nuts, etc. to form a confectionary bar.

Excerpt(s): Many confectionaries are coated with a flavored candy coating. The coating helps to preserve the confectionary, imparts a desired eye-appeal and adds flavor. Bakery produced cakes, ice cream bars and popsicles, candy pieces and candy bars are conventionally coated with such flavored coatings. While these coatings can be flavored with any desired natural or artificial flavor, they are most often flavored with cocoa or chocolate liquor to form a chocolate flavored coating.... Chocolate coatings can be produced in the traditional way of making milk chocolate. This process, however, requires a rather expensive ingredient, i.e., cocoa butter. For this reason and for other reasons, milk chocolate candy coatings are relatively expensive and are not used on popularly priced confectionaries and in lieu thereof a compound coating is used. Compound coatings do not require a cooking step and are, generally speaking, simply a mechanical mixture of principally cocoa, sugar and fat.... As can be appreciated, the solid ingredients and the fat of a compound coating must be so intimately mixed that the texture, mouth feel and taste of the compound coating will approximate that of milk chocolate. The process wherein these ingredients are mixed to that required extent is referred to in the art as the conching step. As is well known in the art, conching must pulverize the sugar, cocoa and other ingredients to the point that the compound coating has no "gritty" texture or mouth feel and to the extent that the cocoa is mechanically worked into the fat.

Web site: http://www.delphion.com/details?pn=US04296141__

- **Conditioning machine for chocolate masses**

  Inventor(s): Sollich; Helmut (Albernbere, DT)

  Assignee(s): Sollich KG (DT)

  Patent Number: 4,059,047

  Date filed: July 20, 1976

  Abstract: A conditioning machine for chocolate masses wherein a pump forces the mass through a stack of cooling stages forming a cylinder, each having cooled top and bottom walls connected to a coolant recirculating system, each stage containing scrapers revolving about the cylinder axis for continuously detaching the mass from the cooling surfaces, each stage having two scrapers axially urged apart by an interposed spring.

  Excerpt(s): The invention relates to a conditioning machine for masses used in the confectionery manufacturing industry and containing fats, particularly chocolate masses.... After leaving the conches such masses must be cooled and conditioned to bring them to the best possible state for further processing. For this purpose use is made of conditioning machines comprising a stack of cooling stages forming a cylinder and each having cooled top and bottom walls connected to a coolant recirculating system, and a pump forcing the mass through all the stages of which each contains scrapers revolving about the cylinder axis. The defect of such machines is their relatively poor throughput and the long time of cooling needed for conditioning the chocolate mass.... It is therefore an object of the present invention to provide a conditioning machine which permits the cooling time to be minimised and a high performance to be achieved.

  Web site: http://www.delphion.com/details?pn=US04059047__

- **Consumer friendly chocolate**

  Inventor(s): Zumbe; Albert (Neuchatol, CH)

  Assignee(s): Jacobs Suchard AG (Zurich, CH)

  Patent Number: 4,963,372

  Date filed: January 19, 1989

  Abstract: A chocolate of good nutritional value offering improved tolerance to consumers who may be allergic to protein in cocoa or milk and/or sensitive to theobromine or caffeine and/or react to bioactive amines present in regular chocolate. It contains no cocoa liquor or cocoa powder or milk powder. Its protein source is protein hydrolysate and/or 1-amino acids, the latter being selected to give good flavor while retaining the essential qualities of the protein.

  Excerpt(s): The invention concerns consumer-friendly chocolate.... In recent years an increase in allergic reactions in all areas of the population has been reported. Many individuals suffer from symptoms after consumption of one of various foods. Among such foods chocolate has been observed to provoke allergic reactions. Symptoms may include mild to severe allergic skin eruptions and respiratory tract allergy. These effects have been attributed to cocoa proteins. Various patentees including Bresnick, U.S. Pat. No. 2,039,884 and Girsh, U.S. Pat. No. 4,078,093 have proposed methods of treating cocoa beans, cocoa liquor or cocoa powder in order to destroy the effect of these proteins. It is clear that consumer-friendly chocolate needs to have no active cocoa proteins present. However at best such treatments eliminate allergic response associated with cocoa protein but leave other substances in cocoa beans, cocoa liquor and cocoa powder which may provoke undesirable effects.... Theobromine and caffeine, reffered to chemically as methylxanthines, are stimulants found in cocoa beans, cocoa liquor and cocoa powder. Such methylxanthines are avoided by an increasing number of consumers as shown for example by the increasing popularity of decaffeinated coffee. A consumer-friendly chocolate should avoid the presence of such methylxanthines. In addition cocoa, together with other foods including cheese, contains small quantities of bioactive amines. These have been suggested as agents, for example, in provoking certain types of migraine. Again such bioactive amines should be effectively absent from consumer-friendly chocolate.

Web site: http://www.delphion.com/details?pn=US04963372__

- **Continuous and automatic apparatus for molding chocolate block having ornamental relief pattern**

Inventor(s): Akutagawa; Tokuji (Tokyo, JP)

Assignee(s): Akutagawa Confectionery Co., Ltd. (Tokyo, JP)

Patent Number: 4,480,974

Date filed: March 25, 1983

Abstract: A continuous and automatic process for molding chocolate blocks each having an ornamental relief pattern of one color and a body portion of different color carrying the relief pattern is provided. Also, there is provided apparatus for continuously and automatically producing such ornamental chocolate blocks. A first chocolate material for forming the ornamental relief pattern is cast into a first mold and scraped to scrape off the excess chocolate material. A second mold is then placed on the first mold and a second chocolate material for forming the body portion is cast into through-openings of the second mold. The second chocolate material inevitably oozing into the interface between the first and second molds adheres only onto a rough surface portion formed around and surrounding the through-openings of the second mold without the second chocolate material adhering onto the first mold. It is thus not necessary to remove the oozing chocolate material from the first mold. Further, the product chocolate block does not have burr.

Excerpt(s): The present invention relates to a process and an apparatus for molding chocolate, and particularly to a process and an apparatus for molding chocolate blocks each including an ornamental relief pattern made of first chocolate material of one color and a body portion carrying the ornamental relief pattern and made of a second chocolate material of different color through a continuous automation system.... In a known process for molding a chocolate block having an ornamental relief pattern, a first chocolate material for forming an ornamental relief pattern is heated to be fluidized and then cast into a first or lower mold having a smooth top face and one or more engraved cavities forming the ornamental relief pattern such as desired design or letters. After scraping the top face of the first mold, the first chocolate material is cooled at some extent, and a second or upper mold having one or more through-openings is placed on the first mold. Before the first chocolate material contained in the engraved cavities of the first mold is not yet solidified, a second chocolate material having a color different from that of the first chocolate material is heated to be fluidized and then cast into the through-openings of the second mold. After the first and second chocolate materials are crystallized and solidified, the upper mold is separated from the lower mold to remove the molded chocolate block from the combined molds. However, the fluidized second chocolate material tends to penetrate into the gap inevitably formed at the interface between the top face of the lower mold and the bottom face of the upper mold. The penetrating second chocolate material adheres on the top face of the lower mold and the bottom face of the upper mold, or adheres to the body portion of the molded chocolate block to form a burr. If an appreciable quantity of the second chocolate material adheres on the top face of the lower mold at the vicinity of the engraved cavity forming the ornamental pattern, the adhering second chocolate material different from the first chocolate material in color and in quality is mixed with the first chocolate material at the scraping step of the next operation cycle, thereby to deteriorate the quality and appearance of the product, resulting in loss of commercial value of the product. In order to remove the residual second chocolate material adhering onto the top face of the lower mold surrounding the engraved cavities for molding the ornamental pattern, the lower mold must be rinsed with warm water followed by drying before it is used repeatedly in the next operation cycle. For this reason, in the conventional process for molding chocolate wherein the ornamental relief pattern is made of a first chocolate material of one color and the body portion is made of a second chocolate material of different color, the process essentially includes the step of rinsing the lower molds with warm water and the step of drying the rinsed lower molds. As a result, it is impossible to realize a simple automation system for continuously and automatically molding chocolate blocks one by one by the recyclic use of the lower molds.... Although it has been contemplated to scrape off the second chocolate material adhering to the lower mold using another scraper after the molded chocolate block is removed therefrom, the lower mold is charged with static electricity by the friction with the scraper to attract fine broken pieces of the second chocolate material. It is thus difficult to remove the once adhering second chocolate material from the lower molds completely by means of the known method. It is not recommendable to scrape off the solidified chocolate material adhering to the first molds, since the top faces of the lower molds are damaged or worn by the scraper or the solidified chocolate material.

Web site: http://www.delphion.com/details?pn=US04480974__

- **Control device for dosing emulsifiers in chocolate mass**

  Inventor(s): Horig; Jurgen (Heidenau, DD)

  Assignee(s): Veb Kombinat Nagema (Dresden, DD)

  Patent Number: 4,587,894

  Date filed: February 19, 1985

  Abstract: A continuous stream of chocolate mass is dosed with lecithin or similar emulsifiers by means of an electronically controlled dosing pump. The throughput or the weight rate of the flow of the chocolate mass is detected by a weighing device and the amount of the emulsifier to be added is adjusted to the changes of the throughput. The percentage of the emulsifier is preselected. The dosing time of each charge of the chocolate mass is determined as a first time interval from the detected weight rate of flow. During the dosing of a charge, a second time interval which is a predetermined fraction of the first time interval, is determined for the next charge during the dosing of a preceding charge. A control unit actuates a time counter for determining the first time interval whose value is stored in an intermediate storage. An operation counter determines the second time intervals and activates a control unit for the emulsifier dosing pump.

  Excerpt(s): The invention relates in general to the manufacture of chocolate and in particular it relates to a method of and a control device for dosing lecithin or similar emulsifier in chocolate mass processed in a continuously operating plant which includes a weighing device for detecting the weight rate of flow of the chocolate mass, and a continuously operating dosing pump arrangement for the lecithin.... For continuous dosing of lecithin in a chocolate mass it has been known to change the dosage by adjusting the rotary speed of a pump operating as a dosing apparatus.... Known are also dosing pumps in which the measured quantity or the dose is changed in dependency on the piston stroke.

Web site: http://www.delphion.com/details?pn=US04587894__

- **Control system for controlling the pressure on chocolate refining machine roll bearings**

  Inventor(s): Ripani; Sergio (Milan, IT), Serafini; Giulio (Milan, IT)

  Assignee(s): Carle & Montanari S.p.A. (Milan, IT)

  Patent Number: 4,620,477

  Date filed: April 22, 1985

  Abstract: A system for controlling the pressure applied on the roll bearings of chocolate refining machines comprises, in addition to a linked multi-pressure control circuit, an additional circuit for applying linked single-pressure control, a selector valve enabling switching of one or the other of the operating modes.The dual-function system imparts refining machines with universal operation capabilities.

  Excerpt(s): This invention relates to a control system for controlling the pressure on chocolate refining machine roll bearings.... As is known, chocolate refining machines require that the pressure exerted on the bearings of the refining rolls downstream of the feeding roll pair be adjustable if the machine is to accommodate chocolate pastes having different percentages of fat. Such fat percentages may vary quite significantly, e.g. within a range up to 4-5%, depending on the chocolate products to be prepared from such pastes.... As is known, by controlling the pressure on the refining roll bearings, the plasticity of the chocolate film delivered can be changed.

  Web site: http://www.delphion.com/details?pn=US04620477__

- **Controlled operation chocolate refiner**

  Inventor(s): Ripani; Sergio (Milan, IT), Serafini; Giulio (Milan, IT)

  Assignee(s): Carle & Montanari S.p.A. (Milan, IT)

  Patent Number: 4,603,815

  Date filed: March 1, 1984

  Abstract: A refiner for mixtures and suspensions having a non-Newtonian rheological characteristic, such as chocolate, which comprises a plurality of power driven refining rollers, and a means of changing the pressure thereof on the respective supports, wherein a means is also provided which is effective to change the actual crowning of the rollers, or the effect of an equivalent crowning, as well as a means of changing the speed of said refining rollers. The crown change is achieved by having the individual rollers supported on an oscillating support adapted to oscillate its respective roller relatively to the associated roller by rotation about an orthogonal midaxis with respect to the roller longitudinal axes, thereby a contact point is established at the roller middle area or circumference while their ends are offset. The speed of the refining rollers is changed through independent and individually operated controls, such as a DC motor. By changing the pressure, crowning, and speed of the rollers, either individually or in combination, the machine may find universal applicability to different viscosity products in desired conditions.

Excerpt(s): This invention relates to chocolate refiner having universal operation characteristics.... As is known in the art, chocolate refiners functions to impart chocolate with a determined fineness or grain size, while making it as homogeneous as possible. The fineness degree aimed at is dictated by the subsequent utilization of the chocolate. For chocolate products of fine quality, degrees of fineness in the order of about 15-30.mu.m are usual. That fineness is achieved by successively squeezing the chocolate through a plurality of refining roller pairs which are spring loaded in succession against each other, the inlet pair forming the feed-in roller pair and the last of the rollers forming the delivery roller.... With such prior machines, one can adjust the pressure on the individual rollers either separately or simultaneously on all rollers. The latter are set apart from each other to form a nip through which the material entrained therealong by adhesion is caused to pass. The speeds of the individual rollers increase from the inlet roller pair to the delivery roller. Conversely, the thickness or depth of the chocolate film will decrease from the inlet roller pair (e.g. at about 100-400.mu.m) toward the delivery roller (e.g. to 15-30.mu.m). The refining action results from a simultaneous compression or squeezing action, and a drawing or shearing action exerted on the chocolate film. The refining rollers are currently quite wide. e.g. up to about two meters wide. Accordingly, it is specially difficult to maintain such small thicknesses over such great widths with those rollers.

Web site: http://www.delphion.com/details?pn=US04603815__

- **Conveying and treatment apparatus for moulds fillable with a castable, solidifying body, such as chocolate mass**

Inventor(s): Bindler; Uwe (Bergneustadt, DE), Schurholz; Theo (Reichshof-Eckenhagen, DE)

Assignee(s): Gebr. Bindler GmbH & Co, KG (Bergneustadt, DE)

Patent Number: 4,822,268

Date filed: February 12, 1988

Abstract: The invention relates of a conveying and treatment apparatus for double moulds for making hollow bodies of a castable, solidifying substance, such as chocolate mass. The double moulds consist of two plate-shaped mould halves which have corresponding mould cavities and are laid one above the other to close the cavities. The apparatus comprises a conveying path via which the double moulds filled with the mass can be fed to a transfer device which takes over the double moulds after the fashion of continuous lift and supplies the moulds to an endless conveyor. During conveying in the transfer device (7), the double moulds are conveyed in parallel and synchronously with supporting and retaining elements of the endless conveyor, being transferred in synchronism by means of a pushing device from the transfer device to the chain conveyor. During conveying in the endless conveyor the double moulds are held together and at the same time rotated around their own axes, more particularly around two axes, so that the castable body gradually solidifies by cooling on the walls of the mould cavities.

Excerpt(s): The invention relates to a conveying and treatment apparatus for moulds consisting of one or two superimposed plates having mould cavities for a castable, solidifying body, such as chocolate mass, the apparatus having a circulating endless conveyor, more particularly constructed in the form of a chain conveyor, which has supporting and retaining elements for receiving and turning the moulds.... For the production of cavities of a castable, solidifying body, for example, chocolate mass, it is common practice to use double moulds having mould cavities whose top and bottom plates are each constructed with mould cavities corresponding to one another. After the castable body has been introduced into the mould cavities in the bottom plate, the cavities are closed by the application of the top plate.... Various apparatuses exist for producing the hollow bodies in this way.

Web site: http://www.delphion.com/details?pn=US04822268__

- **Crimping chocolate, chocolate analog and chocolate substitute articles to prepare containers**

Inventor(s): Jury; Mark (Thirsk, GB)

Assignee(s): Nestec S.A. (Vevey, CH)

Patent Number: 5,882,710

Date filed: November 20, 1996

Abstract: A container, such as a bag or a pouch, is made from a fat-based confectionery material, including such as a chocolate, and is formed by crimping an end or ends of a hollowed tube of the material or crimping edges of a sheet or sheets of the material brought together. The tube or sheet which is crimped is an extrudate which is, upon being obtained from an extruder, temporarily plastically deformable and thereby has a temporary flexibility, and the crimping is carried while the material is plastically deformable.

Excerpt(s): The present invention relates to chocolate products, more particularly to chocolate products having one or more sealed edges to provide thereby a container, including such as a bag or a pouch, which may or may not contain a filling.... It is difficult to close the ends of solid tubular chocolate to form a bag or container by squeezing together to form a crimp-seal because the tube breaks before obtaining a seal owing to the brittleness of the chocolate. Therefore chocolate bags, pouches or similar containers having one or more crimp-sealed edges do not exist.... In European Patent Application Publication No. 0 603 467, the contents of which are hereby incorporated into the present specification, a method is described for the cold extrusion of chocolate or a fat-containing confectionery material in a solid or semi-solid non-pourable form whereby the extruded product has a temporary flexibility or plasticity enabling it to be physically manipulated or plastically deformed, e.g. it can be bent, twisted or forced into a mould. The extruded material is a solid or semi-solid product and may be a hollow profiled product such as a tube.

Web site: http://www.delphion.com/details?pn=US05882710__

- **Crumb products for chocolate production and their preparation**

  Inventor(s): Armstrong; Euan (St. Andrewgate, GB), Carli; Sophie (Heworth, GB), Gibson; Richard (Tadcaster, GB), Jercher; Loreta (Heworth, GB), Samuel; Brian (Wigginton, GB)

  Assignee(s): Nestec S.A. (Vevey, CH)

  Patent Number: 6,261,627

  Date filed: March 1, 1999

  Abstract: Crumb products for preparing chocolate products are prepared by adding together ingredients which include milk solids and a sugar ingredient, particularly sucrose, and which include, optionally, cocoa solids and so that the ingredients added together have a moisture content between 1.2% and 8%, and the ingredients added together are mixed and heated so that the ingredients being mixed are heated-up to a temperature in a range of from 85.degree. C. to 180.degree. C. and so that upon being heated-up to a temperature in the range which is a temperature of at least 85.degree. C. and up to 180.degree. C., the ingredients being mixed are maintained at temperatures in a range of from 85.degree. C. to the heated-up temperature for a period of from 2.5 minutes to 25 minutes to provide a heat-treated reaction product which then is dried. Crumb may be prepared which has, by weight, a milk solids to sugar ingredient ratio of between 1:0.1 and 1:3.

  Excerpt(s): The present invention relates to processes and ingredient formulations for preparing crumb products, particularly chocolate crumb products, which include milk solids and sweetener, for preparing chocolate products and to preparation of chocolate products with the crumb products.... Milk chocolate differs from dark or plain chocolate in that it contains milk solids and the essential part of a process for preparing milk chocolate is the method used to incorporate the milk solids. Milk chocolate is virtually moisture-free in that it contains from 0.5-1.5% water, while full cream milk contains about 87.5% water, the remainder being about 12.5% milk solids including fat.... One method of removing the 87.5% water from milk is by evaporation of the liquid milk and drying to a powder, and a traditional method of producing milk chocolate is by mixing the milk powder together with cocoa liquor or cocoa nibs, sugar, and cocoa butter, followed by refining, conching and tempering.

  Web site: http://www.delphion.com/details?pn=US06261627__

- **Device for conching chocolate compound**

  Inventor(s): Callebaut; Frans (Bambrugge, BE), Bruyland; Rudy (Herdersem, BE)

  Assignee(s): Callebaut N.V. (Lebbeke-Weize, BE)

  Patent Number: 5,657,687

  Date filed: March 29, 1996

  Abstract: A conche for producing chocolate compound consists of a conche container (10) with a main chamber (12) and subsidiary chambers (13, 14). Mixing vanes (22, 23 and 30, 31) are disposed therein on central shafts (19, 20, 21) in order to intimately mix the components fed in from above. In order to improve the mixing effect, additional mixing tools in the form of mixing worms (37, 38) are disposed in the lower part of the conche container (10), in particular in the main chamber (12). Stripping means (24, 25) moved along a cylindrical container wall (15) are supported solely in the region of a central transverse plane on a main shaft (19) in the main chamber (12). The main shaft (19) is provided with a clear cross-sectional thickening (28) which at the same time fills a dead space in the conche container (10).

Excerpt(s): The invention relates to a device (conche) for mixing (conching) components for the production of chocolate compound, with a central main shaft having mixing tools disposed thereon and being rotatable about a horizontal axis in an essentially cylindrical container, especially in a main chamber, and with stripping means revolving along an inner wall surface of the housing in the peripheral direction.... Such a device for conching chocolate compound is known from DE 39 18 813. Such a "classic" conche has a conche container which consists of three axis-parallel cylindrical upwardly open chambers. These are a central main chamber with a greater diameter and two lateral subsidiary chambers. The three chambers merge into one another, thereby forming the conche container. Mixing tools are disposed in each chamber on rotatingly driven shafts.... Heretofore, the conching of chocolate compound has been a time-consuming process. For example, the complete conching of one batch with a conche according to DE 39 18 813 requires 12 h.

Web site: http://www.delphion.com/details?pn=US05657687__

- **Device for continuously feeding (synchronizing) essentially flat articles of the luxury-food or food industry, especially bars or strips of chocolate, to a packaging machine**

  Inventor(s): Lesch; Hans (Garmisch-Partenkirchen, DE)

  Assignee(s): Otto Hansel GmbH (Hanover, DE)

  Patent Number: 4,624,100

  Date filed: August 12, 1985

  Abstract: A device for continuously feeding (synchronizing) essentially flat articles of the luxury-food or food industry, especially bars or strips of chocolate, to a packaging machine, in which carriers in a transport assembly introduce the articles into a tube of wrapping material and shape them into individual packages with it, characterized in that an infeed (25) for the articles (1) that operates transversely with respect to and is synchronized with a transport mechanism (3a) that operates at a constant speed and is equipped with carriers (3) is positioned upstream of the transport mechanism and in that buffers (30) for the articles arriving on the infeed are positioned between the carriers and controlled in such a way that the articles will enter the tube (5) of wrapping material in sequence and in a direction derived from the infeed and transport directions.

  Excerpt(s): The invention concerns a device for continuously feeding (synchronizing) essentially flat articles of the luxury-food or food industry, especially bars or strips of chocolate, to a packaging machine, in which carriers in a transport assembly introduce the articles into a tube of wrapping material and shape them into individual packages with it.... Only a certain packaging output can be achieved with packaging machines of this type, which are known from U.S. Pat. No. 3,283,470 because it is difficult to feed the articles in. Since the tube of packaging material cannot be completely closed, tightly sealed packages cannot be produced. Furthermore, they can be employed only to package solid articles because they are subjected to excessive stress when transported through the machine.... The object of the present invention is to eliminate this defect and provide a device that allows thorough closure of even the most delicate articles in a wrapping that is tightly sealed on all sides at a high packaging output and without noticeable mechanical stress.

Web site: http://www.delphion.com/details?pn=US04624100__

• **Device for controlling and monitoring the thickness of a chocolate film delivered by chocolate refiners**

Inventor(s): Ripani; Sergio (Milan, IT)

Assignee(s): Carle & Montanari S.p.A. (Milan, IT)

Patent Number: 4,519,304

Date filed: January 26, 1984

Abstract: A device for controlling and monitoring the thickness of a chocolate film delivered by chocolate refiners. The chocolate film thickness is controlled by operation of a roller bearing pressure adjustment system of the refiner by way of cut-in signals from an indirect measurement of the instantaneous chocolate film thickness effected by processing representative colorimetric signals for a given mass of chocolate stock of corresponding thickness values emitted by a readout head. The readout head is arranged to reciprocate to measure the film across its entire width. The readout head also enables the integrity of the chocolate film being delivered to be monitored, that is to detect the appearance on the output roller of dry band areas.In the presence of potential causes of refiner roller seizure, the device, after a presettable time delay, will automatically stop the machine.

Excerpt(s): This invention relates to a device for controlling and monitoring the thickness of a chocolate film delivered by chocolate refiners.... As is known in the art, chocolate refiners are machines which comprise essentially a plurality of rollers successively carried for adjustable displacement to and from each other in a supporting frame or stand, to permit the gap between any one roller and the following roller to be adjusted. In this respect, the roller push-aside gap that the material being entrained may create decreases gradually from the input roller pair, arranged side-by-side to form an input chamber, and the last roller pair in the refiner, the last roller being the output or delivery roller. The delivery roller is wrapped over most of its circumference, e.g., 3/4 of its circumference, with the chocolate film being delivered, which will leave said roller onto a doctoring blade associated with the delivery roller. The required chocolate film thickness may vary within a wide range, in general values of 15 to 30.mu.m being those required. Thus, the thickness dimensions handled are very small ones, and are dependent on the thickness dimensions of solid particulates of cocoa, sugar, milk, etc. contained in the film, which comprises, in a conventional manner, a mixture of cocoa, sugar, fatty substance or cocoa butter, milk, and so on. It will be apparent that this mixture is a heterogeneous one through the film of chocolate being delivered, the distribution of the individual ingredients per surface area unit occurring differently and irregularly in a random fashion. With prior refiners, the rollers which are located downstream of the input roller pair have a velocity which increases toward the output roller. This results in a squeezing and entraining action being applied on the chocolate mass to form a filn of decreasing thickness toward the output roller.... In order to resist undesired thickness deviations in the chocolate film being delivered, prior refiners provide for the bearing pressure therebetween to be changed, more specifically the bearing pressure from the input pair to the rollers downstream thereof. This may be achieved substantially in either of two ways, namely, by changing the bearing pressure on all the bearings of the refining rollers, or alternatively, by changing the bearing pressure on individual bearings of said refining rollers, the latter approach enabling the bearing pressure to be varied individually between the rollers. In all cases, the main adjustment is effected on the input roller pair, because, with the refiner in a steady state of operation, the amount per unit of time of the chocolate mass being fed must correspond to the amount by weight of the film being delivered.

Web site: http://www.delphion.com/details?pn=US04519304__

- **Device for filling a mold tray with a thick fluid substance such as chocolate**

Inventor(s): Van Meulenbeke; Pierre (Karel Soetelaan,, 25-2210 Borsbeek, BE)

Assignee(s): none reported

Patent Number: 4,747,766

Date filed: November 25, 1986

Abstract: A device for filling in a single operation of several mould spaces in a mould tray with a thick fluid substance such a chocolate, creme, fondant, and similar. The device consists primarily of a tank; a distribution vessel with filler openings; a transport pipe between the tank and the distribution vessel; a constant-flow pump connected to the tranport pipe and intended for pumping the substance from the tank to the distribution vessel and for pumping the substance out of the filler openings; at least one mould tray located under the distribution vessel with filler openings; a means which switches on and off the pump for pumping the substance; and a means which switches on and off the pump for withdrawing and retaining the substance in the filler openings once the mould tray is filled.

Excerpt(s): The invention is for a device for filling in a single operation of several mould spaces in a mould tray with a thick fluid substance. This thick fluid substance may for example consist of chocolate for moulding pralines (continental chocolates), from creme or fondant for filling the as yet unclosed pralines or confectionery or whatsoever other items placed in the mould spaces.... Known devices for filling the mould spaces in mould trays consist mainly of : a tank filled with a thick fluid substance, such as chocolate for example; a number into a single row placed and simultaneously controlled switch cocks which are connected on the one hand to the said tank and on the other hand to an equal number of suck and blow units, whereby the filler openings of these cocks are in turn located above one of the rows of mould spaces in a mould tray underneath. The cocks are first turned in such a way that the substance is first sucked from the tank into the suck and blow units, the pistons of which can be adjusted in order to dertermine the volume of the sucked-up substance and are then turned so that the sucked-up substance is pushed from the suck and blow units via the filler openings of the cocks into a single row of mould spaces in the mould tray underneath. This procedure is then repeated in order to fill each following row of mould spaces in the mould tray, the mould tray being moved for every filling.... This known device has, however, as chief disadvantage that only a single row of mould spaces can be filled at a time and not all rows of mould spaces of the mould tray are filled simultaneously. The mould tray must therefore be moved each time the next row of mould spaces is to be filled, until all the rows of mould spaces are filled. Other disadvantages are that the device is bulky, complicated and of an expensive construction, that the pistons in the suction and compression units are difficult to set accurately and that the entire device requires quita a lot of maintenance.

Web site: http://www.delphion.com/details?pn=US04747766__

- **Device for preparing chocolate**

  Inventor(s): Tadema; Jan C. (Bergen, NL)

  Assignee(s): Wiener & Co. B.V. (Amsterdam, NL)

  Patent Number: 4,380,193

  Date filed: February 25, 1981

  Abstract: A device for treating a mixture for the manufacture of chocolate, said device comprising a cyclic course of a milling vessel and a mixing vessel each having a driving motor for driving the milling members and the mixing members respectively and means connected with the cycle for supplying the mixture to be treated and means for the delivery of the ready product provided with means for adding to the cycle a viscosity-reducing agent.

  Excerpt(s): The invention relates to a device for treating a mixture for the production of chocolate, said device comprising a cycle including a milling vessel and a mixing vessel, each having a driving motor for driving the milling members and mixing members respectively, and means connected with said cycle for the supply of the mixture to be treated and means for delivering the ready product. Such a device is known from Dutch patent application No. 69.01227.... In this so-called "Wiener"-process the mixture to be treated is constantly circulated through the cyclic system and subjected to milling and mixing operations.... Irrespective of the ratios between the constituents chocolate always contains sugar, milk powder, cocoa powder and cocoa butter. Dependent upon the desired kind of chocolate substances are added such as glucose, vanilla, flavourings, dried fruit and candied rind. Among these substances cocoa butter is for the major part determinative of the taste. However, it is the most expensive of the ingredients. Therefore, the manufacturer tends to minimize the amount of cocoa butter. A limiting factor is, however, the required taste. A further limiting factor is the workability. If the amount of cocoa butter is comparatively small, the mixture will be tough and can be stirred only with difficulty. The ratio between the constituents of the mixture is the manufacturer's trade secret. It is, however, very likely for a given, desired taste to be obtained by a minor amount of cocoa butter, but the mixture may then become unworkable. The invention has for its object to provide a solution for this problem. In the device according to the invention this is achieved by means of supplying a viscosity reducing agent to the cycle. It is thus possible, if desired, to add a given amount of viscosity-reducing agent in order to enhance the stirring effect, whilst the amount of expensive cocoa butter may be kept low. The means for supplying the viscosity-reducing agent may be formed by a dosing device connected with a supply vessel. The dosing device may be actuated when it is assessed by a monitoring member that the workability has dropped below a given level. The viscosity-monitoring member may be the driving motor of the mixing vessel or the milling vessel.

  Web site: http://www.delphion.com/details?pn=US04380193__

- **Device for processing chocolate mass**

  Inventor(s): Tadema; Jan C. (Bergen, NL)

  Assignee(s): Wiener & Co. Apparatenbouw B.V. (Amsterdam, NL)

  Patent Number: 5,297,743

  Date filed: July 2, 1992

Abstract: Chocolate is ground in order to obtain a very small average particle size. A determined viscosity is necessary for further processing. In order to keep as small as possible the fraction with particle size lying above the desired value and having an adverse effect on the taste of the final product, according to the invention the process mass is circulated in a cycle incorporating a grinding device and a ball mill. This has the result of accelerating the grinding process and reducing the inconsistency in the distribution of the particle size.

Excerpt(s): The invention relates to a method and device for mixing and grinding chocolate, fats or the like, wherein a process mass of cacao and/or cacao powder, cacao butter, edible fat, sugar and the like are pre-mixed and ground in a grinding device and a ball mill.... Up until the present the components for processing were pre-mixed in a pre-mixer and ground in a grinding device. The pre-mixer and grinding device can also be unified to one unit. After grinding the mass is then ground in a ball mill to make it still finer as required until the final desired particle size is obtained.... In a ball mill it is possible to grind the process mass to a very small average particle size and to therein obtain the desired viscosity, although the uniformity in the distribution of the particle size leaves something to be desired. Unless grinding continues to a very small particle size, which is very time-consuming and moreover produces an adverse viscosity value, it can occur that the process mass still has a fraction with particle sizes lying far above the desired value. Such a fraction has an adverse effect on the taste of the final product.

Web site: http://www.delphion.com/details?pn=US05297743__

- **Device for producing chocolate shells**

Inventor(s): Bindler; Uwe (Bergneustadt, DE)

Assignee(s): Gebr. Bindler Maschinenfabrik GmbH & Co. KG (Bergneustadt, DE)

Patent Number: 6,244,851

Date filed: December 23, 1998

Abstract: A device for producing a chocolate article, in particular a shell for hollow chocolate bodies, comprises a conveyor device having a first collecting line, from which chocolate molds can be discharged, and a second collecting line, which is parallel to the first collecting line, to receive the discharged molds. Each mold has at least one alveolus for receiving a liquid chocolate preparation, and at least one ram element for immersion into the alveolus. Each mold is conveyed along with its corresponding ram element from the first collecting line to the second collecting line.

Excerpt(s): This invention concerns a device for producing a chocolate article, in particular a shell for hollow chocolate bodies, with a conveyor device for conveying molds, each having at least one alveolus for metering a liquid chocolate preparation, with each mold having at least one ram element by means of which a cooled ram element can be advanced to the minimum of one alveolus for immersion in the chocolate preparation while it is still liquid.... German Utility Model No. 9,419,672 G discloses a device for producing a chocolate article having a conveyor device for conveying molds. The molds have at least one alveolus for metering a liquid chocolate preparation and at least one ram element.... It is known from British Patent No. 207,974 to provide a cooled ram which is immersed in the liquid chocolate preparation in a chocolate mold, resulting in a hollow chocolate body of the desired thickness. Another device for producing chocolate articles is known from European Patent No. 589,820, where the ram which is immersed in the chocolate preparation is cooled to a temperature of at least 0.degree. C.

Web site: http://www.delphion.com/details?pn=US06244851__

- **Device for tempering chocolate masses and the like**

Inventor(s): Blum; Gunter (Quickborn, DE)

Assignee(s): Blum & Co., Maschinen- und Apparatebau GmbH (Kaltenkirchen, DE)

Patent Number: 4,648,315

Date filed: November 19, 1985

Abstract: A device for tempering chocolate masses comprises a casing and a sequential series of cooling sections in the casing for cooling and working a chocolate mass to produce a stable, homogeneous chocolate product. Each of the cooling sections includes a pair of cooled upper and lower cooling surfaces and a pair of rotating upper and lower working elements which are received between the cooling surfaces therein. The working elements have helical scraping elements on the surfaces thereof which face the adjacent cooling surfaces, and the scraping elements are constructed so that as the working elements are rotated, the scraping elements on the lower working elements move chocolate outwardly along the lower cooling surfaces and the scraping elements on the upper working elements move chocolate inwardly along the upper cooling surfaces.

Excerpt(s): The instant invention relates to devices for tempering and cooling chocolate masses and the like and more particularly to a device wherein chocolate is effectively cooled and worked as it is passed through a series of sequential cooling sections.... It is generally known that in order to effectively cool chocolate, it must be cooled in a tempering process which induces the formation of stable.beta. crystals in the chocolate. In this connection, although tempering devices have been heretofore available for cooling and working chocolate in a plurality of sequential cooling steps to produce suitably-cooled chocolate products, the heretofore available devices have generally required large numbers of cooling steps; and as a result, they have generally been highly expensive.... The instant invention provides a highly effective device for cooling a chocolate mass in a plurality of cooling steps, wherein highly effective mass flow and heat transfer is achieved in each cooling step, and wherein a high percentage of the chocolate is formed into.beta. crystals as it is cooled. However, the device of the instant invention is also adapted to be made in relatively inexpensive constructions since it can be made with substantially fewer cooling sections than the hertofore available devices for cooling and tempering chocolate. More specifically, the device of the instant invention comprises a casing having an inlet adjacent the lower end thereof and an outlet adjacent the upper end thereof, and a series of cooling sections in the casing through which chocolate passes as it flows from the inlet of the casing to the outlet thereof. Each of the cooling sections comprises a pair of opposed, cooled upper and lower cooling surfaces which are defined by cooling elements in the casing and which are positioned so that they cooperate to define a cooling chamber therebetween, and a pair of rotating concentric upper and lower working elements in the cooling chamber. Each pair of working elements and the respective cooling chamber in which they are received are constructed so that chocolate enters the chamber adjacent the hub of the lower working element and passes outwardly between the lower working element and the lower cooling surface and then inwardly between the upper working element and the upper cooling surface toward the hub of the upper working element. Each of the working elements preferably comprises a disc portion and at least four helical scraping elements on the side thereof which faces the adjacent cooling surface. Further, the helical scraping elements are preferably constructed and oriented so that as the working elements in a chamber are rotated, the helical scraping elements on the lower working element move chocolate outwardly, whereas the helical scraping elements on the upper working element in the same chamber move chocolate inwardly. Still further, the working elements preferably each further comprise at least four substantially radially extending mixing elements on the side thereof which is opposite from the scraping elements thereon and which therefore faces the adajcent working element, and the mixing elements on adjacent working elements are preferably disposed at angles of approximately 45.degree. with respect to each other. Even further, the disc portions of the working elements are preferably formed with outlets or notches along the outer peripheral edges thereof which allow chocolate to be transferred from the area between the lower working element and the lower cooling surface to the area between the upper working element and the upper cooling surface.

Web site: http://www.delphion.com/details?pn=US04648315__

- **Dextrose-containing chocolate products with sucrose fatty acid polyester fat substitutes**

Inventor(s): Surber; Kevin J. (Lombard, IL), Miller; Mark S. (Arlington Heights, IL)

Assignee(s): Kraft Foods, Inc. (Northfield, IL)

Patent Number: 5,474,795

Date filed: August 19, 1994

Abstract: Low-fat or reduced-fat chocolate products containing sucrose fatty acid polyesters and dextrose are provided which have texture and mouthfeel properties similar to conventional chocolate products. The sweetener used is dextrose or blends of dextrose and sucrose. These chocolate products are prepared using a sucrose fatty acid polyester or a blend of sucrose fatty acid polyesters in place of the conventional cocoa butter constituent and dextrose or blends of dextrose and sucrose in place of the convention sucrose sweetener. The preferred form of dextrose is dextrose monohydrate. The sucrose fatty acid polyesters used do not necessarily mimic the rheological and thermal properties of cocoa butter. The improved chocolate products have similar texture and mouthfeel properties of conventional chocolate with significantly fewer calories and lower fat content. Moreover, the texture and mouthfeel properties can be varied for various uses by varying the relative proportions of the sucrose fatty acid polyesters and the relative proportions of the dextrose and sucrose in the sweetener. The use of dextrose results in chocolate compositions having improved mouthfeel and significantly reduced levels of waxiness.

Excerpt(s): The invention generally relates to the field of chocolate products, especially low-fat or reduced-fat chocolate products. More specifically, this invention relates to low-fat or reduced-fat chocolate products having texture and mouthfeel similar to conventional chocolate products. The chocolate products of this invention are prepared using a sucrose fatty acid polyester or a blend of sucrose fatty acid polyesters in place of the conventional cocoa butter constituent. The sweetener used is dextrose (i.e., glucose) or a blend of dextrose and sucrose. The preferred form of dextrose is dextrose monohydrate.... Chocolate is a highly desirable confection product which has unique texture and flavor release properties in the mouth. Many of these desirable properties are generally attributable to the fat component of chocolate--cocoa butter--which has a narrow melting point range just slightly below normal body temperature and a sharp melting curve. Accordingly, the desirable flavor release and organoleptic sensations of chocolate occur rapidly as the chocolate melts in the mouth.... Conventional chocolate products generally contain about 30 to 60 percent sugar, about 10 to 70 percent chocolate liquor (which normally contains about 50 percent cocoa butter), about 20 to 25 percent added cocoa butter, and about 1 percent flavor and other constituents. Typically, such chocolate products contain about 30 to 34 percent total fat in the form of cocoa butter. Unfortunately, therefore, conventional chocolate products are generally high in undesirable saturated fats and calories. Due to the relatively recent interest in reducing calorie and saturated fat intake in the diet, there has been an increased interest in providing reduced-calorie and/or reduced-fat chocolate products. Most of these efforts have attempted to provide a substitute for the cocoa butter component in conventional chocolate products.

Web site: http://www.delphion.com/details?pn=US05474795__

- **Dietetic chocolate composition**

Inventor(s): Riesen; Alfred (6405 Immensee, CH)

Assignee(s): none reported

Patent Number: 4,011,349

Date filed: September 24, 1975

Abstract: Dietetic chocolate compositions having a specific proportion of ingredients and a combination of sorbitol and cyclamate or saccharin which results in an extremely appealing taste.

Excerpt(s): This invention relates to new chocolate compositions, and more particularly, dietetic chocolate compositions.... Attempts at production of dietetic chocolate candy with reduced caloric content and/or low sugar content have led to products which mostly are poor substitutes, with a small percentage achieving what might be classified as even palatable, leaving much to be desired by the chocolate candy consumer who for reasons of health, e.g., latent diabetes, is restricted from the well-known chocolate products of high caloric and carbohydrate content.... Chocolate flavored beverages and frozen deserts of low carbohydrate content have been described in the prior art, as in U.S. Pat. Nos. 2,876,104 and 3,806,607, in which natural sugar is replaced by synthetic sweetners, e.g. saccharin and cyclamate sweetners. Sorbitol has been employed in the production of solid sugarless confections as described in U.S. Pat. Nos. 3,438,787 and 3,738,845. The use of soya as a complex with lecithin in long-lasting confections has been described in U.S. Pat. No. 2,740,720. Chocolate products made with skim milk are described in U.S. Pat. Nos. 2,760,867 and 2,851,365.

Web site: http://www.delphion.com/details?pn=US04011349__

- **Dry chocolate flavored beverage mix**

Inventor(s): Dolan; Kenneth M. (The Procter & Gamble Company, 6071 Center Hill Ave., Cincinnati, OH 45224-1703), Hughes; Donald L. (The Procter & Gamble Company, 6071 Center Hill Ave., Cincinnati, OH 45224-1703), Leavell; Kimberly A. (The Procter & Gamble Company, 6071 Center Hill Ave., Cincinnati, OH 45224-1703), Swaine, Jr. Robert L. (The Procter & Gamble Company, 6071 Center Hill Ave., Cincinnati, OH 45224-1703), Hayes; Mariaelena Z. (The Procter & Gamble Company, 6071 Center Hill Ave., Cincinnati, OH 45224-1703)

Assignee(s): none reported

Patent Number: H1,620

Date filed: June 6, 1995

Abstract: Disclosed is a dry chocolate-flavored beverage mix and a process for making it. The dry beverage mix comprises from about 3% to about 13% by weight of cocoa powder, from about 40% to about 60% by weight of particulate sugar, from about 3% to about 5% by weight of caramel powder, from about to about 20% by weight of malt extract, from about 0.25% to about 1.0% by weight of flavor enhancing salt, from about 10% to about 32% by weight of a powdered non-dairy creamer wherein the non-dairy creamer contains from about 40% to about 60% vegetable fat by weight of the non-dairy creamer, from about 0.02% to about 3.0% by weight of a thickening agent, from 0 to about 1.0% by weight of added lecithin, an effective amount of an antioxidant, less than about 6% by weight of moisture, from 0 to about 20% by weight of an added protein source, and nutritionally supplemental amounts of vitamins and minerals.

Excerpt(s): The present invention relates to a dry chocolate flavored beverage mix and a process for making it. Such a dry beverage mix does not require substantial amounts of added milk or whey solids, and can be reconstituted with tap water to deliver a chocolate flavored beverage with certain milk-like organoleptic properties.... Many chocolate flavored milk-based beverage formulations are known. Among these formulations are dry beverage mixes which can be diluted prior to consumption to form a chocolate flavored milk-based beverage. These chocolate flavored milk-based beverages, referred to generically by consumers as "chocolate milk," are especially popular among children. Given the potential level of protein, mineral and vitamin fortification possible in such beverages, these beverages can be an excellent source of nutrition for children, especially children in developing countries where daily nutrition is a serious, ongoing concern.... Chocolate flavored milk-based beverages are normally marketed as chilled chocolate flavored milk or as dry chocolate-flavored beverage mixes which can be reconstituted with milk, powdered milk and water, or water. Such reconstituted chocolate flavored beverages will normally contain milk solids in order to provide milk-like organoleptic properties and protein fortification. Milk solids, however, are relatively expensive and add substantially to the cost of the dry beverage mixes. Such costs can be reduced by replacing some or all of the milk solids in the dry beverage mixes with whey solids. Whey can provide protein fortification to the dry beverage mixes and it is an inexpensive, abundant raw material. Whey solids, however, often contribute an objectionable off-flavor to beverages. Whey-based beverages also have a watery texture that is readily distinguishable from that of the more desirable, creamy, milk-based beverages. Accordingly, consumers have rejected whey-based beverages or have simply added whole milk or milk solids to the product prior to consumption to improve its organoleptic profile. The addition by consumers of such milk solids, e.g., dehydrated milk, is expensive and inconvenient. Manufactures have responded by making whey-based chocolate flavored beverage mixes with enough milk solids to satisfy consumer tastes. Consumers prefer these products but many cannot easily afford them.

Web site: http://www.delphion.com/details?pn=US0H1620__

- ## Dry drink mix and chocolate flavored drink made therefrom

  Inventor(s): Kealey; Kirk S. (Lancaster, PA), Snyder; Rodney M. (Elizabethtown, PA), Romanczyk, Jr. Leo J. (Hackettstown, NJ), Geyer; Hans M. (Hershey, PA), Myers; Mary E. (Lititz, PA), Whitacre; Eric J. (Elizabethtown, PA), Hammerstone, Jr. John F. (Nazareth, PA), Schmitz; Harold H. (Branchburg, NJ)

  Assignee(s): Mars Incorporated (McLean, VA)

  Patent Number: 6,599,553

  Date filed: November 5, 2001

  Abstract: A dry drink mix which is rich in cocoa polyphenols such as catechin, epicatechin, and cocoa procyanidins contains a cocoa polyphenol rich cocoa powder, an alkalized cocoa powder, and a sweetener. The dry mix contains other conventional ingredients such as vanillin an emulsifier. A chocolate flavored drink can be prepared from the dry drink mix by adding milk, for example a low fat milk. The cocoa polyphenol rich cocoa powder is prepared from non-roasted cocoa beans or blends thereof having a fermentation factor of 275 less, i.e., slaty and/or purple cocoa beans. The alkalized cocoa powder is prepared from roasted cocoa beans.

  Excerpt(s): The invention relates to cocoa components having enhanced levels of cocoa polyphenols, processes for producing the same, methods of using the same and compositions containing the same. More specifically, the invention provides a method of producing cocoa components having an enhanced content of cocoa polyphenols, in particular procyanidins. The cocoa components include partially and fully defatted cocoa solids, cocoa nibs and fractions derived therefrom, cocoa polyphenol extracts, cocoa butter, chocolate liquors, and mixtures thereof.... The invention also relates to versatile novel processes for extracting fat from cocoa beans and/or processing cocoa beans to yield a cocoa component having a conserved level of polyphenols, in particular procyanidins. The invention provides a significantly less complex process with respect to total cost of process equipment, maintenance, energy and labor, with the concomitant benefit of obtaining components having conserved concentrations of polyphenols relative to the starting materials.... Documents are cited in this disclosure with a full citation for each. These documents relate to the state-of-the-art to which this invention pertains, and each document cited herein is hereby incorporated by reference.

  Web site: http://www.delphion.com/details?pn=US06599553__

- ## Dry stable chocolate beverage containing iron and vitamin C

  Inventor(s): Mehansho; Haile (Fairfield, OH), Saldierna; Maria E. Z. (Echegaray, MX)

  Assignee(s): The Procter & Gamble Company (Cincinnati, OH)

  Patent Number: 5,002,779

  Date filed: November 7, 1989

  Abstract: The present invention relates to nutritional improvements in vitamin C and iron supplemented chocolate powders or flavored beverage mixes which preferably contain nonfat milk solids. Other vitamins such as vitamin A, B, D or E and encapsulated.beta.-carotene (vitamin A-precursor) can be added to the dry beverage mix. The supplement can contain other minerals, such as calcium, zinc and copper. In particular, methods for fortifying dry beverage mixes with highly bioavailable iron compounds and stable vitamin C without producing undesirable color or flavor in the mix are disclosed.

Excerpt(s): The present invention relates to nutritional improvements in vitamin C and iron supplemented chocolate powders or flavored beverage mixes. In particular, methods for preparing stable iron and vitamin C fortified dry beverage mixes having enhanced iron bioavailability and stable vitamin C without affecting flavor or color of product are disclosed.... Vitamin and mineral supplements for human and veterinary use are commonplace. The medical management of certain anemias can be handled rather well by increasing the daily intake of iron Some diets, or heavy physical exercise, may require the intake of considerable quantities of minerals apart from those generally obtained through what otherwise would be considered a balanced diet.... Vitamin supplementation is important primarily for those who have inadequate diets, including growing children. In developing countries where the dietary intake of minerals and vitamins are low in the general population, such a nutritional supplement would have great value.

Web site: http://www.delphion.com/details?pn=US05002779__

- **Fat blends for chocolate compositions**

Inventor(s): Weyland; Mark (London, GB3), Cebula; Deryck J. (Bushmead Fields, GB3), Dekker; Willem (Hoorn, NL)

Assignee(s): Van den Bergh Foods Co., Division of Conopco Inc. (New York, NY)

Patent Number: 5,171,604

Date filed: April 5, 1991

Abstract: The invention concerns with fat blends comprising cocoa butter and butter olein and optionally cocoa butter equivalent and butter fat.These blends can be used in chocolate compositions. In the processing of chocolate compositions they are used to lower the viscosity at temper of these compositions.

Excerpt(s): The invention concerns new fat blends, that can be used in chocolate compositions. So far cf. for example EP No. 0 006 034, fat blends are known for this application that contain cocoa butter and butter fat, whereas part of the cocoa butter may be replaced by a cocoa butter equivalent (CBE). These fat blends possess a certain hardness as e.g. can be defined by the Stevens texture. When in these blends the butter fat is at least partly replaced by an oil, while the total fat content remains the same, it was expected that the Stevens hardness would become too low. However we have found new fat blends in which at least part of the butter fat is replaced and in which yet the Stevens hardness remains satisfactory, whereas the performance of such fat blends, when used in chocolate compositions is good both in continuous and in batch temper processes, especially the viscosity of these compositions at temper is very satisfactory, e.g. expressed as the viscosity difference between the viscosity at temper and at 50.degree. C. This is in particular advantageous because a too high viscosity leads to problems in the processing of the chocolate compositions. Another advantage of a lower viscosity is, that many chocolates at temper would benefit from a greater flexibility, because of the lower viscosity, in different applications e.g. depositing, enrobing etcetera, wherein a different flow behavior is required.... In the fat blends according to the invention at least part of the butter fat is replaced by a butter olein (=Bu-f).... Therefore the invention concerns in the first place fat blends, comprising 50-75 wt % cocoa butter (=CB), 10-35 wt % of butter olein with a melting point of maximum 20.degree. C., 0-25 wt % of a cocoa butter equivalent (=CBE) and 0-25 wt % of butter fat. The butter olein has preferably an N.sub.20 value of less than 5.0. In particular butter olein with an N.sub.10 value of 5-15 and an I.V. of more than 35 are used.

Web site: http://www.delphion.com/details?pn=US05171604__

- **Flavor system having high chocolate flavor impact**

Inventor(s): Haynes; Louis V. (Cincinnati, OH), Pflaumer; Phillip F. (Ross, OH), Rizzi; George P. (Cincinnati, OH), Roberts; Bruce A. (Batavia, OH)

Assignee(s): The Procter & Gamble Co. (Cincinnati, OH)

Patent Number: 4,707,365

Date filed: June 5, 1985

Abstract: A natural chocolate flavor system having high chocolate flavor impact is disclosed. This system has: (1) a high level of cocoa solids; (2) a high level of a mixture of pyrazines; and (3) high ratios of certain dimethyl pyrazines to trimethyl and tetramethyl pyrazines. This chocolate flavor system is useful in formulating chocolate chips and chocolate coatings for storage-stable crisp and chewy cookies.

Excerpt(s): This application relates to a flavor system having high chocolate flavor impact useful in formulating chocolate chips and other chocolate flavored products for baked goods. Fresh, home-baked cookies are the standard of excellence in the cookie world. The dominant characteristic of such cookies is the texture, specifically, a crisp outside surface and a chewy interior. The interior contains pockets of super-saturated sugar solution (syrup) which are ductile and are sometimes visible as strands when the cookie is pulled apart. Unfortunately, within a few weeks or less, such home-baked cookies undergo a spontaneous and irreversable process of degradation, becoming hard and crumbly throughout.... The problem of storage-stability for these dual-textured cookie products has been solved. In particular, U.S. Pat. No. 4,455,333 to Hong et al., issued June 19, 1984, discloses cookie products having distributed therein discrete regions having a crisp texture and discrete regions having a chewy texture. Most importantly, these crisp and chewy regions remain storage-stable over time, i.e., the process of degradation occurring in fresh, home-baked cookies does not occur or occurs much more slowly. Other examples of these storage-stable, dual-textured cookies are disclosed in U.S. Pat. No. 4,344,969 to Youngquist, et al, issued Aug. 17, 1982 and U.S. Pat. No. 4,503,080 to Brabbs et al., issued Mar. 5, 1985.... The storage-stable, dual-textured cookies of the Hong et al. patent can contain chocolate chips. It has been found that the chocolate chips previously used in such cookies lose chocolate flavor impact on aging. This aging problem has been found to be due to the higher water activity of the cookie crumb relative to the much lower water activity of the chocolate chips. Specifically, the moisture in the cookie crumb diffuses into the chips and desorbs the chocolate flavor compounds present therein. These desorbed compounds then diffuse back into the cookie crumb.

Web site: http://www.delphion.com/details?pn=US04707365__

- **Flavored nut spreads having milk chocolate flavor and creamy soft texture**

Inventor(s): Wong; Vincent York-Leung (Hamilton, OH), Schmidt; Michael Charles (Reading, OH), Chen; Jing (West Chester, OH), Bruno, Jr. David Joseph (Hamilton, OH)

Assignee(s): The Procter & Gamble Company (Cincinnati, OH)

Patent Number: 5,942,275

Date filed: October 27, 1997

Abstract: Chocolate flavored nut spreads, especially chocolate flavored peanut butters having a milk chocolate like flavor without a bitter aftertaste and with desirable spreadability. Cocoa solids substantially free of dairy solids that are encapsulated by sugar are dispersed substantially homogeneously throughout the spread. The level of cocoa butter is also below the point where it can crystallize out (i.e., typically about 20% or less on a total fat basis).

Excerpt(s): This application relates to flavored nut butters, especially peanut butters, having milk chocolate flavor without the use of dairy solids. This application particularly relates to chocolate flavored nut butters that have a creamy soft texture.... Conventional peanut butter and other nut butters typically comprise cohesive, comminuted mixtures of solid nut particles suspended in oil (nut paste), a sweetener such as sugar, high fructose corn syrup or honey, salt and a stabilizing agent (e.g., a high melting point fat or hardstock) to prevent separation of the oil and particulates. The primary component of peanut butter, peanut paste, is formed by roasting, blanching, and grinding shelled peanuts. During the grinding step, the cellular structure of the peanuts is ruptured, releasing the peanut oil in which the pulverized peanut solids become suspended.... Chocolate can be an especially complimentary flavor to peanut flavor and is often used to enrobe peanut flavored centers or nougats or to form an exterior cup that is then filled with peanut flavored material. Indeed, the concept of flavoring nut butters and especially peanut butter with chocolate flavored bits is know in the art. See, for example, U.S. Pat. No. 5,079,027 (Wong et al), issued Jan. 7, 1992, which discloses adding chocolate chips or other flavored bits to peanut butter.

Web site: http://www.delphion.com/details?pn=US05942275__

- **Food composition and method of making a cookie or a chocolate shell containing a fermented filling based on a dairy product**

Inventor(s): Saintain; Michel (Fontenay Les Briis, FR)

Assignee(s): Compagnie Gervais Danone (FR)

Patent Number: 5,573,793

Date filed: February 23, 1995

Abstract: A food composition of the type containing a cookie or a chocolate shell and a filling based on a dairy product wherein the filling is fermented and contains live lactic acid bacteria, has a water activity (Aw) of between 0.75 and 0.81·and wherein the fat content of the filling is such that it makes it possible to obtain a water-in-oil type emulsion.

Excerpt(s): The present invention relates to a food composition based on a dairy product, and in particular yoghurt.... There have been for some time in the sector of food compositions products called food bars based on various pastry products filled with chocolate products and/or various sweet products.... This type of product is perceived by the consumer as being a long-life product in the same way as plain cakes for example.

Web site: http://www.delphion.com/details?pn=US05573793___

- **Fruit-containing chocolate products and process of their preparation**

Inventor(s): Vajda; Gabor (Budapest, HU), Ravasz; Laszlo (Budapest, HU), Vajda; Gaborne (Budapest, HU), Karacsonyi; Bela (Budapest, HU)

Assignee(s): Agro-Industria Innovacios Vallalat (Budapest, HU)

Patent Number: 4,837,042

Date filed: July 24, 1987

Abstract: The invention relates to the preparation of mouldable or smearable fruit-containing chocolate products. According to the invention one part by mass of chocolate optionally containing an emulsifier is melted at 32.degree. to 40.degree. C., the melt is homogenized with 0.5 to 1.0 parts by mass of a fruit concentrate containing at least 8% by mass of fruit dry substance, which has previously been admixed with sugar or any other carbonhydrate and 0.2 to 8.0% by mass of a lyophilic additive, and concentrated to 62 to 68 Ref%, and the homogeneous mixture is filled into moulds, containers or used for coating corpora. The pH of the fruit employed is adjusted to 5.0 to 6.8. To obtain a creamy consistence vegetable fats are added to the chocolate. As a lyophilic additive for example sodium alginate, carrageen, soluble starch, carboxymethyl starch, carboxymethyl cellulose, casein, agar-agar and sodium citrate or mixtures thereof can be used.

Excerpt(s): The invention relates to fruit-containing chocolate products and a process for their preparation. More particularly, the invention concerns fruit-containing chocolate products which are mouldable or smearable. In this connection, the term "smearable" is a physical state of the chocolate product which is paste-like such that it can easily be applied, by spreading, smearing, etc. onto an edible substrate, for example, crackers, bread, etc. or the product can be consumed by itself, by spoon, for example. Also, the smearable product of the present invention can be used to fill pastry in much the same way that presently available chocolate products are used, which, however, do not contain fruit.... The basic material of chocolate is the cocoa mass prepared from cocoa bean by roasting, husking, reduction in size and refinement. The most important components of cocoa mass are cocoa butter and cocoa dry substance. Cocoa butter is the fatty component of cocoa, while the dry substance includes the protein, carbohydrate and alkaloid pigment and mineral components of cocoa. From the cocoa mass, chocolate is prepared by adding sugar. The character of chocolate is determined by the ratio of cocoa butter, cocoa dry substance and sugar.... The dipping chocolate, also known by its well-known German name "Tunkmasse" is prepared for further processing and contains 44% by weight, the bitter chocolate 30 to 43% by weight, the sweet chocolate 50 to 55% by mass and the usual "household" chocolate 66% by mass of sugar.

Web site: http://www.delphion.com/details?pn=US04837042___

- **Gas-incorporated chocolate and its production**

  Inventor(s): Asama; Koji (Izumisano, JP), Yamada; Kazuhisa (Izumisano, JP), Nago; Atsushi (Izumisano, JP)

  Assignee(s): Fuji Oil Company, Limited (Osaka-Fu, JP)

  Patent Number: 6,482,464

  Date filed: April 11, 2001

  Abstract: There is disclosed gas-incorporated chocolate, in particular, air-incorporated chocolate whose chocolate material requires tempering and comprises a polyglycerin fatty acid ester and lecithin, said chocolate material being subjected to tempering with a seed agent. Its production is also disclosed. The gas-incorporated chocolate has light mouthfeel without an oily taste and can be produced with a simple apparatus.

  Excerpt(s): The present invention relates to gas-incorporated chocolate, in particular, air-incorporated chocolate such as so-called "air chocolate" or "whipped chocolate", and its production. More specifically, it relates to gas-incorporated chocolate of a tempering-requiring type which can be produced by using a simple apparatus such as a vertical mixer, and its production.... Recently, for giving light mouthfeel to chocolate, many chocolate products which are combined with other confectionery such as baked confectionery, e.g., biscuit, have been marketed. In addition, there are so-called "air chocolate" and "whipped chocolate" whose chocolate material itself contain bubbles (cells) so that its specific gravity is lowered to give light mouthfeel to the chocolate.... For giving light mouthfeel to chocolate by incorporation of bubbles into a chocolate material, several methods have been proposed. For example, a chocolate material is agitated to incorporate air into the chocolate material to some extent, followed by maintaining it at reduced pressure to lower specific gravity of the chocolate material (JP-A 63-202341), or gas is incorporated in a chocolate material under pressurized conditions, followed by depressurization to atmospheric pressure to lower specific gravity of the chocolate material (JP-A 63-49040). Further, whipped shortening is mixed with a chocolate material to lower specific gravity thereof (JP-A 63-28355), or a fat containing a certain amount or more of triglycerides whose constituent fatty acid residues have 58 or more carbon atoms in total is formulated in a chocolate material so that bubbles formed by whipping are stabilized by crystals of the fat to lower specific gravity of the chocolate material (JP-A 3-201946).

  Web site: http://www.delphion.com/details?pn=US06482464__

- **Hard fat replacer and chocolate containing same**

  Inventor(s): Soeters; Cornelis J. (Rotterdam, NL), Paulussen; Cornelis N. (Maasland, NL), Padley; Frederick B. (Welwyn Garden City, GB2), Tresser; David (London, GB2)

  Assignee(s): Lever Brothers Company (New York, NY)

  Patent Number: 4,283,436

  Date filed: December 16, 1976

  Abstract: Hard fat replacers, particularly for cocoa-butter, are provided comprising mixtures of mid-fraction from palm oil and at least 85% pure SOS, POS or SOS/POS. SOS is 1,3-distearyl-2-oleyl glycerol and POS is 1-palmityl-2-oleyl-3-stearyl glycerol. Using these hard fat replacers hardened milk chocolate and plain chocolate suitable for tropical use can be prepared as well as excellent normal plain and milk chocolates.

Excerpt(s): The invention relates to fats, particularly to hard fats, often called hard butters.... Hard fats are specially important in confectionery, bakery and pharmaceutical products. Such fats have the special property that at room temperature they are hard but melt quickly at body temperature in the mouth. The most important example of a hard fat is cocoa-butter. Because of such very special properties, although also because of long association, cocoa-butter can command high prices. There has been a long-standing need for fats to take the place of the generally expensive hard fats. As more fully explained below, fats have been developed that partly meet this need. But all these fats suffer from one or more disadvantages.... A further problem with hard fats is that, although they indeed have special properties particularly fitting them for their use in specialty products such as confectionery, bakery and pharmaceutical products, the theoretical optimum behaviour is far from met by the available fats. For instance there is a need for a fat that would enable chocolate to be prepared that would show less finger-imprinting than chocolate made from cocoa-butter but would still display sharp melting characteristics in the mouth. Further instances are the need for a fat that is more bloom resistant than cocoa-butter and a fat that would enable chocolate to be stored under tropical or semi-tropical conditions; such conditions occur in centrally heated buildings as well as in tropical countries. General needs are for fats that provide more flexibility and for more reliable fats, i.e. fats of more consistent quality, than the hard fats at present available. Such a fat should preferably be compatible with most hard fats, particularly with cocoa-butter.

Web site: http://www.delphion.com/details?pn=US04283436__

- **Heat resistant chocolate and production method thereof**

Inventor(s): Takemori; Toshio (Tokyo, JP), Tsurumi; Toshinobu (Saitama, JP), Takagi; Masahiro (Chiba, JP), Ito; Masanori (Saitama, JP)

Assignee(s): Lotte Company Limited (JP)

Patent Number: 5,232,734

Date filed: January 29, 1991

Abstract: A heat-resistant chocolate is obtained by adding an O/W type emulsion which is an emulsion of fine particles of oils and fats in water as the continuous phase, to a chocolate, thereby to impart heat resistance to the chocolate while maintaining good taste and a good property of dissolving in the mouth. The O/W type emulsion contains 20-70% water, and is used in an amount from 1 to 10% of the final chocolate.

Excerpt(s): The present invention relates to a chocolate having heat resistance, in particular relates to a heat resistant chocolate and a production method thereof which can be obtained by adding an O/W type emulsion which is an emulsion of water and oils and fats to chocolate and maintains a quality of good taste and good dissolving in the mouth without causing deterioration in quality due to heat.... Generally, the chocolate has such a structure in which fine particles such as cacao, milk, and sugars are dispersed in oils and fats. Namely, a general chocolate uses oils and fats which easily dissolve on account of increase in temperature as a dispersing base. Therefore, the chocolate is no heat stable, and as the oils and fats dissolve, deterioration in quality takes place such as sticking to hands, blooming and the like.... In order to improve such properties of the chocolate, many studies have been hitherto done to achieve a heat resistant chocolate.

Web site: http://www.delphion.com/details?pn=US05232734__

- **Heat-resistant chocolate and a method for producing it**

Inventor(s): Takemori; Toshio (Urawa, JP), Tsurumi; Toshinobu (Urawa, JP), Takagi; Masahiro (Urawa, JP)

Assignee(s): Lotte Company Limited (Tokyo, JP)

Patent Number: 5,160,760

Date filed: February 22, 1990

Abstract: There is disclosed a heat-resistant chocolate which is formed by dispersing and mixing a water-in-oil emulsion and a chocolate base material, wherein an oil phase and a water phase in which a hydrophilic substance is contained are mixed and emulsified with an emulsifying agent to form said water-in-oil emulsion. There is also disclosed a method for producing a heat-resistant chocolate, wherein a water-in-oil emulsion is mixed and dispersed which is formed by mixing and emulsifying an oil phase and a water phase in which a hydrophilic substance is contained using a emulsifying agent into a chocolate base material which is temperature-tempered by an usual mean, which is cooled to form a solid, after which increase in heat-resistance depending on time is contemplated.

Excerpt(s): The present invention relates to a chocolate having heat-resistance, and more particularly relates to a chocolate and a method for producing it in which a framing structure is gradually formed with solids other than oils and fats to give a smooth melt feeling in mouth and a soft mouth-feel keeping a good quality level equivalent to that of a conventional good chocolate, and with shape retention at a temperature above 40.degree. C. such that it is not sticky to the direct touch.... Chocolate has the disadvantage that the better the quality of the chocolate, the more easily the influence of temperature affects it. Conventional chocolate becomes soft at above 28.degree. C., and loses shape retention at above 32.degree. C. Thus, in order to overcome such disadvantage, a number of investigations on heat-resistant chocolate have conventionally been carried out.... (2) a framing structure is formed with solids other than oils and fats.

Web site: http://www.delphion.com/details?pn=US05160760__

- **Heat-resistant chocolate and method of making same**

Inventor(s): Kealey; Kirk S. (Long Valley, NJ), Quan; Nancy W. (Budd Lake, NJ)

Assignee(s): Mars, Inc. (McLean, VA)

Patent Number: 5,149,560

Date filed: March 25, 1991

Abstract: This invention concerns a heat-resistant or thermally robust chocolate and method for making same. The inventive method provides a means of adding moisture to chocolate through use of lipid microstructure technology such as reverse micelle technology to form a stable water-in-oil emulsion, for example, hydrated lecithin. The stable water-in-oil emulsion is added to tempered chocolate during processing, and upon aging and stabilization, thermal robustness develops in the chocolate product. The heat-resistant chocolate of the instant invention is suitable for use in the same manner and for the same purposes for which ordinary chocolate is used. The invention provides a heat-resistant chocolate product having the desired taste, texture, mouth feel and other characteristics of ordinary chocolate.

Excerpt(s): This invention relates to a heat-resistant or thermally robust chocolate and method for making same. More particularly, this invention relates to a chocolate and method of manufacturing the chocolate, which involves the addition of moisture to chocolate. This is done by initially creating a stable water-in-oil emulsion, for example, a hydrated lecithin, and then adding the emulsion to tempered chocolate. Upon aging and stabilization, thermal robustness develops in the chocolate product.... The heat-resistant or thermally robust chocolate of this invention is suitable for use in the same manner and for the same purposes as ordinary chocolate. For example, it can be roll formed molded into bars shell molded, co-sprayed or used to coat, or enrobe, other confectioneries or other food products.... Ordinary chocolate is composed primarily of fats or fatty substances, such as cocoa butter, in which there are dispersed non-fat products such as cocoa components, sugars, proteins, etc. Therefore, since chocolate is primarily constituted by fat bodies, its melting temperature is relatively low. This means that ordinary chocolate is not particularly resistent to summer temperatures or the heat of tropical countries. Therefore, a need exists for a chocolate which is resistant to relatively high ambient temperatures.

Web site: http://www.delphion.com/details?pn=US05149560__

- **Heat-resistant chocolate composition and process for the preparation thereof**

Inventor(s): Alander; Jari (Karlshamn, SE), Warnheim; Torbjorn (Bromma, SE), Luhti; Erwin (Karlshamn, SE)

Assignee(s): Karlshamns Oils & Fats AB (Karlshamn, SE)

Patent Number: 5,486,376

Date filed: August 2, 1994

Abstract: A heat-resistant or thermostable chocolate composition is prepared by mixing a chocolate mass, commonly used for preparing chocolate compositions, with a solution mainly consisting of a water-in-oil microemulsion comprising water, fat and an emulsifier, and optionally small amounts of one or more other phases, the water in the microemulsion being present in the form of droplets having a size of 10-1,000.ANG..In a process for preparing the heat-resistant chocolate composition, a chocolate mass commonly used for preparing chocolate compositions is mixed with a solution mainly consisting of a water-in-oil microemulsion comprising water, fat and an emulsifier, and optionally small amounts of one or more other phases, the water in the microemulsion being present in the form of droplets having a size of 10-1,000.ANG..

Excerpt(s): The present invention relates to a heat-resistant or thermostable chocolate composition and a process for the preparation thereof.... For consumer appeal, a chocolate bar should have a very special consistency. It should snap brittly at room temperature but melt quickly in the mouth, where the temperature is about 35.degree. C. In warmer countries, for instance, it may, however, be difficult to maintain the texture of the chocolate up to the moment the chocolate is to be eaten. The problem then is to keep the brittleness of the chocolate without impairing its other properties.... By the use of various additives, sometimes combined with special processes of preparation, chocolate can be made to keep its texture also at temperatures at which it would otherwise have melted or at least softened excessively. Chocolate thus stabilised is referred to as heat-resistant or tropicalised chocolate.

Web site: http://www.delphion.com/details?pn=US05486376__

- **Heuchera Chocolate Ruffles**

  Inventor(s): Heims; Dan M. (Portland, OR)

  Assignee(s): Terra-Nova Nurseries, Inc. (Portland, OR)

  Patent Number: PP8,965

  Date filed: December 30, 1993

  Abstract: A new and distinct hybrid of Heuchera characterized by unique, ruffled leaves of chocolate coloration showing the burgundy underside through the ruffles.

  Excerpt(s): The present invention relates to a new and distinct hyrbid of Heuchera which originated as a cross-pollination of Heuchera "Pewter Veil" and Heuchera micrantha "Ruffles" in the Saxifragaceae family.... (1) Summer, fall and winter: Chocolate-Olive coloration on the ruffled foliage. Reverse shown.... (2) Spring: Foliage of a warm Chocolate Brown on ruffled foliage with a Burgundy reverse.

  Web site: http://www.delphion.com/details?pn=US0PP8965__

- **Home chocolate processing apparatus**

  Inventor(s): Snyder, Jr. Francis H. (Danbury, CT)

  Assignee(s): Olaf Kayser (Stamford, CT), Meyerie; George (Brookfield, CT)

  Patent Number: 4,907,502

  Date filed: October 5, 1987

  Abstract: A bowl, which accommodates a coating, is removably mounted in a casing. A moving device in the casing is coupled to the bowl for rotating said bowl. A heater is positioned in the casing in operative proximity with the bowl for melting the chocolate. A cooling unit is positioned in the casing in operative proximity with the bowl for cooling the coating. A control circuit is electrically connected to the heater and cooling unit for controlling the heating and cooling of the coating.

  Excerpt(s): The present invention relates to home chocolate processing apparatus and the novel method of making chocolate candies.... The techniques for processing pure chocolate into chocolate candies are taught in industry, but such techniques have not been made available to the consumer, due in part to the high cost, large size, and required expertise in the use of such equipment.... The interest in chocolate world-wide has intensified over the past years. This interest is manifested best by the emergence and success of the so-called gourmet chocolate shops and store boutiques. Some of these products are selling for up to $32 per pound! During 1984, a new magazine "Chocolatier" was introduced which deals exclusively with the subject of producing chocolate-based delicacies in the home. This magazine is enjoying high growth, thereby indicating that the public is very interested in processing this relatively exotic material in the home. A great many people around the world love chocolate.

  Web site: http://www.delphion.com/details?pn=US04907502__

- **Homogeneous, storage-stable chocolate milk comestibles and process of making**

  Inventor(s): Schuppiser; Jean-Luc (Claye Souilly, FR), Coutant; Antoine (Paris, FR), Bozetto; Jean-Claude (Chilly Mazarin, FR)

  Assignee(s): Rhone- Poulenc Chimie (Courbevoie, FR)

  Patent Number: 5,066,508

  Date filed: January 22, 1990

  Abstract: Essentially homogeneous and storage-stable liquid chocolate milk products, having viscosities ranging from 10 to 100 mPa.s, are formulated from milk bases including a suspension of cocoa particulates and a suspension stabilizing amount of a xanthan/galactomannan admixture adapted for the formation of an aqueous gel therefrom, wherein the ratio by weight of xanthan/galactomannan ranges from 80/20 to 20/80.

  Excerpt(s): More particularly according to the present invention, a xanthan gum is a heteropolysaccharide having a molecular weight of several millions, produced by the fermentation of carbohydrates under the action of bacteria of the genus Xanthomonas and more particularly Xanthomonas campestris, or other species, as is very well known in this art.... Galactomannans are natural gums derived from seeds of the legume family. They include Dgalactose and Dmannose units. Among the galactomannans which form, in an aqueous medium, continuous gels with xanthan gum in a concentration of at least 0.1%, carob gum, Tara gum and Cassia gum are especially representative.... All of these gums are readily commercially available in different grades, depending upon the production and processing techniques employed. Any foodgrade material is suitable for use according to the invention.

  Web site: http://www.delphion.com/details?pn=US05066508__

- **Hypoallergenic chocolate**

  Inventor(s): Girsh; Leonard S. (Benjamin Fox Pavilion, Old York and Township Line Rds., Jenkintown, PA 19046)

  Assignee(s): none reported

  Patent Number: 4,078,093

  Date filed: October 12, 1976

  Abstract: A hypoallergenic chocolate is prepared by treating cocoa powder so as to denature substantially all of the protein allergens which cause chocolate allergies. The cocoa powder with its denatured protein allergen is then mixed with sugar, cocoa butter, and other flavoring additives and further heat treated (and denatured) to produce the hypoallergenic chocolate. The hypoallergenic chocolate may be used itself or as a flavoring ingredient in various food products and other edible materials, including specifically prescribed hypoallergenic food substitutes and/or anti-allergic medications and other medicinal preparations.

  Excerpt(s): Many persons suffer from various allergies, many of which are caused by ingesting food containing allergens.... Although the biochemistry is not precisely understood, it is believed that the allergen causes a specific reagin to be formed in the bloodstream upon ingestion or other contact of the allergen with the body. The ability to produce reagins in response to a given allergen is thought to be an inherited characteristic that differentiates an allergic from a non-allergic person. The specificity of the allergen-reagin reaction and its dependence on molecular configuration of the allergen and reagin is similar to the antigen-antibody reaction. In this respect, the allergen molecule, which is often a protein, may be regarded as a key which exactly fits the corresponding structural shape of the reagin molecule, which may be likened to a lock. When this occurs, an allergic reaction results.... Different materials contain different allergens. Not all persons can form the appropriate reagin with which the allergen from a specific source can react and are therefore not allergic to that particular allergen containing substance. When someone does produce a particular reagin in response to the presence of the specific allergin, an allergic reaction results. Allergic reactions range from very mild symptoms, such as minor skin rashes (allergic eczema and urticaria), dermal, respiratory, including allergic rhinitis and bronchial asthma, gastro-intestinal, migraine allergic type symptoms, to violent manifestations of these illnesses. Violent illnesses have been known to even include shock-like reaction, vascular collapse, allergic anaphylaxis, and for some people under certain conditions, death.

Web site: http://www.delphion.com/details?pn=US04078093__

- **Installation for preparing a chocolate paste**

  Inventor(s): Chaveron; Henri (Paris, FR), Pontillon; Jean (Meulan, FR), Billon; Michel (Unieux, FR), Adenier; Herve (Compiegne, FR), Kamoun; Ahmed (Sfax, ZA)

  Assignee(s): Clextral (Paris, FR)

  Patent Number: 4,679,498

  Date filed: January 30, 1986

  Abstract: Apparatus for preparing a chocolate paste in which the various ingredients comprising at least cocoa and powdered sugar are subject to operations of grinding to a predetermined degree of particle size, of fluidification by dispersion of the particles of sugar and of cocoa into a continuous fatty phase and of degasification for the removal of water and undesirable volatile compounds. At least part of the treatment is carried out in a conveyor with several screws and an arrangement for regulating the temperature of the entrained material. After preliminary grinding of the ingredients to obtain a refined paste having the desired degree of particle size in the screw conveyor, dry-conching of the refined paste is carried out and then the liquefaction of the paste is obtained by the incorporation of additives in accordance with the receipe.

  Excerpt(s): The invention relates to a process and installation for preparing a chocolate paste.... Generally, to produce plain chocolate, a pasty mass of cocoa is first prepared which is mixed with sugar previously ground to a very small particle size, of the order of 100 microns. The pasty mass of cocoa and sugar, and optionally, in the case of milk chocolate, the dehydrated milk powder, are mixed in suitable proportions with a minimum of cocoa butter and the chocolate paste thus-prepared then undergoes refining in a device constituted by a plurality of cylinders, generally five, between which the particle size is again reduced until a refined paste is obtained in flake or very fine powder form, of the order of 10 to 20 microns, which can then be mixed with a predetermined proportion of cocoa butter.... For producing quality chocolate, the refined mass is subjected to the process long known under the name of conching and which consists of causing the paste to undergo prolonged kneading, carried out in special vessels called conches. It is in the course of this conching treatment that the aroma is produced and that the desired rheological properties of the chocolate are obtained.

Web site: http://www.delphion.com/details?pn=US04679498___

- **Isothermal preparation of chocolate products**

  Inventor(s): Mackley; Malcolm R. (Cambridge, GB)

  Assignee(s): Nestec S.A. (Vevey, CH)

  Patent Number: RE36,937

  Date filed: August 5, 1997

Abstract: Chocolate products are formed by feeding solid set chocolate to an extruder and passing the chocolate through the extruder at a temperature below the pour point of the chocolate to deform and extrude the chocolate.

  Excerpt(s): The present invention relates to extrusion of fat-containing confectionery products and particularly to extrusion of chocolate.... Fat-containing confectionery products, generally, are prepared from fats, including fat fractions and fat-substitutes, and may include sugar, milk-derived components, and solids from vegetable or cocoa sources in various proportions.... In general, chocolate products, which may be divided into groups of plain, or dark, chocolate and milk chocolates, including white chocolate, have a moisture content less than about 5% by weight. Plain chocolate typically is obtained by mixing sugar, cocoa butter (and optionally other fats and/or fat fractions and/or fat substitutes) and cocoa mass. Milk chocolate contains milk fat and non-fat milk solids (and optionally vegetable fat and/or fat fractions and/or fat substitutes) as additional ingredients. White chocolate contains milk fat and non-fat milk solids, sugar and cocoa butter (and optionally other fats and/or fat fractions and/or fat substitutes) without with addition of cocoa mass.

  Web site: http://www.delphion.com/details?pn=US0RE36937___

- **Leak-resistant feeding chamber for chocolate refining machines**

  Inventor(s): Ripani; Sergio (Milan, IT), Serafini; Giulio (Milan, IT)

  Assignee(s): Carle & Montanari S.p.A. (IT)

  Patent Number: 4,627,337

  Date filed: April 15, 1985

Abstract: A lateral end upright for the feeding roll pair in chocolate refining machines is formed by two half-uprights in mutual abutment relationship and individually mounted to one of the feeding rolls. The abutment sides of the half-uprights have a thickness dimension which is selected to ensure continuity thereof even with the feeding roll axles tilted to their full oscillated positions. A flexible insert may be interposed to the upright halves.Offsetting play due to wear can be taken up, as can differences in the working lengths of the feeding rolls.

  Excerpt(s): This invention relates to lateral end uprights for the feeding roll pair in chocolate refining machines.... As is known, in chocolate refining machines, chocolate paste is fed into the machine by means of a pair of feeding rolls. The feeding chamber is formed by the juxtaposed upper portions of said feeding rolls, and at the sides, by lateral end uprights or legs having a substantially wedge-like configuration wherein the sloping sides are replaced by arcuate portions bearing on said juxtaposed feeding rolls. More specifically, the uprights are made to bear on the rolls and an end stepped-down portion of said rolls, so that the sealing surface area is increased while forming an abutment shoulder on the roll against which springs or pneumatic device can be urged by means of wedges to improve the upright sealing. In the radial direction, said uprights bear on the rolls by gravity. Thus, a seal is achieved both against the radial and axial pressures.... In fixed axle roll refining machines, prior lateral end uprights can only provide a proper seal with the feeding rolls held truly in parallel and having exactly the same working lengths. In the instance of some slight differences in length, in fact, the uprights would only bear axially in the abutment step of the longer roll, to leave at the shortest roll a gap whereat product leakage occurs. Such leakage paths would also be formed in the event that the axes of the feeding rolls are not truly parallel to each other.

Web site: http://www.delphion.com/details?pn=US04627337__

- **Low calorie chocolate**

    Inventor(s): Takemori; Toshio (Tokyo, JP), Tsurumi; Toshinobu (Saitama, JP), Ito; Masanori (Saitama, JP), Kamiwaki; Tatsuya (Saitama, JP)

    Assignee(s): Lotte Co., Ltd. (Tokyo, JP)

    Patent Number: 5,629,040

    Date filed: November 10, 1994

    Abstract: A chocolate includes a glucide that comprises a hydrogenated isomaltulose and a sugar showing a hygroscopic property and an emulsifying agent that comprises a lecithin and any of lipophilic emulsifying agents except for the lecithin. The chocolate may further includes at least one selected from the group consisting of calcium salts, calcium containing materials, magnesium salts and magnesium containing materials.

    Excerpt(s): The invention relates to a low calorie chocolate, and more particularly to a chocolate having improved softness and pleasantness with a lowered calorie.... It has been well known in the art that calcium and magnesium have functions to suppress an internal absorption of a cocoa butter that may be used as oils and fats of chocolates. When, however, the cocoa butter contained in the chocolate is absorbed, it has been still unclear whether calcium and magnesium are capable of displaying an appreciable degree of the function for suppressing the internal absorption of the cocoa butter.... Recently, in place of sugars, developments of various sweeteners that are commercially available have been a great success. A hydrogenated isomaltulose has been known as one of low calorie sweeteners. The hydrogenated isomaltulose comprises a mol-equivalent mixture of isomers, for example, alpha-D-glucopyranosil-1, 6-mannitol (GPM) and alpha-D-glucopyranosil-1, 6-glucitol (GPG). The hydrogenated isomaltulose is commercially available in the name of "PALATINIT" as a registered trademark. The hydrogenated isomaltulose exhibits a low efficiency in conversion into energy and an anticarious function that is useful to prevent teeth from decaying. It is disclosed in the Japanese laid-open patent application No. 5-260894 to add chocolates with the hydrogenated isomaltulose as a sweetener.

    Web site: http://www.delphion.com/details?pn=US05629040__

- **Machine for filling chocolate-box trays and the like**

  Inventor(s): Klug; Telesforo (Porto-Ronco, CH), Hofmann; Armin (Renens, CH)

  Assignee(s): SAPAL Societe Anonyme des Plieuses Automatiques (FR)

  Patent Number: 3,977,160

  Date filed: April 24, 1975

  Abstract: A machine for delivering different chocolates or other objects to selected positions on trays comprises, for each type of chocolate, a distribution head receiving chocolates along a waiting line. Yokes of an intermittent chain conveyor laterally displace a number of chocolates to be delivered to a tray, and these chocolates are blown down respective channels leading to the selected positions, where they are taken up by vertically moving suction cups and lowered into the respective position in a tray carried by an intermittently driven conveyor. Synchronized drive of the various members is provided by a directly-linked kinematic chain.

  Excerpt(s): The invention relates to machines for filling container units with different objects, for example chocolate-box trays with wrapped or unwrapped chocolates, in which objects of one type are delivered to an object-distribution head in a column along a waiting line from a loading conveyor belt and from said head to a respective distribution station for the different objects.... Several automatic machines have already been proposed for placing chocolates or other products of different types in selected positions in trays or similar container units. For example, a box of chocolates may include one tray holding 250g of chocolates, or two or three trays respectively with 500 or 750g of chocolates.... In known machines, each distribution station includes suction members which take up a chocolate and deliver it to the desired location in a tray. These suction members are either pivoted by 180.degree. to deliver the chocolates from the input of the distribution station to the tray, or are moved vertically and in translation by a cam and lever system.

  Web site: http://www.delphion.com/details?pn=US03977160__

- **Machine for forming chocolate shaving spirals**

  Inventor(s): Hanson; Douglas R. (Anoka, MN)

  Assignee(s): Bake Star, Inc. (Anoka, MN)

  Patent Number: 5,226,353

  Date filed: August 17, 1992

  Abstract: A machine for automatically shaving a large bar of chocolate for forming a thin chocolate shaving that curls into a spiral, for use for decorative purposes. The machine has cutters that will cut an end of a chocolate bar in three separate spirals, on each stroke of the cutter. The chocolate bar is moved a desired distance for new cuts. The knives are partly curved in cross section and have cutting edges that are angled to insure a smooth separation of a thin shaving to form the curl around the curvature of the individual knife. The chocolate temperature is important in cutting, and generally is maintained in the range of 88 to 90 degrees Fahrenheit. The machine itself can be placed in a suitable environment or chamber to maintain that temperature.

  Excerpt(s): The present invention relates to a machine which will shave off an end of a standard industry bar of chocolate into thin shavings that are curled, and which curls have sufficient structural strength to be used for topping on pies, cakes, for and other decorative items utilizing chocolate curls.... At the present time, chocolate bar shavings are manually made, by operators utilizing various types of knives that shave off curls from chocolate bars. This of course, is quite slow and time consuming, and does not provide for a precisely repeatable shaving thickness and curl. The use of chocolate shavings and various chocolate confectionery items is desirable because of taste and appearance, and thus a way of making the shavings on a uniform, automatic basis is desirable.... The present invention relates to a machine for simultaneously cutting precise size and shape shavings off an end of a confectionery or candy type bar, such as a standard chocolate bar. The shavings curl as they are sliced off and for use in decorations of confectionery items. The machine supports a chocolate bar in the proper position, and has a gang of three knives that are positioned to shave off material from one end of the chocolate bar. The two corners are shaved at a chamfer or angle, and the center section surface generally perpendicular to the longitudinal bisecting plane of the bar is shaved as well. The knives are operated in a repeatable path, and between each cutting stroke, the knives retract from the chocolate bar slightly and the chocolate bar will be advanced to its cutting position. The chocolate bar is held in a support which relieves the holding pressure during the return stroke of the knives while the chocolate bar is being advanced. The parts which come in contact with the chocolate can be removed for reloading and cleaning. The knives are arranged at angles to insure smooth cutting during one stroke. The machine is relatively compact, and maintains the shavings from a chocolate bar at uniform thickness and a substantially uniform curl under controlled conditions.

Web site: http://www.delphion.com/details?pn=US05226353__

- **Machine for treating chocolate paste and method for producing crumb**

Inventor(s): Schulte; Manfred (Enger, DE), Hartsieker; Martin (Bad Oeynhausen, DE), Mechias; Bernd (Braunschweig, DE), Muntener; Kurt (Bad Salzuflen, DE)

Assignee(s): Richard Frisse GmbH (Bad Salzuflen, DE)

Patent Number: 5,419,635

Date filed: March 10, 1993

Abstract: Machine for treating chocolate masses in which solid matter can be fed in and comminuted if so desired. The arrangement is designed such that in addition to a mixing and kneading device, at least one feeding screw is employed, with which a cutting procedure is carried out, preferably in simultaneous operation. The feeding screw can be made up of different individual screw elements, which are convenient for the material to be treated. This treatment is particularly suited for producing crumb.

Excerpt(s): The invention relates to a device for treating chocolate paste in a trough comprising one at least partly cylindrical inner surface, in which there is provided at least one treating rotor with radially extending treating tools, with the treating rotor running concentrically to the cylinder walls; and to a method for producing chocolate crumb Whose ingredients are subjected at least in part to a mixing procedure.... Treating machines for mixing operations have become known in various forms and are disclosed e.g. in the DE-OS 17 82 585 and also in the DE-PS 964 131.... A problem in treating chocolate masses may arise when also solid matter is to be kneaded in, for example nuts. The same problem may arise when the paste itself should have formed hard, cloddy particles by way of agglomeration. It has become apparent that the number of revolutions of the treating rotor, which, to a certain extent, also determines the treating performance of the device, will then be limited, particulary in such a case. At times, an accumulation of the solid matter or agglomerates to be kneaded in can then be observed on the trough wall, so that the homogeneity will no longer be completely assured. Hitherto, this manifestation has been tolerated, at the most one has taken the measure to reduce the number of revolutions of the treating rotor.

Web site: http://www.delphion.com/details?pn=US05419635__

- **Malt-infused cocoa and chocolate formulations**

  Inventor(s): Miller; Van (P.O. Box 100, Norval Ontario, CA L0P 1A0)

  Assignee(s): none reported

  Patent Number: 6,521,273

  Date filed: July 26, 2002

  Abstract: A malted-infused chocolate formulation comprises from 19% to 50% by weight of cocoa liquor and from 81% to 50% by weight of a non-fat, cereal based cocoa extender; or alternatively the formulation comprises from 11% to 29% by weight of cocoa butter, and from 89% to 71% by weight of non-fat, cereal-based cocoa extender. The non-fat, cereal based cocoa extender consists of finely ground toasted malted cereal chosen from the group consisting of barley, wheat, rye, buckwheat, rice and mixtures thereof. Methods of making the chocolate formulations include the steps of toasting the cereal to a desired color and flavor, grinding the toasted cereal, cooling, and adding the requisite amount of cocoa liquor or cocoa butter.

  Excerpt(s): This invention relates to malt-infused cocoa and chocolate formulations. In effect, the present invention relates to chocolate formulations having cereal-based cocoa extenders, where the cocoa extenders are derived from toasted malted cereals.... The present discussion assumes a working knowledge by the reader and practitioner of this invention of the basics of chocolate formulations in general, and of the manner in which cereals, such as barley, are malted.... Nonetheless, for purpose of understanding certain terminology used herein, a brief review of those technologies now follows.

  Web site: http://www.delphion.com/details?pn=US06521273__

- **Method and a machine for removing from their molds moldings of confectionery masses which have been formed into chocolate centers, bars or other single or continuous moldings**

  Inventor(s): Sollich; Helmut (Kalletal-Talle, DT)

  Assignee(s): Sollich AG (Bad Salzuflen, DT)

  Patent Number: 4,059,378

  Date filed: July 20, 1976

  Abstract: A machine for molding confectionery masses into chocolate centers which includes a feed hopper which feeds a molding cylinder having molding recesses, a single intake cylinder between the feed hopper and the molding cylinder for pressing the mass into the recesses, and a suction belt embracing part of the circumference of the molding cylinder for the removal of the finished moldings.

  Excerpt(s): The invention relates to a method of removing from their molds moldings of confectionery masses in the form of chocolate centers, bars, or other single or continuous moldings. The invention also proposes a machine for performing the method.... Centers for chocolates have in the past been produced by extrusion or on an automatic molding machine, usually by employing two generally milled intake or pressure cylinders which force the mass either through a die or into molding recesses in a moulding cylinder. It has been found that in these machines especially masses which are soft and have a high fat content suffer damage, and that in the case of automatic moulding machines they fail to detach themselves from the molding recesses. Another drawback of these known machines is that the frictional engagement of the mass by the pressure and intake rollers is excessive and causes the mass to become hot, resulting in a considerable quantity of fat being squeezed out of the mass.... On the other hand, it is the practice when processing hot masses after cooking and mixing first to cool these masses on cooling tables or in cooling tunnels to a temperature at which they can be extruded and cut, a procedure which not only requires long cooling zones and an extruder but also very expensive cutting equipment which first cuts an extruded blanket into strips, separates the strips and finally by cross cutting chops them to length.

Web site: http://www.delphion.com/details?pn=US04059378__

- **Method and a system for producing articles of chocolate-like mass in a continuous production-plant**

  Inventor(s): Aasted; Lars (Charlottenlund, DK)

  Assignee(s): Aasted-Mikroverk ApS (Farum, DK)

  Patent Number: 6,159,520

  Date filed: March 11, 1999

  Abstract: A method and a system for producing articles of fat-containing, chocolate mass in a continuous production-plant having a conveyor for mould elements with mould cavities. The production-plant comprises steps of initially filling mould cavities with liquid mass, cooling of the articles, and releasing the articles from the mould cavities. The number of mould elements per unit time leaving the cooling step is regulated to deviate from the number of mould elements per unit time entering the cooling step. The resulting advantage is that it is possible to regulate the residence time for a certain mould element in a cooling step without changing the residence time in the steps prior to the cooling step. A manufacturer of chocolate articles is thereby provided an easy way of adapting the cooling time to the specific article being produced without influencing other steps of production.

  Excerpt(s): The present invention concerns a method for producing articles of a fat-containing, chocolate mass in a continuous production-plant having throughgoing conveying means for mould elements with mould cavities, comprising steps of initial filling of mould cavities with liquid mass, cooling of the articles, and releasing the articles from the mould cavities.... The invention also concerns a system for use in the performance of the method for producing articles of a fat-containing, chocolate mass in a continuous production-plant having throughgoing conveying means for mould elements with mould cavities, comprising means for initial filling of mould cavities with liquid mass, means for cooling of the articles, and means for releasing the articles from the mould cavities.... Production-plants performing methods of the above mentioned art are known and have been marketed a substantial number of years. In these plants the liquid mass is continuously filled into the mould cavities. The mould cavities are formed in mould elements, which are conveyed through the production-plant by means of the throughgoing conveying means. After the mould cavities are filled, the mould elements are conveyed through a cooling step at a predetermined travel speed. This speed always corresponds to the actual travel speed of the throughgoing conveying means. In the cooling step the articles are allowed to sufficiently solidify.

Web site: http://www.delphion.com/details?pn=US06159520__

- **Method and a system for the production of chocolate articles**

Inventor(s): Aasted; Lars (Charlottenlund, DK)

Assignee(s): Aasted-Mikroverk ApS (Farum, DK)

Patent Number: 5,705,217

Date filed: October 3, 1996

Abstract: A method for producing chocolate articles having an outer shell (5) of solid chocolate, wherein a mould cavity (2) is filled with a tempered chocolate mass (3). Then a "supercooled" cooling member (1) is immersed into the chocolate mass (3) and lifted clear of it again after a residence time of 2 to 3 seconds. The produced chocolate shells (5) have a completely uniform wall thickness and an accurately predetermined shell volume.

Excerpt(s): The present invention concerns a method for producing outer shells of fat-containing, chocolate-like masses in particular for chocolate articles, wherein a mould cavity is filled with a tempered chocolate-like mass which, under crystallisation, solidifies from the mould cavity and inwardly to form the outer shape of the shell, the temperature of the mould cavity being lower than the temperature of the tempered mass.... Methods of this type are known wherein the mould cavity has to be filled with a tempered chocolate mass in an amount which is at least twice as large as the amount required for the finished chocolate shell. After the tempered chocolate mass has been filled into the mould cavity, the mould cavity is shaken for a subsequent period of time during which the chocolate mass solidifies under crystallisation from the mould cavity and inwardly. Then the mould cavity is inverted, and the excess chocolate mass is shaken out of the solidified shell-forming chocolate mass in the immediate vicinity of the mould cavity and is collected to be tempered and used again in the manufacturing process. When the shell has obtained a "leather-like" consistency during its solidification, the excess chocolate amount at the upper annular edge of the shell can be cut off. The chocolate shell can subsequently be filled with a center, e.g. in the form of cremes or the like before it is removed from the mould cavity after having solidified completely.... The obtained thickness and uniformity of the shell produced depends completely on the prepared state and thus viscosity of the chocolate as well as on how long the mould cavity is shaken and on how uniform the heat release of the chocolate to the mould cavity is. The prepared state of the chocolate depends in particular upon how finely and uniformly the cocoa beans have been prepared as well as on the fat content of the mass. Before the chocolate mixture is filled into the mould cavity, it must be tempered within a very limited temperature range between 27.degree. C. and 32.degree. C. to avoid undesirable crystal growth in the mixture. The viscosity of the chocolate mixture in the tempered state depends mainly on the composition of the mixture and thus on the fat content. A relatively high content of fat is therefore frequently necessary for the desired viscosity to be obtained.

Web site: http://www.delphion.com/details?pn=US05705217__

- **Method and an apparatus for continuous tempering of chocolate-like masses**

Inventor(s): Aasted; Lars (Charlottenlund, DK)

Assignee(s): Aasted-Mikroverk ApS (DK)

Patent Number: 5,514,390

Date filed: June 9, 1994

Abstract: The present invention concerns a method and an apparatus (1) for continuous tempering of chocolate-like masses, said apparatus (1) comprising at least two cooling zones (Z1, Zk) and a subsequent reheating zone (Z2) for the mass. Each of the zones has its own separately controllable cooling medium circuit and heating medium circuit, respectively (10, 11 and 12, respectively) for controlling temperature and/or flow amount of the cooling medium and the heating medium. A first cooling zone (Z1) comprises initial and final cooling surfaces (A1' and A1"), between which the cooling surfaces (Ak) of a second cooling zone (Zk) are positioned, seen in the flow direction (M) of the mass. In operation, the cooling surfaces (Ak) of the second cooling zone (Zk) can constitute the crystallization zone. It is hereby possible to control the tempering process and in particular the heat energy transport in a defined zone, such as the crystallization zone, to obtain a predetermined number of stable.beta.-crystals in the mass. Further, a particularly simple, compact and efficient apparatus in relation to its dimensions is provided.

Excerpt(s): The present invention concerns a method and an apparatus for continuous tempering of a flowing, fat-containing chocolate-like mass, said apparatus comprising at least two cooling zones having a plurality of cooling surfaces, and a subsequent reheating zone having a plurality of heating surfaces for the mass, seen in the flow direction of said mass, each cooling zone and heating zone comprising an associated, separately controllable cooling medium circuit and heating medium circuit having sensors for measuring medium and/or mass temperature as well as an associated control unit for controlling temperature and/or flow amount of the cooling medium and the heating medium during the passage thereof across the cooling surfaces and heating surfaces of the zone concerned and a first cooling zone of said zones comprising initial and final cooling surfaces, seen in the flow direction of the mass.... Devices of this type have been known for a large number of years, and their basic structure still corresponds to the first devices which were marketed protected by a plurality of patents, including CH-B-261 118. All of the devices have a structure with mass chambers and medium compartments which are arranged alternately on top of each other, and which are separated by intermediate plates having the cooling or heating surfaces concerned at opposed mass sides and medium sides, respectively. The mass is pumped continuously through the mass chambers and is mixed and distributed over the surfaces by means of mixing blades mounted on a through drive shaft. Both mass chambers and medium compartments, in particular cooling medium compartments, have been provided with thermometers, as described in the CH patent specification, so that the development in the cooling of the mass in the tempering machine can be monitored exactly. A heater has simultaneously made it possible to adjust the temperature of the cooling water accurately for the cooling medium compartment concerned. All the separately controllable cooling or heating medium circuits are usually connected with a common medium inlet and outlet. Further, the devices may also include a common pump which applies pressure to the circuits. However, nowadays the devices are frequently provided with a pump in each separate circuit.... In the operation of the tempering devices at the manufacturers of articles made of a tempered mass, usually at least one cooling section has been set to maintain a constant cooling water temperature.

In practice, large amounts of cooling water having a temperature corresponding to the important crystal formation temperature of the chocolate mass concerned were conveyed through the cooling zone. It was believed that when passing the cooling surfaces of the cooling zone concerned, the mass would be cooled to the cooling water temperature concerned with certainty so that the formation of the important stable.beta.-crystals took place precisely in the zone concerned. Thus, in practice the temperature was set according to the crystal formation temperature of the mass concerned. It is common to the known devices having the said basic structure corresponding to the apparatus described in the CH patent that temperature and/or flow amount of the cooling medium in any cooling zone--which is not the first cooling zone, seen in the flow direction of the mass--can be controlled and in particular to achieve a constant cooling medium temperature independent of the temperature and amount of the mass which flows through the apparatus. The said cooling zone will in practice constitute precisely the crystal formation zone.

Web site: http://www.delphion.com/details?pn=US05514390__

- **Method and apparatus for continuous tempering of chocolate-like mass**

  Inventor(s): Haslund; Henning (Bj.ae butted.verskov, DK)

  Assignee(s): Aasted-Mikroverk ApS (Farum, DK)

  Patent Number: 6,164,195

  Date filed: March 15, 1999

  Abstract: Method and apparatus for continuously tempering a fat-containing, chocolate-like mass. The mass is subjected to a cooling creating crystals in the mass as it passes over crystal creating cooling surfaces, and a final reheating (H). For any raise or drop in the cooling medium temperature or flow, the temperature of the crystal creating cooling surfaces is controlled to be lower than, or equal to a predetermined, maximum temperature value, which creates crystals in the mass.

  Excerpt(s): The invention concerns a method of continuously tempering a fat-containing, chocolate-like mass, whereby the mass is subjected to a cooling creating crystals in the mass as it passes over crystal creating cooling surfaces, and a final reheating.... The invention further concerns an apparatus for continuously tempering a fat-containing, chocolate-like mass, comprising a cooling section with crystal creating cooling surfaces and a final reheating section.... For many years, the method has been used extensively for production of a great variety of chocolate-like masses. Before tempering, the chocolate-like mass is warmed up to around 40-60.degree. C. After tempering, the mass typically has a temperature of around 29-33.degree. C., whereafter it is being used for many purposes, such as being filled in moulds, deposited on top of other articles, etc.

  Web site: http://www.delphion.com/details?pn=US06164195__

- **Method and apparatus for making chocolate-coated ice cream cookie sandwiches**

  Inventor(s): Jones; John F. (140 Summit Rd., Prospect, CT 06712)

  Assignee(s): none reported

  Patent Number: 4,580,476

  Date filed: April 27, 1984

Abstract: A low labor, highly efficient process and system for manufacturing chocolate coated ice cream cookie sandwiches is achieved by incorporating a conveyor system for transporting the ice cream cookie sandwich through the various stages of its manufacture along with uniquely constructed ice cream brick slicing machines and a unique chocolate coating machine. In addition, a pass-through freezer is preferably employed prior to the chocolate coating, in order to assure a high quality, tasty product. The ice cream slicing machine of the present invention employed in the process and manufacturing system of this invention is constructed for receiving a plurality of ice cream bricks and cutting each brick into a plurality of slices in an efficient, automatic, integrated operational procedure and presenting each ice cream slice to a holding zone for placement on a cookie moving along the conveyor system. In addition, the chocolate coating machine of the present invention incorporated into the process and manufacturing system of this invention incorporates a plurality of clamps controllably driven about the coating machine and positioned for receiving the ice cream cookie sandwich and automatically submerging the sandwich in a chocolate bath and automatically releasing the chocolate-coated ice cream cookie sandwich when the chocolate coating has completely cooled and dried.

Excerpt(s): This invention relates to a process and to machines for making ice cream cookie sandwiches and, more particularly, to the process and machines employed in making chocolate-coated ice cream cookie sandwiches.... Although ice cream sandwiches and ice cream cookie sandwiches have existed for many years and have been manufactured using a variety of alternate methods, no prior art system has been developed which is capable of employing ice cream bricks by cutting the bricks into a plurality of smaller slices, and then assembling the slices between two cookies in an efficient manner wherein labor costs are maintained at a minimum.... Furthermore, no prior art apparatus or process is capable of providing chocolate-coated ice cream cookie sandwiches, wherein the chocolate coating is achieved efficiently, with all used chocolate being recycled. In addition, prior art systems typically require a high degree of handling, thereby reducing production efficiency and causing increased production costs.

Web site: http://www.delphion.com/details?pn=US04580476__

- **Method and apparatus for refining chocolate mass**

Inventor(s): Muntener; Kurt (Bad Salzuflen, DE)

Assignee(s): Richard Frisse GmbH (Bad Salzuflen, DE)

Patent Number: 5,814,362

Date filed: May 30, 1997

Abstract: In a method and an apparatus for refining chocolate mass within a trough, the trough contains at least one trough compartment wherein the chocolate mass is treated or conched. After entering the trough and after begin of operation of the machine, at least one additive, such as fat (cocoa butter), is added at a certain moment. Addition of the at least one additive is done into one compartment of the continuously operated conching machine. The composition of the chocolate mass is monitored after adding the additives by means of a spectrometer. An output signal of the spectrometer is used to control the added amount of the respective additive.

Excerpt(s): The invention relates to a method for refining chocolate mass within a trough comprising at least one trough compartment wherein the chocolate mass is treated by known conching tools exerting a rheological shearing and mixing action. In such a conching process, at least one additive, such as lecithin, cocoa butter, milk or the like, is added to the cocoa containing mass at a certain moment after having begun the conching treatment.... The invention concerns also a conching arrangement comprising a conching machine for continuous operation which includes an inlet, at least one compartment for receiving said chocolate mass to be conched, and an outlet. Furthermore, at least one feeding device is provided to supply the at least one additive which has to be added in a metered amount to the cocoa containing mass (optionally containing already sugar or the like).... A method of this kind has become known from U.S. Pat. No. 5,351,609. In this document, a continuous conching machine is described having a plurality of compartments. The addition of the ultimate amount of additives, such as milk powder or the like, is only done subsequently to the conching operation in at least two quasi-continuously working badge mixers that are alternately filled and discharged. The reason for using badge mixers is that the amount of additives can better be kept under control in such an operation. Of course, this will result in additional expenditure, since in addition to the conching machine, that would be able to admix the additives, not only the mixers have to be purchased, but have to be accommodated within the space available so that further two cost factors will arise. Therefore, it is an object of the invention to reduce the expenditure in an arrangement comprising a continuous conching machine.

Web site: http://www.delphion.com/details?pn=US05814362__

- **Method and device for producing thin pieces of chocolate**

Inventor(s): Van Dyck; Jan (Toekomstlaan 4, B-2200 Herentals, BE), Van Dyck; Kris (Kasterleesesteenweg 77, B-2460 Lichtaart (Kasterlee)

Assignee(s): none reported

Patent Number: 6,303,171

Date filed: October 13, 2000

Abstract: The present invention concerns a method for producing thin pieces of chocolate, in particular slices of chocolate, whereby the chocolate is melted and is provided in the shape of flat, thin pieces of chocolate, which are put one after the other, on at least one endless, flexible conveyor belt of a conveying device, whereby the conveyor belt is subsequently bent crosswise so that it forms a trough before the pieces have stiffened, and the conveyor belt is kept in this bent position until the pieces lying in the trough and which are bent along with the conveyor belt have sufficiently stiffened so as to keep their bent shape.

Excerpt(s): The present invention concerns a method for producing thin pieces of chocolate, in particular slices of chocolate, whereby the chocolate is melted and is provided in the shape of flat, thin pieces on a conveying device and is made to stiffen thereupon.... According to a known method, chocolate is melted, provided on an endless conveyor belt in the shape of thin slices and finally cooled down until the slices have stiffened.... It is clear that, as the slices are provided on a conveyor belt, they will have a flat side after they-have stiffened and will have a flat look as a whole.

Web site: http://www.delphion.com/details?pn=US06303171__

- **Method for coating confectionery articles with chocolate**

Inventor(s): Kreuter; Walter (Norderstedt, DT)

Assignee(s): Kreucoha AG (Zug, CH)

Patent Number: 4,032,667

Date filed: May 5, 1976

Abstract: Confectionery articles are coated with precrystallized, molten tempered chocolate by forcing the chocolate under pressure through a nozzle onto a veil plate to produce a downwardly descending film of chocolate under gravitational force, passing the confectionery article through said film, collecting unused chocolate and recirculating the unused chocolate through said nozzle.

Excerpt(s): Flowable compositions containing cocoa butter display a relatively complicated behaviour which is to be attributed to the fact that in a very narrow temperature range between about 30.degree. and about 40.degree. C., the cocoa butter can assume and pass through very different states of crystallisation; both the properties of the flowable composition, especially its viscosity, and the properties of the chocolate or chocolate coatings produced therefrom by cooling and setting are very greatly dependent upon the state of crystallisation present in each case. Although the processes have not yet been clarified in detail, nevertheless, on the basis of experience and the theoretical concepts available hitherto it has been possible to develop specific methods of treatment of compositions containing cocoa butter, in which it is possible to combine good processibility of the composition with favourable properties of the solidified chocolate produced therefrom, especially as regards gloss and stability against the formation of fat bloom. These preparation processes in the case of chocolate are known in the art under the name "tempering" or "pre-crystallisation". By a well-tempered chocolate composition there is to be understood relatively thin liquid composition which on cooling forms a high-gloss surface which does not tend to the formation of fat bloom in storage.... Special difficulties arise if a flow of cocoa butter-containing composition after tempering or pre-crystallisation is not caused to solidify as a whole, as is the case for example in the production of block chocolate, but only a fraction is consumed in one cycle and the remainder undergoes further cycles. In this case the quantity consumed in each cycle can be made up by the supply of a corresponding additional quantity. This process is encountered predominantly in so-called coating machines, in which any articles, for example pieces for confectionary, are coated with the composition. In this case the procedure is generally adopted whereby a many times too large flow of the composition is poured over the articles and the major part of the proportion which runs away unused is returned in the cycle for renewed use. In such applications the composition must be kept over considerable periods of time as far as possible without change in the state of crystallisation which is most favourable for working. In order to achieve the highest possible uniformity of the coatings, it is sought to keep the viscosity practically constant as far as possible over the entire working period (normally one day). In most cases the thinnest possible coatings and correspondingly low viscosities are desired, and frequently for the purpose of adjustment and regulation of the thickness of the coatings a regulatable blower is also provided. With the ordinary methods of tempering or pre-crystallisation, the viscosity cannot be kept constant over the relatively long periods of time in the desired manner; instead one observes an irreversible increase of the viscosity despite the temperature being kept constant, and it is very difficult to obtain a constantly thin coating layer by other means, for example by increasing the output of the said blower. Moreover once the composition has become thicker more unfavourable properties appear after cooling;

more especially the gloss of the produced coatings deteriorates. Therefore, frequently in practice the whole composition is tempered in the cycle afresh at relatively short time intervals or even at every circulation, as a whole or at least a considerable part. Since the tempering operation itself is also quite complicated a considerable expense for procedure and apparatus is incurred.... Methods for pre-crystallisation (tempering) are also known in which it is possible to obtain compositions the viscosity of which remains constant over lengthy periods of time (if the temperature is kept constant accordingly), so that these compositions can be stored without re-tempering over lengthy periods of time. According to present day knowledge this is based on the fact that, in these methods, cocoa butter crystals are obtained in the stable, so-called.beta.-modification, while in the methods known earlier which were based predominantly upon the principle of seeding with solid chocolate, predominantly crystals of the unstable so-called.beta.'-modification were formed. It has appeared that with the use of the described compositions of constant viscosity a considerably longer and more trouble-free operation is possible even of coating apparatuses. Since however in such and other apparatuses where the composition is conducted in the cycle and used repeatedly, greatly varied influences act upon the composition, for example acceleration, retardation, reversal, contact with various materials, especially the articles to be coated, contact with air, division of the surface, etc. Even if compositions practically of constant viscosity per se are used, troubles can arise the causes of which are mostly complex and the elimination of which is accordingly difficult. However, even in the case of compositions which are tempered in accordance with older methods and accordingly have a viscosity which per se is not constant, due to the described and possibly also other influences in the cycle conducted, there is a considerable number of sources of potential troubles, so that even with these compositions, additional difficulties and variations of the viscosity can occur, the cause of which is difficult to perceive.

Web site: http://www.delphion.com/details?pn=US04032667__

- **Method for continuous production of chocolate mass**

   Inventor(s): Berkes; Klaus (Dresden, DD), Forster; Helmut (Heidenau, DD), Huth; Wolfgang (Dresden, DD), Ritschel; Gunter (Heidenau, DD), Schebiella; Georg (Heidenau, DD), Scholz; Norbert (Dresden, DD), Thomas; Frank-Gerhard (Dresden, DD)

   Assignee(s): Veb Kombinat Nagema (Dresden, DD)

   Patent Number: 4,440,797

   Date filed: April 30, 1981

   Abstract: A method of continuous production of refined chocolate mass from a non-refined cocoa mass composed of a mixture of components reduced in size to a fineness required for the final mass but still containing undesired aromatic substances and moisture and being processed into a low fat, friable or pulverized chocolate mass, is mixed in a plasticator with a preheated air stream which is admitted in the same feeding direction, simultaneously externally heated for a time interval between 5 and 8 minutes while being intensively mixed by shearing stresses until the mass becomes plasticized; thereupon the fluidity of the mass is increased by an emulsifier, then the entrained gas is separated from the mass, the latter is weighed and supplemented according to a final recipe by additional fat content, and the final mass is collected in a container and subjected to an additional homogenizing treatment and in a cooled condition is forwarded for the final processing.

Excerpt(s): The invention relates in general to the production of chocolate, and in particular to a method of and a device for the continuous production of a chocolate mass from a non-refined cocoa mass which still contains undesired aromatic substance and moisture, finally ground and mixed to a degree required by the final prescription and also contains all usual constituents except fat, water and emulsifier.... These constituents, as known, are sugar only when producing dark chocolate, or sugar, milk powder and cocoa butter in the case of milk chocolate mass.... In producing chocolate masses it is conventional to grind and mix raw stocks and, in order to create the desired aromatic and tasty quality as well a favorable processing quality of the pretreated mass, the latter is subjected to a simultaneous mechanical and heat treatment. This refining process, which is called a tumbling treatment in a conche represents with respect to the quality of the final product the essential part in the technological process in the manufacture of chocolate mass.

Web site: http://www.delphion.com/details?pn=US04440797__

- **Method for continuously producing milk chocolate masses**

Inventor(s): Schmitt; Armin (6056 Heusenstamm, Birkeneck 88, DE)

Assignee(s): none reported

Patent Number: 4,156,743

Date filed: March 10, 1976

Abstract: A process for continuously producing milk chocolate masses, wherein the roasted cocoa kernel fragments are finely ground and, with the addition of cocoa butter, lecithin, sugar and powdered milk, are kneaded, rolled, homogenized and refined, in which the finely ground cocoa kernel fragments are subjected continuously and alternately to a batch mixing or kneading, and in this alternate batch treatment, cocoa butter and powdered milk are added, while, during the treatment of one batch, the other batch which has been mixed or kneaded is continuously removed and the mass already containing the powdered milk is subsequently subjected to a thin layer treatment for desiccation and evaporation while, subsequently, cocoa butter, lecithin and sugar are added to the mass and the mass is continuously subjected to alternate batch homogenization, from which the finished mass of one batch is continuously removed while the other batch undergoes homogenization.

Excerpt(s): The invention relates to a process for continuously producing milk chocolate masses, whereby the roasted cocoa kernal fragments are finely ground and, with the addition of sugar, lecithin, cocoa butter and powdered milk, are kneaded, rolled, homogenised and refined.... Preliminary mill, fine mill, thin layer treatment apparatus, Konti kneader, rollers and conche. The conche treatment has to be carried out in batches, in order to eliminate the water necessarily introduced by means of the powdered milk added in advance of the Konti kneader, i.e., fairly late, until only the permissible proportion remains, since the water should only be present in a certain percentage in the end product, and thus also to expel any undesirable flavours which are also introduced by the powdered milk.... The total expenditure of energy and also the expenditure on machines are correspondingly high in traditional processes, and also in the semi-continuous process, particularly as a result of the necessary use of a conche. On the one hand, it had long been known that the conche time required could be reduced by increasing the energy concentration, but on the other hand one was forced to acknowledge that, for constructional reasons, it is no longer possible to increase the throughput density (KW/m.sup.3) substantially. Nor does another possible method, namely first liquifying a crude chocolate mass consisting of cocoa, sugar, powdered milk and cocoa butter, in a suitable apparatus and subsequently subjecting it to a thin layer treatment, have the desired success. Indeed, extensive tests have shown that, although such a treatment is possible, the degree of success is too small and therefore is not an economical solution. Tests were able to show that the sensory properties of the chocolate mass are indeed noticeably changed from the better by the thin layer treatment, but that it was not possible to dehydrate and improve the viscosity of the mass to the desired final state under economical conditions and without forfeiting the quality of the mass in the short thin layer process. The great absorption characteristics of the sugar already contained in the mass are responsible for this.

Web site: http://www.delphion.com/details?pn=US04156743__

- **Method for extending the shelf-life of chocolate confectionery products containing peanuts and the product produced therefrom**

  Inventor(s): Patterson; Gordon (Hershey, PA), Stuart; David A. (Hershey, PA), Thomas; Paula (Harrisburg, PA), Lehrian; Douglas W. (Hummelstown, PA)

  Assignee(s): Hershey Foods Corporation (Hershey, PA)

  Patent Number: 5,585,135

  Date filed: August 24, 1995

  Abstract: The present invention is directed to chocolate confectionery containing roasted high oleic acid peanuts, in whole, or in part, and a process for making same.

  Excerpt(s): The present invention relates to chocolate confectionery products containing peanuts, either whole or in part, having high oleic acid content.... Candies, confections and snack foods are consumed for their eating enjoyment. The food properties responsible for giving the enjoyable sensation, the tastes, aromas and textures are often measured as a group often referred to as the organoleptic property of a food composition. This global measurement can be defined by quantitative sensory value, defined as likability or acceptability. The value is the sum total of sensory perception of the food as determined by trained experts who taste the food. While the measurement of likability or acceptability may appear subjective, when done under controlled conditions and with scientific methods, these measures can be determined with great precision and accuracy. In the food industry, the overall sensory likability or acceptability is used as a prediction of the commercial success of a new product and is the basis for multi-million dollar decisions regarding the product introduction.... The fat and oil components of most confectionery products greatly influence the perception of quality and overall likability or acceptability. The fats and oils become part of the system as a constituent of raw materials, such as cocoa beans, milk and the like. When nuts, such as peanuts, are added to the confectionery, the fats and oils therein also become part of the system.

  Web site: http://www.delphion.com/details?pn=US05585135__

- **Method for improving the yield of chocolate cake**

  Inventor(s): Chung; Frank H. Y. (Norwalk, CT)

  Assignee(s): Nutrisearch Company (Cincinnati, OH)

  Patent Number: 4,421,777

  Date filed: March 27, 1981

  Abstract: A process for preparing a chocolate flavored cake comprising mixing together and baking cake ingredients, the improvement, comprising adding to the ingredients of about 3% to about 15% on a flour basis of (1) a defined whey protein-containing composition in combination with (2) an amount of sodium bicarbonate sufficient to elevate the pH of the cake crumb to a pH within the range of about 7.5 to about 9.

  Excerpt(s): The present invention relates to a process for improving the yield and texture characteristics of chocolate cake and particularly chocolate sponge cake.... Chocolate cake is a well known item of dessert in this country as well as other countries in the world. Chocolate cakes are usually prepared by recipes somewhat different than recipes needed to prepare an ordinary plain cake because the addition of chocolate or cocoa to the recipe makes the batter thicker, more acid and less sweet. Since the color of chocolate cake varies greatly with pH, extra soda is usually added to maintain the pH. In the same vein, cocoa is often treated with an alkali during its manufacture to make it darker in color, less acid in flavor and less likely to settle in a cup. Alkali treated cocoa is generally called Dutch process cocoa (Foods, An Introductory College Course by G. E. Vail, 5th edition, Houghton Mifflin Company at page 104).... The pH is also responsible for flavor characteristics. A chocolate product with an acidic pH loses its typical flavor notes. An alkaline pH is required to develop the full flavor of the chocolate. A typical pH value for a chocolate cake ranges between about 7.5 and 8.0 whereas a typical pH for a devil's food cake ranges from about 8.0 to 9.0. The use of excess alkali to develop extremely dark color in a chocolate provides a soapy taste and is to be avoided (see an article entitled "The Role of pH in Cake Baking" by D. J. Ash and J. C. Colmey, The Baker's Digest, February 1973, pages 38 et seq. and Experimental Cookery 4th Edition, E. Lowe, John Wiley and Sons (1966) at page 492). Also of interest to the question of pH in cakes is an article entitled "Observations on the Hydrogen-ion Concentration of Cakes," Cereal Chem. 16 419-423 (1939).

  Web site: http://www.delphion.com/details?pn=US04421777__

- **Method for making chocolate and chocolate flavored materials**

  Inventor(s): Szegvari; Andrew (Akron, OH)

  Assignee(s): Union Process International, Inc. (Akron, OH)

  Patent Number: 4,224,354

  Date filed: September 22, 1978

  Abstract: A method is provided for making chocolate and chocolate flavored materials. A pump means repeatedly circulates a liquid continuum containing chocolate solids through conducting means to comminuting means formed of a bed of agitated grinding elements where the solids are comminuted, and through conducting means back to the pump means at a rate of at least about 30 and preferably between 50 and 500 volumes of liquid continuum containing solids in the comminuting means per hour. Chocolate and chocolate flavored materials having substantially greater particle size uniformity and other superior and unique properties are thus produced. Also in processing, the temperature is controlled during processing to liberate undesirable components, such as acetic acid, from the composition while retaining other desired components.

Excerpt(s): This invention relates to a method for comminuting particulate solids, and particularly chocolate and chocolate flavored compositions in a liquid continuum.... Various methods and apparatus have been known for grinding particulate solids in a liquid media. They include ball mills, pebble mills, roll mills, sand mills and agitated-media mills. Illustrative art is believed to be U.S. Pat. Nos. 1,577,052, 2,764,359, 3,903,191, 3,008,657, 3,131,875, 3,298,618, 3,149,789, 3,204,880, 3,337,140, 3,432,109, 3,591,349, British Pat. Nos. 716,316 and 1,038,153, and German Pat. Nos. 1,214,516 and 1,233,237.... An agitated-media comminuting apparatus commutes the solids in liquid suspension by subjecting them to generally random contact in a bed of agitated grinding elements. In an agitated-media comminuting apparatus, the grinding is usually performed in a vertical cylindrical stationary tank or vessel with a rotatable agitator disposed on a substantially vertical axis. The agitator has one or more solid protuberances such as arms or discs extending out from the axis thereof into a mass of grinding media or elements such as pebbles, ceramic balls or metal balls that occupies a substantial portion of the vessel. The rotation of the protuberances through the mass of grinding media causes the media to occupy an increased apparent volume with the result that the grinding elements have a substantial free space between them and impinge on each other in a manner somewhat similar to the classic model of a gas. The particulate material to be ground and the liquid, which serves as a carrier and dispersing media for the material, occupy the spaces between the grinding media. The material is ground by the action of the agitated grinding media. A built-in pumping action may be used to maintain circulation within the comminuting means during comminution.

Web site: http://www.delphion.com/details?pn=US04224354__

- **Method for manufacturing a jelly confectionery coated with chocolate**

Inventor(s): Yoon; Young-No (Seoul, KR)

Assignee(s): Crown Confectionery Co. (Seoul, KR)

Patent Number: 4,563,363

Date filed: August 25, 1983

Abstract: A novel structural jelly confectionery product is provided. This confectionery product is prepared by providing a jelly having a lower level of sugar content, enrobing a baked biscuit with said jelly and then coating the enrobed product with chocolate.

Excerpt(s): The present invention relates to a novel method for manufacturing a jelly confectionery and more particularly to a jelly confectinery coated with chocolate.... 2. In a process in which the biscuits are moisturized by a mechanical processing, the process was suffered from a rise of the production costs in the aspects of the installation as well as the operation conditions.... Thus, in the art, there has long been desired an appearance of a novel confectionery in which the aforementioned prior art darwbacks have effectively been eliminated.

Web site: http://www.delphion.com/details?pn=US04563363__

- **Method for manufacturing deaerated chocolate products**

  Inventor(s): Hachiya; Iwao (Kanagawa, JP), Joyama; Norio (Kanagawa, JP)

  Assignee(s): Meiji Seika Kaisha Ltd. (Tokyo, JP)

  Patent Number: 4,572,835

  Date filed: June 21, 1984

  Abstract: A method for manufacturing a deaerated fatty confectionaries, specifically, chocolate blocks, chocolate blocks with a confectionary center, chocolate covered products, white chocolate or colored chocolate blocks, and the like, having a substantially reduced air content without requiring excessive shaking. In accordance with the invention, the fatty confectionary mass in a fluidal state and flowing in the form of a film is subjected to a reduced pressure, preferably, within a range of 10 to 350 Torr. Tempering can be carried out either prior to, during, or subsequent to the deaerating treatment. The deaerated mass can then be used for manufacturing chocolate products by molding, shell-molding, or covering.

  Excerpt(s): The present invention relates to a method for manufacturing fatty confectionaries such as chocolates, white chocolates or the like which contain substantially no air therein and which have an excellent color, gloss and flavor.... Fatty confectionaries formed of chocolate mass used for chocolate blocks, chocolate-covered candies or cookies and the like and chocolate-like mass used for white chocolates, colored chocolates and the like have been susceptible to the admission of air therein when the latter is stirred in a chocolate reservoir associated with a blender, storage tank, tempering machine, depositor, or enrober or other coating apparatus in chocolate processing and molding steps, and a portion of this air is formed into bubbles distributed in the mass.... For forming fatty confectionaries such as chocolate blocks and the like with the use of molds, the chocolate or chocolate-like mass is filled into the mold by a filling apparatus such as a depositor or the like and then subjected to shaking or tapping. This causes a portion of the air bubbles contained therein to float on the top surface (bottom surface of the finished product) of the fatty mass or the area adjacent the top surface. The bubbles are then burst and scattered from the mass, thereby achieving partial deaerating. However, many fine bubbles are still left, dispersed in the mass, when the mass is cooled and solidified. The larger residual bubbles have a diameter of typically 20 to 50 microns, while the smaller residual bubbles have a diameter of typically 2 to 10 microns. The chocolate blocks and the like during molding are solidified with the bottom surface thereof having many bubble venting traces due to the removal of the bubbles during cooling and solidification. Hence, the products tend to have a rough surface due to the residual bubbles and bubble venting traces at the bottom surface and the area adjacent thereto.

  Web site: http://www.delphion.com/details?pn=US04572835__

- **Method for manufacturing water-containing chocolates and chocolate compositions produced thereby**

  Inventor(s): Morikawa; Kazutoshi (Izumisano, JP), Kurooka; Akira (Izumisano, JP)

  Assignee(s): Fuji Oil Co., Ltd. (Izumisano, JP)

  Patent Number: 6,159,526

  Date filed: October 26, 1999

Abstract: The present invention is a method for manufacturing a water-in-oil type water-containing chocolates by mixing chocolate foodstuff with aqueous components, wherein sucrose-fatty acid ester, whose HLB value is 3 or less and the number of carbon atoms in its main constituent fatty acid is 16-18, and polyglycerin polyricinoleate is each used in the range of 0.05 wt. % to 5.0 wt. % with respect to the chocolate foodstuff.

Excerpt(s): The present invention relates to methods for manufacturing water-containing chocolates, as well as to water-containing chocolate compositions. In particular, the present invention relates to a method for manufacturing water-containing chocolate, and to chocolate compositions that even with moisture added is not gritty from clumping of its solid content, nor is elevated in viscosity, and that has satisfactory workability and is moreover good tasting. Although there are water-in-oil type and oil-in-water type emulsion systems for water-containing chocolates, the present invention relates to methods for manufacturing water-in-oil type water-containing chocolates.... Various water-containing chocolates exist, from those whose moisture content is slight to those containing a large amount of moisture. For instance, the emulsion system of ganache, which is manufactured by mixing ordinary chocolate with different creams, is generally an oil-in-water type and hence, when used as a coating material, has the drawbacks of drying slowly and sticking to paper wrapping or of its moisture dehydrating. Further, a method that with a lipophilic emulsifier makes high moisture-containing components into a water-in-oil type emulsion added to chocolate, as a substance that can be mold-formed like ordinary chocolate, has been advocated (Japanese Laid-Open Gazette Pat. Appl. No. 60-27339). Nevertheless, making the moisture-containing components into the water-in-oil type emulsion is complicated by the need for exclusive processing facilities, and increases the work another step.... Still further, methods for adding aqueous components directly to chocolate have been advocated (Japanese Laid-Open Gazette Pat. Appl. Nos. 56-28131 and 3-164137). Such methods, however, limit the aqueous components to liquid sugar or enriched fresh cream. Moreover, methods for adding aqueous components, not particularly limited, directly to chocolate by using specific emulsifiers have been advocated (Japanese Laid-Open Gazette Pat. Appl. Nos. 3-151831, 6-062743, 6-189682, 6-237694, 8-070776, 9-140332, and 9-248132.) Water-containing chocolate in accordance with these suggestions is to an extent satisfying; nonetheless research toward improving quality further is ongoing.

Web site: http://www.delphion.com/details?pn=US06159526__

- **Method for pouring quantities of chocolate into molds**

  Inventor(s): Cerboni; Renzo (Milan, IT)

  Assignee(s): Carle & Montanari S.p.A. (Milan, IT)

  Patent Number: 5,534,283

  Date filed: May 5, 1994

  Abstract: Method of pouring a liquid mass of chocolate into an elongated mold by depositing greater quantities of the mass at both shorter end regions of the mold, and by depositing a lesser quantity of the mass at a longer central region of the mold.

  Excerpt(s): The present invention relates to a method and to an apparatus for pouring quantities of chocolate into forming molds.... The introduction of quantities of chocolate into molds for the production of bars of different sizes by a "tongue" pouring method is known in the art.... For this purpose a molding machine which translates relative to the mold and so deposits a "tongue" of pasty product in the wells of the mold, is used.

Web site: http://www.delphion.com/details?pn=US05534283__

- **Method for processing chocolate mass**

Inventor(s): Tadema; Jan C. (Bergen, NL)

Assignee(s): Wiener & Co. Apparatenbouw B.V. (Amsterdam, NL)

Patent Number: 5,156,878

Date filed: December 28, 1990

Abstract: Chocolate is ground in order to obtain a very small average particle size. A determined viscosity is necessary for further processing. In order to keep as small as possible the fraction with particle size lying above the desired value and having an adverse effect on the taste of the final product, according to the invention the process mass is circulated in a cycle incorporating a grinding device and a ball mill. This has the result of accelerating the grinding process and reducing the inconsistency in the distribution of the particle size.

Excerpt(s): The invention relates to a method and device for mixing and grinding chocolate, fats or the like, wherein a process mass of cacao and/or cacao powder, cacao butter, edible fat, sugar and the like are pre-mixed and ground in a grinding device and a ball mill.... Up until the present the components for processing were pre-mixed in a pre-mixer and ground in a grinding device. The pre-mixer and grinding device can also be unified to one unit. After grinding the mass is then ground in a ball mill to make it still finer as required until the final desired particle size is obtained.... In a ball mill it is possible to grind the process mass to a very small average particle size and to therein obtain the desired viscosity, although the uniformity in the distribution of the particle size leaves something to be desired. Unless grinding continues to a very small particle size, which is very time-consuming and moreover produces an adverse viscosity value, it can occur that the process mass still has a fraction with particle sizes lying far above the desired value. Such a fraction has an adverse effect on the taste of the final product.

Web site: http://www.delphion.com/details?pn=US05156878__

- **Method for producing molded chocolate product having complicated concaved and convexed decorative pattern thereon**

Inventor(s): Akutagawa; Tokuji (Tokyo, JP), Otani; Uichi (Tokyo, JP)

Assignee(s): Akutagawa Confectionery Co., Ltd. (Tokyo, JP)

Patent Number: 5,443,856

Date filed: June 15, 1994

Abstract: A method for producing a molded chocolate product having a complicated concaved and convexed decorative pattern thereon involves the steps of: (a) charging a low viscosity fluidized chocolate material into a complicated concaved and convexed decorative pattern portion of an elastic mold in bag form for forming the complicated concaved and convexed decorative pattern of the chocolate product so that air bubbles necessarily incorporated into the low viscosity fluidized chocolate material ascend therethrough so as to be removed, (b) charging an ordinarily tempered fluidized chocolate material into the elastic mold to form a main body of the chocolate product, and (c) solidifying the low viscosity fluidized chocolate material and the ordinarily tempered fluidized chocolate material charged into the elastic mold followed by taking the molded chocolate product out of the elastic mold.

Excerpt(s): This invention relates to a method for producing a molded chocolate product, and more particularly to a method for producing a molded chocolate product from which air bubbles can be removed especially when producing such a product having a complicated or intricate concaved and convexed decorative pattern at which air bubbles are formed.... A variety of methods for removing air bubbles incorporated into a chocolate material in the chocolate production process have been known. For example, it has been well known to vibrate a chocolate mold into which a fluidized chocolate material having approximately 60,000 centipoises after ordinary tempering is performed is charged. Although in the conventional methods it is possible to remove air bubbles incorporated into the chocolate material charged into a chocolate mold having a simple shape for producing a plate-shaped chocolate product, there arises a problem with such conventional methods in that it is only insufficiently possible to remove air bubbles incorporated into an ordinarily tempered chocolate material having a viscosity of approximately 60,000 centipoises present in complicated concaved and convexed decorative portions formed within a bag shaped elastic mold such as finely shaped decorative portions or inverted tapered decorative portions thereof. The chocolate products having decorative patterns on which air bubbles are present are commercially less valuable or can not be sold depending on the bubbles being formed. Accordingly, with the conventional methods decorative patterns of chocolate products are necessarily simple and limited in designing.... It is, therefore, an object of the present invention to provide a method for producing a molded chocolate product in which it is possible to readily remove air bubbles incorporated into a chocolate material in complicated concaved and convexed decorative pattern portions of a chocolate mold, the inside of which the complicated patterns such as fine or inverted tapered configurations are formed.

Web site: http://www.delphion.com/details?pn=US05443856__

- **Method for production of chocolate**

Inventor(s): Lipp; Eberhard (Altrip, DE)

Assignee(s): Lipp Mischtechnik GmbH (Mannheim, DE)

Patent Number: 5,945,150

Date filed: May 12, 1998

Abstract: A process for manufacturing chocolate includes premixing a charge of cocoa paste, sugar, and optionally powdered milk under application of heat, subsequently conveying the charge to a first grinder, and thereafter treating the resulting paste by tumbling in at least one stirring device under temperature control. In this process, removal of the volatile components as well as the reactions of the charge are conducted in a first operation, the paste is then pulverized, and after that the addition of fat and emulsifiers, and the dispersion and the liquefaction of the paste are implemented in a further operation.

Excerpt(s): The invention concerns a method for producing chocolate in which a charge of cocoa paste and sugar, and optionally powdered milk, are mixed in a premixer with application of heat. The charge is subsequently fed into a first grinder and there prepulverized. Thereafter, the paste so obtained is subjected to conching treatment in at least one stirring device under temperature control, while substantially removing volatile components in the form of water and organic acids by means of a gas, particularly air, passed through the stirring device. Reactions between the organic components and the reactive carbohydrates of the cocoa paste or milk for the development of taste, addition of fat and emulsifiers, especially in the form of cocoa butter and lecithin, dispersion of fat and emulsifiers and flavorings, as well as the final liquefaction of the paste, are conducted in further steps. Furthermore, the invention concerns an apparatus for implementing this method.... Such a process for manufacturing chocolate is generally known, for which reason this will not be repeated here again in detail. Temperature and other operating conditions are especially known which are a precondition for the process of working the paste in the stirring device, also designated as the conche.... Such a stirring device consists in a known case of a horizontal mixing drum in which is arranged a rotor driven by an electric motor, optionally with a reversible direction of rotation, on which essentially radially directed mixing tools are axially distributed for axial and radial product movement. These mixing tools are so installed that they serve to scrape the paste from the mixing drum wall in one direction of rotation of the rotor, while promoting the unguent-like and paste-like consistency of the paste in the other direction of rotation. Moreover, the jacket on the mixing drum is constructed as a double jacket to which, for example, water can be fed as a heating or cooling liquid , depending on whether in the current stage of the tumbling process in the conche cooling of the paste is indicated for energy elimination or heating of the paste is indicated for maintaining the necessary operating conditions. Finally, the interior of the stirring device is ventilated with the aid of a blower for removal of volatile components accumulating during the operating process, whose presence in the finished chocolate is undesirable.

Web site: http://www.delphion.com/details?pn=US05945150__

- **Method for rapidly producing chocolate forms**

  Inventor(s): Kaupert; Guenther (Erndtebrueck, DE)

  Assignee(s): none reported

  Patent Number: 4,426,402

  Date filed: August 11, 1982

  Abstract: In a method and apparatus for producing chocolate forms, the molding tools are provided with chocolate retaining and handling elements which are disposed in the molds before the molding process and which define part of the molding cavity. During and after injection of the hot chocolate into the cavity, the molding tool top part is cooled to a temperature much lower than the bottom part, whereby the top part can be rapidly and easily lifted from the bottom part and the retaining and handling element can be removed from the molds with the chocolate forms supported thereon, which forms can then be further cooled outside the molding tool. The molding tool is then available for the next molding step. The retaining and handling element may remain with the chocolate forms and may become part of the packaging, thereby greatly facilitating handling and accelerating production of delicate chocolate forms.

  Excerpt(s): The invention relates to a method and apparatus for producing chocolate forms in molding tools consisting of several parts which together define a molding cavity corresponding to the chocolate form to be produced, the cavity being closed except for an inlet opening through which heated chocolate is injected under pressure until the cavity is completely filled with chocolate. Solidifying of the chocolate is achieved by cooling of the molding tool.... It is known for example from German Pat.

No. 462,968 to provide a molding cavity by combining two shell-shaped mold parts such that they define therebetween a molding cavity with an inlet opening through which chocolate of a pasty consistency is injected under pressure. When the mold is filled, the pressure is maintained for some time in order to improve the density of the chocolate within the mold cavity. The mold is then removed from the injection station and, after a stem is inserted into the inlet opening into the chocolate form within the cavity, the mold is conveyed through a cooling chamber. At the exit end of the cooling chamber the mold is opened and the chocolate form is removed from the mold.... This method, however, has not been successful in practice; first, because the achievable molding rate is relatively low when compared with competing methods since, with the use of shell-type molds, the applicable molding pressure is relatively low for mechanical reasons so that the filling process itself already is relatively time-consuming. Second, since the chocolate form can be removed from the mold only after the mold has been conveyed through a cooling chamber, each mold is needed for a relatively long time in the production of every single chocolate form such that, for mass production, a large number of relatively expensive molds is required.

Web site: http://www.delphion.com/details?pn=US04426402_

- **Method for reducing the viscosity of chocolate**

  Inventor(s): Cully; Kevin John (Lake Bluff, IL), Carvallo; Federico De Loyola (Wheeling, IL), Abdallah; Qadri Mustafa (Lake Villa, IL), Gaim-Marsoner; Gunther Rudolf (Hauterive, CH)

  Assignee(s): Kraft Foods, Inc. (Northfield, IL)

  Patent Number: 5,676,995

  Date filed: February 3, 1997

  Abstract: The present invention is directed to a method for reducing the viscosity of melted chocolate. In the method, a chocolate mixture is provided which includes a chocolate source, a fat source and a sweetener. The chocolate mixture is subjected to refining and conching or other processing. Thereafter, the liquified chocolate mixture, which is liquified during conching, is subjected to high shear mixing while the chocolate mixture is still in the molten state.

  Excerpt(s): The present invention is directed to a method for reducing the viscosity of melted chocolate. More particularly, the present invention is directed to a method for reducing the viscosity of melted chocolate which results in an improvement in the smoothness of the chocolate. As used herein, the term chocolate means confectionery masses containing cocoa butter and/or other vegetable fats.... The essential components of a conventional chocolate formulation are cocoa "nib", i.e., the roasted cocoa bean with shell and germ removed, sugar and cocoa butter additional to that contained in the nib. Cocoa nib is approximately 50% cocoa butter, the balance being proteins, carbohydrates, tannins, acids, etc. The cocoa butter content of the chocolate controls its setting characteristics and largely governs its cost, and while the ratio of cocoa nib to sugar determines the type of chocolate, the cocoa butter content varies according to the application. Thus, bitter sweet chocolate has a ratio of nib to sugar of 2:1 while sweet chocolate has a ratio of 1:2. Molding chocolate may have a fat content of 25% to 40%, covering chocolate 33 to 36%, chocolate for hollow goods 38 to 40% and chocolate for covering ice cream 50 to 60%.... The typical preparation of chocolate involves four stages. In the first stage, the ingredients are mixed together in a process which also involves grinding or rubbing, e.g., on a multiple roll press to provide a smooth fluid paste. The ingredients may be added sequentially and in particular the cocoa butter may be added stepwise to control the viscosity of the composition. The sugar may also be preground to a smaller particle size to reduce the length of time required in the grinding/rubbing of the chocolate mixture. Most chocolate, and certainly all good quality product, is subjected after mixing to the process of "conching" in which the chocolate mixture is subjected to temperature treatment and mechanical working to give the chocolate an improved texture and a fuller and more homogeneous flavor. Other ingredients such as flavors, e.g., vanilla and extra cocoa butter may be added at this stage if desired. A frequently added additional ingredient is lecithin or other emulsifier which improves the flow properties of the chocolate and thereby enables the amount of fat to be reduced. The third stage of the chocolate preparation is called "tempering" in which nuclei are provided in the liquid chocolate composition to facilitate the rapid crystallization of selected stable fat crystals on cooling. The final appearance of the chocolate, its texture and keeping properties depend upon correct tempering stage conditions. After tempering, the chocolate may finally be cast into molds to set or may be used in an enrobing process to produce chocolate coated confectionery, etc.

Web site: http://www.delphion.com/details?pn=US05676995__

- **Method for wrapping essentially flat products of the luxury-item or foodstuffs industry, especially squares or bars of chocolate, in packaging foil**

Inventor(s): Lesch; Hans (Garmisch-Partenkirchen, DE)

Assignee(s): Otto Hansel GmbH (Hanover, DE)

Patent Number: 4,670,279

Date filed: April 3, 1984

Abstract: Methods and devices for wrapping essentially flat products of the luxury-comestibles or foodstuffs industry, especially squares or bars of chocolate, in packaging foil or film. The object is tubular packaging, especially the inner wrapping of squares or bars of chocolate at high machine output without especially stressing the particular packaging foil while maintaining a low level of packaging-material consumption. This is attained in that the webs of foil are transported by means of an intermittently direct connection between foil web and pushers.

Excerpt(s): The invention concerns a method of wrapping essentially flat products of the luxury-comestibles or foodstuffs industry, especially squares or bars of chocolate, in packaging foil or film and simultaneously discloses a device for carrying out the method. Machines called tubular machines, in which packaging film runs from a supply roll in the form of a web to which the pieces to be wrapped are conveyed one following another at an interval by pushers resting on a transport traveling in the same direction as the web of film, subsequent to which the film is wrapped around each individual piece and sealed at its longitudinal and transverse edges, have been employed up to now to package all types of packaged goods. The plastic films employed in this process must be especially rugged and pliable because they have to be drawn over shaping tools of the widest range of types during the operation. Considerable wrapping-material overlap must be provided in order to make the package conform with the requisite tightness standards. This leads to high material consumption and low machine output. Very thin aluminum foil, which is especially amenable to heat-sealing can hardly be employed. Still, metal foils of this type are just the materials that are particularly intended for packaging candy, especially squares or bars of chocolate.... The object of the present invention is to eliminate the aforesaid drawback and create a method and device that allow tubular packaging to be carried out, especially for the inner wrapping of flat articles like squares or bars of chocolate, without specially stressing the particular packaging foil and simultaneously reducing the consumption of packaging material.... Packages in which a longitudinal seam is produced at the narrow end are intended in particular to be manufactured and foils, especially thin metal foils amenable to heat sealing, that are not processed over the type of shaping shoulder ordinarily used in conventional tubular machines are employed, ensuring seams that are particularly tight.

Web site: http://www.delphion.com/details?pn=US04670279__

- **Method of casting chocolate**

Inventor(s): Cerboni; Renzo (Milan, IT)

Assignee(s): Carle & Montanari S.p.A. (Milan, IT)

Patent Number: 4,588,599

Date filed: August 21, 1984

Abstract: A forming machine for chocolate has a distributor bottom plate formed with a discharge manifold channel into which there open, through interconnecting grooves, the blind holes aligned with overlying delivery holes in the forming machine. The discharge manifold channel is connected to an excess chocolate recovery portion selectively conducting to either an intermediate storage or feeding hopper of the forming machine. In the course of the casting process implemented thereby, all of the pistons, irrespective of their being reciprocating or rotary ones, are fed at all times independently of the molds being used. In moving from one mould to another, only the distributor bottom plate is replaced and no pistons need be manipulated.

Excerpt(s): This invention relates to a method of casting chocolate, cream, and the like products, and to a forming machine and bottom plate for implementing the method.... As is known, for casting chocolate, cream, candy, and the like products with either of the two most commonly used methods, i.e. spot and continuous casting, it has been heretofore possible to employ forming machines of two types, namely reciprocating piston and rotary piston forming machines.... Irrespective of its design, each forming machine is provided with an equal number of chocolate delivery holes to the number of reciprocating or rotary pistons it comprises. In order to be able to use one forming machine with different master molds, i.e. molds having either a different number of receptacles or the same number of differently patterened receptacles, or again, to produce different chocolate articles with one master mold, it is known to associate with the bottom delivery end of the forming machine distributor bottom plates having inlet holes which correspond by number and arrangement to the forming machine delivery holes. Also known is to arrange said holes of the bottom plates in a branched pattern such that a greater number of mold receptacles can be filled with respect to the forming machine delivery holes, and accordingly, the product can be distributed more evenly to the mold receptacles, especially where large surface receptacles are used, as for bars and the like. In each case, those pistons which happen to be in communication with forming machine delivery holes not controlled to deliver chocolate for the time being, must be stopped or somehow prevented from delivering chocolate while the machine is in operation.

Web site: http://www.delphion.com/details?pn=US04588599__

- **Method of conching bulk chocolate in a mixing apparatus**

  Inventor(s): Lucke; Roland (Paderborn, DE), Meyer; Thomas (Paderborn, DE), Luke; Bernhard (Paderborn, DE)

  Assignee(s): Gebrueder Loedige Maschinenbau-Gesellschaft mbH (Paderborn/Fed., DE)

  Patent Number: 5,707,145

  Date filed: June 20, 1996

  Abstract: Bulk chocolate is added into a mixing apparatus whereby a plurality of conching tools (10) is fixed together with several others, on a shaft (11). The shaft (11) is rotatably mounted in end walls (21) of a horizontal drum (12). The ends of the mixing tools (10) are located a short distance from the inside wall (18) of the drum, and the shaft (11) has a drive which turns the direction of rotation of the shaft (11), the clearance between the leading edge (19) of each tool (10) and the inside wall (18) of the drum is greater than the clearance between the trailing edge (20) of the tool and the inside wall (18) of the drum. The shaft (11) is rotated to press the bulk chocolate between a bottom wall of mixing tools (10) and the inside surface of the drum (12) whereby the bulk chocolate first enters the leading edge (19) to experience a pressing force as it travels across from the leading region to the trailing region of the mixing tool (10).

  Excerpt(s): The invention concerns the use of a mixing apparatus comprising a drum with a shaft having a drive mechanism rotatably mounted therein for conching, in particular of bulk chocolate, wherein a plurality of mixing tools are attached to the shaft.... Mixing tools of this kind are known in the art through German patent manuscript 1 276 986.... This type of mixing tool has been known in the art for decades, and they are utilized in largely horizontal drums in order to mix solid and liquid bulk materials of all kinds. The tools are attached to a shaft which is mounted in a rotatable fashion in the drum. When installing the mixing tools one must pay particular attention to the installation location of the mixing tools relative to the inner wall of the drum since the mixing tools should have a small separation from the drum inner wall. Material deformation can lead to a blocking of the centrifuge mechanism in the drum in the event of improper configuration of the centrifuge mechanism (shaft and mixing tools) and their positioning relative to the drum. That is to say, even without any product in the mixing device, it is possible for material deformation (of the drum and/or the centrifuge mechanism) to occur and due to the intrinsic weight of the centrifuge mechanism, individual mixing tools can seat on the drum surface to block the centrifuge mechanism in the drum. This problem can always be addressed if one arranges the mixing tools sufficiently far from the inner surface of the drum such that even under unfavorable circumstances, direct contact between the mixing tools and the drum is not possible.

  Web site: http://www.delphion.com/details?pn=US05707145__

- **Method of creating painted chocolate**

  Inventor(s): Waters; Peter B (2 Split Oak Dr., East Norwich, NY 11732)

  Assignee(s): none reported

  Patent Number: 6,376,000

  Date filed: January 3, 2000

  Abstract: A method of forming chocolate mold having an image printed thereon. The method includes the steps of forming a piece of edible paper, releasably securing a first side of the edible paper to a backing sheet, printing an image on a second side of the edible paper and securing the edible paper to the chocolate mold. The image is printed on the edible paper by a printer using food coloring loaded into a cartridge of the printer. The step of securing the edible paper to the chocolate mold may include placing the edible paper within a mold with the image facing a side of the mold, pouring chocolate into the mold and atop the edible paper, allowing the chocolate poured into the mold to harden and removing the hardened chocolate and edible paper from the mold. The hardening of the chocolate forms a bond between the chocolate and the edible paper it is poured atop. Alternatively, the step of securing the edible paper to the chocolate mold may include pouring chocolate into a mold, allowing the chocolate poured into the mold to harden, removing the hardened chocolate from the mold and securing the edible paper to a desired position on the hardened chocolate. In this instance, the edible paper is secured to the hardened chocolate with an edible adhesive such as gum arabic.

Excerpt(s): The present invention relates generally to methods of forming chocolate and, more specifically, to a method of forming art work on a chocolate mold without causing the chocolate to become unstable and flake.... Numerous methods of placing art work on chocolate molds have been provided in the prior art. An examples of such a method includes hand painting the chocolate bar with a desired image. However, creating a chocolate mold in this manner was very time consuming, labor intensive and tedious. Another attempt at placing art work on a chocolate mold centered around printing a desired image directly on the chocolate. This method printed the image on chocolate which is the wrong color for the image, is oily and has an uneven surface. Thus, this method did not provide consistent and desirable results. Still other methods centered around silk screening images on rice paper and gluing the rice paper to the chocolate. This method required large runs of numerous units and also created chocolate which was unstable and flaked.... While these methods may be suitable for the particular purpose to which they address, they would not be as suitable for the purposes of the present invention as heretofore described.

Web site: http://www.delphion.com/details?pn=US06376000__

- **Method of dosing emulsifiers in chocolate mass**

  Inventor(s): Horig; Jurgen (Heidenau, DD)

  Assignee(s): Veb Kombinat Nagema (Dresden, DD)

  Patent Number: 4,563,361

  Date filed: July 2, 1984

  Abstract: A continuous stream of chocolate mass is dosed with lecithin or similar emulsifiers by means of an electronically controlled dosing pump. The throughput or the weight rate of the flow of the chocolate mass is detected by a weighing device and the amount of the emulsifier to be added is adjusted to the changes of the throughput. The percentage of the emulsifier is preselected. The dosing time of each charge of the chocolate mass is determined as a first time interval from the detected weight rate of flow. During the dosing of a charge, a second time interval which is a predetermined fraction of the first time interval, is determined for the next charge during the dosing of a preceding charge. A control unit actuates a time counter for determining the first time interval whose value is stored in an intermediate storage. An operation counter determines the second time intervals and activates a control unit for the emulsifier dosing pump.

Excerpt(s): The invention relates in general to the manufacture of chocolate and in particular it relates to a method of and a control device for dosing lecithin or similar emulsifier in chocolate mass processed in a continuously operating plant which includes a weighing device for detecting the weight rate of flow of the chocolate mass, and a continuously operating dosing pump arrangement for the lecithin.... For continuous dosing of lecithin in a chocolate mass it has been known to change the dosage by adjusting the rotary speed of a pump operating as a dosing apparatus.... Known are also dosing pumps in which the measured quantity or the dose is changed in dependency on the piston stroke.

Web site: http://www.delphion.com/details?pn=US04563361__

- **Method of forming a multi-color chocolate product**

  Inventor(s): Newsteder; Robert (Utica, NY)

  Assignee(s): Chocolate Pix, Inc. (Utica, NY)

  Patent Number: 4,778,683

  Date filed: December 4, 1986

  Abstract: A method of forming a multi-color chocolate product, includes the steps of applying a first color chocolate into a chocolate mold having a planar upper surface and recesses formed therein which form a sharp angle at the junction of the recesses with the planar upper surface; squeegeeing the first color chocolate across the planar upper surface such that the first color chocolate fills the recesses and is scraped from the planar upper surface; permitting the first color chocolate to at least partially harden; applying a second color chocolate into the chocolate mold on the planar upper surface thereof; permitting the second color chocolate to harden to form the multi-color chocolate product; and removing the multi-color chocolate product from the chocolate mold.

  Excerpt(s): The present invention relates generally to producing multi-color chocolate products with fine definition.... The chocolate candy industry dates back two hundred years to the time in which cocoa or chocolate was first converted into a solid edible substance. Since that time, a wide variety of methods have been developed for casting the chocolate into blocks having different configurations. For the most part, however, these molding techniques have remained virtually unchanged.... At the present time, the chocolate industry is generally limited to the reproduction of letters, such as the addition of the trademarks "Hershey's" or "Nestles" with a single chocolate color, which is in very broad detail. This is generally accomplished by casting the chocolate bar with the appropriate markings, or by using expensive molds which create very fine detail but are limited to one color, the expense of which can easily be accounted for in view of the mass production of such chocolate bars. Reference is also made to U.S. Pat. No. 4,200,658 which discloses a method of making a single color chocolate bar with a detailed design.

  Web site: http://www.delphion.com/details?pn=US04778683__

- **Method of forming an image with photographic likeness on chocolate**

  Inventor(s): Newsteder; Robert (Utica, NY)

  Assignee(s): Chocolate Pix, Inc. (Utica, NY)

  Patent Number: 4,668,521

  Date filed: August 1, 1986

  Abstract: A method of forming an image with photographic likeness on a chocolate material is disclosed. The image is "developed" on the chocolate material by means of an edible developer.

  Excerpt(s): This invention relates to a process for producing a photographic quality likeness of a photographic image on the surface of a chocolate candy.... Images are typically created in castable materials by simply casting the material against a mold surface having a pattern cut or otherwise formed therein. The mold pattern is a reversal of the desired image to be reproduced. The quality of the final image is to a large extent dependent upon the amount of detail that is contained in the mold pattern. High quality molds require a good deal of fine detail and are very expensive to construct. Because of the mold costs involved, these quality molds are typically used in the manufacture of high priced items, or those that can be mass produced and sold on a high volume basis.... U.S. Pat. No. 4,200,658 issued to Sandra Katzman, et al. on Apr. 29, 1980 discloses a method for making candy (hereinafter "the Katzman patent"). The Katzman patent is intended to make novelty chocolate items but simply is not up to the task of making chocolate having a photographic likeness image formed thereon which can be "developed" at will by a person.

  Web site: http://www.delphion.com/details?pn=US04668521__

- **Method of forming an image with photographic likeness on chocolate and product thereof**

  Inventor(s): Newsteder; Robert (Utica, NY)

  Assignee(s): Chocolate Pix, Inc. (Utica, NY)

  Patent Number: 4,832,966

  Date filed: May 20, 1987

  Abstract: A method of reproducing in chocolate a selected image, comprising the steps of optically scanning the image, laser etching the selected image in a surface of a plate in response to the optical scanning such that peaks and valleys are created in the surface of the plate corresponding to the selected image, controlling the laser etching by a scanning laser or a displayed frame of the image, casting a deformable transfer blanket against the surface of the etched plate surface to record in a surface of the transfer blanket peaks and valleys corresponding to the selected image, casting a chocolate material against the surface of the transfer blanket to record the selected image by peaks and valleys in a surface of the chocolate, and removing the cast chocolate material from the transfer blanket.

  Excerpt(s): This invention relates to a process for producing a photographic quality likeness of a photographic image on the surface of a chocolate candy.... Images are typically created in castable materials by simply casting the material against a mold surface having a pattern cut or otherwise formed therein. The mold pattern is a reversal of the desired image to be reproduced. The quality of the final image is to a large extent dependent upon the amount of detail that is contained in the mold pattern. High quality molds require a good deal of fine detail and are very expensive to construct. Because of the mold costs involved, these quality molds are typically used in the manufacture of high priced items, or those that can be mass produced and sold on a high volume basis.... U.S. Pat. No. 4,200,658 issued to Sandra Katzman, et al. on Apr. 29, 1980 discloses a method for making candy (hereinafter "the Katzman patent"). The Katzman patent is intended to make novelty chocolate items but simply is not up to the task of making chocolate having a photographic likeness image formed thereon which can be "developed" at will be a person.

Web site: http://www.delphion.com/details?pn=US04832966__

- **Method of making a reduced fat agglomerated chocolate**

  Inventor(s): Dubberke; Karin (Dublin, OH)

  Assignee(s): Nestec S.A. (Vevey, CH)

  Patent Number: 6,117,478

  Date filed: March 12, 1998

  Abstract: A low fat agglomerated chocolate having an average particle size up to 5 mm and containing from 18 to 24% by weight fat based on the total weight of the chocolate and a reduced fat milk chocolate bar comprising a mixture of from 60 to 90% of a reduced fat chocolate containing less than 27% fat and from 40 to 10% of a reduced fat agglomerated chocolate having an average particle size up to 5 mm and containing from 18 to 24% by weight fat based on the total weight of the chocolate. The products have a unique crunchy texture, melt easily and have a smooth texture in the mouth.

  Excerpt(s): The present invention relates to a reduced fat agglomerated chocolate and to a process for its preparation.... Conventional milk chocolate contains about 30-31% fat. It may contain more or less but rarely less than 27% fat. Calorie-conscious consumers demand a chocolate with lower calories and one way of reducing the calories in chocolate is by reducing the fat content. However, there are technical difficulties in reducing the fat content of milk chocolate causing the quality, taste and texture to be inferior to that of conventional milk chocolate. For example, reduced fat milk chocolates usually give a dry and coarse mouthfeel and the viscosity is too high for normal handling during preparation.... In U.S. patent application Ser. No. 09/038,937, filed on Mar. 12, 1998 the entirety of which is hereby incorporated by reference, I have described a reduced fat milk chocolate which has the same or better physical characteristics such as texture, mouthfeel (lubrication), snap, viscosity, handling (tempering, mould, enrobing), and gloss than a conventional milk chocolate, e.g. containing 30-31% by weight fat.

  Web site: http://www.delphion.com/details?pn=US06117478__

- **Method of making chocolate candy sculpture of photo image**

  Inventor(s): Syrmis; Victor (New York, NY)

  Assignee(s): Chocolate Photos (New York, NY)

  Patent Number: 4,455,320

  Date filed: September 30, 1982

Abstract: A chocolate candy having its upper surface sculpted as the image of a person's face and a method for sculpting a person's face from a photograph onto a chocolate candy by adapting a photographic image of a person's face, converting the adapted image onto a transfer medium or die, and then embossing such adapted image onto chocolate candy.

Excerpt(s): This invention is in the combined fields of manufacturing chocolate candy and psychiatry. Chocolate is obviously one of the most popular condiments for complex reasons of taste, various positive attributes persons often associate with chocolate and the act of eating chocolate, and certain real or alleged favorable body chemistry or mental reactions from eating chocolate candy. The actual manufacture of chocolate in its various chemical compositions is known in the prior art. The new invention herein disclosed concerns the creation on the surface of a chocolate candy of a sculpture or embossed image of a person's face adapted from a photographic image of same.... The concept of creating and embossing a design or manufacturer's name on the surface of a chocolate or other candy is well known. The novelty herein is sculpting a person's image in chocolate by taking a person's own photographic image, adapting it in a manner to render it transferrable onto a chocolate candy surface, and carrying out the steps to complete such a process and simultaneously creating a sealed container for each candy where the container top also bears the person's image.... While it is obvious that a person's facial appearance is of great concern to him or her, it was surprising to discover that many persons are very favorably disposed to having their images sculpted on a chocolate candy that will be seen and eventually eaten by themselves and others. It was also discovered, however, that a photographic image, when transferred directly onto a mold as by photo-etching, for example, and thence onto chocolate often produces a very unattractive and inaccurate replication of the photographic image and impression. It is due to the color, composition and texture of chocolate that direct photo-transfer processes, which might be obvious in the paper products industry, are wholly intolerable in making chocolate photo embossments. For example, freckles, eyes and dimples which usually comprise beauty features, are likely to appear on chocolate as blemishes, pits or worse.

Web site: http://www.delphion.com/details?pn=US04455320__

Patent Applications on Chocolate

As of December 2000, U.S. patent applications are open to public viewing.[10] Applications are patent requests which have yet to be granted. (The process to achieve a patent can take several years.) The following patent applications have been filed since December 2000 relating to chocolate:

- **Apparatus and method for producing ice-creams or similar products with stick, covered with chocolate or similar products**

    Inventor(s): Grigoli, Franco Albino Luigi; (Milano, IT)

    Correspondence: NOTARO & MICHALOS P.C. Empire State Building; Suite 6902; 350 Fifth Avenue; New York; NY; 10118-6985; US

    Patent Application Number: 20020146496

    Date filed: January 4, 2002

---

[10] This has been a common practice outside the United States prior to December 2000.

Abstract: The invention relates to an apparatus and the relevant method for producing ice-creams with stick, covered, providing for:filling the moulds, become cold by means of previous production cycles, with the covering product, for example chocolate;suction of chocolate from the moulds so that only the desired layer of frozen product adheres to said moulds;filling of the mould with ice-cream or other edible product;insertion of the stick before the starting of the freezing of the top or during or soon afterwards for obtaining the best results;gas freezing of the product top for obtaining a closing "plug" of the tub;starting of brine freezing that will end after the dosage of the closing plug;optionally measure such a chocolate layer or other edible product as to obtain a total covering.Said method according to the invention allows to obtain ice-creams or similar covered products, by accurately giving to the covering layer the desired shape and above all by using a brine (or similar liquids) linear or rotary tank type system, quick and inexpensive.

Excerpt(s): optionally measure such a chocolate layer or other edible product as to obtain a total covering.... Said method according to the invention allows to obtain ice-creams or similar covered products, by accurately giving to the covering layer, the desired shape and above all by using a brine (or similar liquids) linear or rotary tank type system, quick and inexpensive.... In addition, it is also possible to make use of existing apparatuses, without the need to produce ad hoc equipment, but by completing the apparatus with components already in use in the same sector.

Web site: http://appft1.uspto.gov/netahtml/PTO/search-bool.html

- **Apparatus and method for producing particles from a food material, in particular a chocolate material**

Inventor(s): Tilz, Wolfgang; (Schwetzingen, DE), Schnoor, Lars; (Heidelberg, DE)

Correspondence: MARSHALL, GERSTEIN & BORUN; 6300 SEARS TOWER; 233 SOUTH WACKER; CHICAGO; IL; 60606-6357; US

Patent Application Number: 20020197387

Date filed: February 15, 2002

Abstract: Described is an apparatus and a method for producing particles from a food material, in particular a chocolate material. The material is heated with a melting device up to flowability and supplied to a shaping device which includes at least one nozzle for dripping the flowable material as well as a cooling device for solidifying the material drops in particle form. To make such an apparatus and such a method more efficient in a constructionally simple way, it is suggested that the cooling device should contain a cooled contact surface which is movable relative to the nozzle.

Excerpt(s): The present invention relates to an apparatus and a method for producing particles from a food material, in particular a chocolate material, of the type explained in the preambles of claims 1 and 14.... Such an apparatus and method are known from EP 976 333. The known apparatus contains a downpipe which is arranged with a vertical central axis and in the upper portion of which a dripping device is arranged for the flowable chocolate material. The dripping device includes a nozzle block which substantially covers the cross section of the downpipe and consists of a plurality of individual dripping nozzles from which material drops exit and freely fall through the downpipe. The nozzle block is heated to prevent chocolate material from solidifying already during the dripping process and from clogging the nozzles. A cooled gas, preferably nitrogen, is used as the sole coolant. The nitrogen should have a temperature of at least -60.degree. C., preferably -160.degree. C. when introduced and -80.degree. C. when leaving the downpipe. Nevertheless, this still requires a downpipe length of a total of about 20 m. The coolant is preferably passed in countercurrent fashion relative to the fall path of the drops and leaves the downpipe in the area of the nozzle block. It can thus not be avoided that the heated nozzle block also comes into contact with the coolant. In the most advantageous case this results in waste of energy and in the most disadvantageous case chocolate material may already harden in the area of the nozzles and thus clog the nozzles.... If in the case of the known apparatus the shape of the particles to be produced thereby is to be varied, this must be carried out in a rather troublesome way by a correspondingly changed gas guidance of the coolant in order to produce a specific turbulence of the gas that will yield the desired result. This turbulence is preferably achieved by a tangential inflow of the gas, whereby a twist component is to be produced in the pipe flow; i.e., by a constructionally entirely different solution which requires a separate downpipe.

Web site: http://appft1.uspto.gov/netahtml/PTO/search-bool.html

- **Apparatus for continuously molding chocolate products**

Inventor(s): Collins, Thomas M. (Nazareth, PA), Willcocks, Neil A. (Flanders, NJ), Martin, John M. (Glendale, CA), Suttle, James M. (East Stroudsburg, PA), Camporini, Alfred V. (Hackettstown, NJ)

Correspondence: FITZPATRICK CELLA HARPER & SCINTO; 30 ROCKEFELLER PLAZA; NEW YORK; NY; 10112; US

Patent Application Number: 20010041205

Date filed: February 1, 2001

Abstract: Methods for continuously molding finished chocolate tablets, pieces and the like are disclosed. Apparatus for use with the method, comprise a chilled rotating mold having at least one recess into which liquid chocolate is deposited. Liquid chocolate, is held in place by a retaining/casting belt as the rotating mold turns. The liquid chocolate cools and partially sets while in contact with the rotating mold and retaining/casting belt, and a molded chocolate is removed from the recess. Novel finished chocolate molded products made by the methods and with the apparatus, having detailed surface design and surface gloss are also disclosed.

Excerpt(s): The invention relates to the molding of chocolate. Specifically, the disclosed method and apparatus are directed to the continuous molding of chocolate tablets, pieces and the like on a rotary mold.... Finished chocolates having a desired three-dimensional shape or having an image or design imprinted on a surface are conventionally produced by molding, and are herein referred to as "molded chocolate." The finished chocolate may be a solid block, a hollow shell, or a shell filled with a confectionery material such as fondant, fudge or soft caramel (Chocolate, Cocoa and Confectionery: Science and Technology by Bernard W. Minifie, Third Edition, page 183, herein incorporated by reference in its entirety). Whatever the particular form of the finished chocolate, all are characterized by attributes such as detailed finishes and high surface gloss. Further, these finished chocolates do not require further processing such as enrobing with chocolate, which only provides a home-made look to a product and lacks high gloss and fine surface detail.... Conventional molding typically employs very large numbers of molds, usually made of polycarbonate. These polycarbonate molds are typically flat, approximately 1 inch in height and anywhere from 1 to 2 feet long and 1 to 5 feet in width.

Web site: http://appft1.uspto.gov/netahtml/PTO/search-bool.html

- **Cacao endoproteinases and production of cocoa flavor from same**

Inventor(s): Laloi, Maryse; (Tours, FR), Bucheli, Peter; (La Ville aux Dames, FR), McCarthy, James; (Noizay, FR)

Correspondence: WINSTON & STRAWN; PATENT DEPARTMENT; 1400 L STREET, N.W. WASHINGTON; DC; 20005-3502; US

Patent Application Number: 20030148417

Date filed: January 10, 2003

Abstract: The present invention pertains to novel aspartic endoproteinases from Th. cacao which are involved in the production of cocoa flavor and DNA sequences coding for them. These enzymes are advantageously used in the manufacture of cocoa flavor.

Excerpt(s): This application is a continuation of the US national phase designation of International application PCT/EP01/07255 filed Jun. 26, 2001, the content of which is expressly incorporated herein by reference thereto.... The present invention pertains to novel endoproteinases involved in the production of cocoa flavor and the DNA coding for them. In particular, the present invention relates to the use of said enzymes for the manufacture of cocoa flavor.... It is known that in processing cacao beans the generation of the typical cocoa flavor requires two steps--the fermentation step, which includes air-drying of the fermented material and the roasting step. Though roasting seems to be the key stage of obtaining cocoa flavor subjecting non fermented beans to a roasting step does not yield cocoa flavor suggesting that during the fermentation step precursors are produced that are essential for flavor generation (Rohan J. Food Sci. 29 (1964), 456-459).

Web site: http://appft1.uspto.gov/netahtml/PTO/search-bool.html

- **Chocolate confectionery having high resolution printed images on an edible image-substrate coating**

Inventor(s): Suttle, James M. (East Stroudsburg, PA), Narine, Suresh S. (Bethlehem, PA), Shastry, Arun V. (Neshanic Station, NJ), Collins, Thomas M. (Nazareth, PA), Ben-Yoseph, Eyal M. (Stroudsburg, PA), Willcocks, Neil A. (Flanders, NJ)

Correspondence: FITZPATRICK CELLA HARPER & SCINTO; 30 ROCKEFELLER PLAZA; NEW YORK; NY; 10112; US

Patent Application Number: 20020114878

Date filed: December 15, 2000

Abstract: A chocolate confectionery is disclosed having on a surface thereof a chocolate base layer, a non-delaminating integral substantially white or light colored edible image-substrate coating disposed on at least a portion of a surface of the chocolate base layer and a high resolution edible black and/or colored print image disposed on at least a portion of the edible image-substrate coating. A method is also disclosed for preparing the confectionery.

Excerpt(s): This invention is directed to a chocolate confectionery having a black or colored high resolution edible image deposited on an image-substrate coating that is dispersed on a surface of the chocolate confectionery. Preferably, the chocolate is milk or dark chocolate and the image-substrate coating is substantially white or light colored, which provides for excellent image contrast when edible high resolution images are printed thereon using edible inks applied by ink jet printing.... It is known to form highly detailed images on milk and dark chocolates using pad printing with a white ink. However, the formation of high resolution colored images on milk and dark chocolate has been difficult due in part to the lack of contrast between the chocolate and the colored food dyes. Attempts to avoid this problem have included printing colored images on white chocolate. However, the typical dull white of white chocolate does not provide a very good contrast background for printing high resolution black or colored images. In addition, when you print directly on the chocolate surface the image tends to be prone to smearing and the image resolution is poor. Moreover, milk chocolate and dark chocolate have a much greater presence in the market place.... Frosting sheets have been used in the cake industry to provide a means of placing an ink jet printed color image on a cake. The frosting sheet is printed and then either placed on or bound to the top of the cake. There has, however, been no suggestion of printing on chocolate confectionery.

Web site: http://appft1.uspto.gov/netahtml/PTO/search-bool.html

- **Chocolate crumb flavor manipulation**

  Inventor(s): Sievert, Dietmar; (Epalinges, CH), Armstrong, Euan; (Leeds, GB), Kochhar, Sunil; (Savigny, CH), Budwig, Christopher; (Dublin, OH), Hansen, Carl Erik; (Epalinges, CH), Juillerat, Marcel Alexandre; (Lausanne, CH)

  Correspondence: WINSTON & STRAWN; PATENT DEPARTMENT; 1400 L STREET, N.W. WASHINGTON; DC; 20005-3502; US

  Patent Application Number: 20030129276

  Date filed: October 23, 2002

  Abstract: A process for manipulating the flavor of a chocolate crumb which comprises treating one or more of the crumb ingredients to enhance the flavor and preparing the crumb. The flavor of a milk or white chocolate prepared from chocolate crumb can be manipulated by adding the flavor-modified chocolate crumb to other chocolate ingredients to prepare the chocolate.

  Excerpt(s): The present invention relates to processes for the manipulation of the flavor of chocolate crumb and in the preparation of chocolate using such a crumb.... The process of making chocolate is described in "Industrial Chocolate Manufacture and Use", edited by S. T. Beckett, (Third Edition, 1999, Blackwell Science). One of ordinary skill in the art is familiar with and understands the contents of this text as it represents the background to the present invention.... Chocolate is generally obtained by mixing sugar and cocoa butter with cocoa liquor or cocoa nibs, followed by refining, conching and tempering. Milk chocolate is prepared in a similar way but with the addition of milk. White chocolate is prepared in a similar way to milk chocolate but without the addition of cocoa liquor. One traditional method of producing milk chocolate (i.e., the dry process) is by mixing milk powder together with cocoa liquor or cocoa nibs, sugar, and cocoa butter, followed by refining, conching and tempering. White chocolate may be prepared in a similar way to the above method of preparing milk chocolate but in the absence of cocoa liquor and cocoa nibs.

  Web site: http://appft1.uspto.gov/netahtml/PTO/search-bool.html

- **Chocolate production by super-cooling and press-forming**

Inventor(s): Kirtley, Nigel; (Rhode-St-Genese, BE), Ebbinghaus, Lars; (Sollentua, SE), Wutz, Harald; (Munchen, DE), Demmer, Thomas; (Munchen, DE), Baxter, John F. (Munchen, DE)

Correspondence: FITCH EVEN TABIN AND FLANNERY; 120 SOUTH LA SALLE STREET; SUITE 1600; CHICAGO; IL; 606033406

Patent Application Number: 20020015775

Date filed: April 27, 2001

Abstract: The present invention relates to a process for producing chocolate wherein liquid chocolate mass is subjected to tempering, super-cooling and press-forming. This process allows a quick and simple production of chocolate products having a good and glossy surface appearance.

Excerpt(s): The present invention relates to a novel process for the production of chocolate. The invention moreover pertains to the use of stamps for the press-forming of chocolate.... Chocolate is undoubtedly one of the most popular types of confectionary. This is reflected by the enormous amounts of chocolate consumed. In 1989 the consumed amount per person was as high as 6.9 kg on average, which sums up to several hundred thousand tons each year.... Given these huge amounts of chocolate, the industry is continuously trying to improve existing chocolate production processes or to invent new methods for manufacturing. The driving force behind such research and development activities is the need for quick and simple production processes which allow the production of high -quality chocolate.

Web site: http://appft1.uspto.gov/netahtml/PTO/search-bool.html

- **Chocolate-based fat system having improved organoleptic properties**

Inventor(s): Choy, Edward; (Thornhill, CA), Miller, Vladimir; (Thornhill, CA), Miller, Van; (Norval, CA)

Correspondence: MARKS & CLERK; 350 BURNHAMTHORPE ROAD WEST; SUITE 402; MISSISSAUGA; ON; L5B 3J1; CA

Patent Application Number: 20020081359

Date filed: February 4, 2002

Abstract: An edible anhydrous chocolate-based fat system is provided, having a significant granulated sugar component. This provides an unusual mouth sense, and allows for significantly different organoleptic properties of the chocolate-based fat system--which otherwise emulates chocolate. The chocolate may be light or dark, or white chocolate. An additional sweet flavor may be added to the chocolate-based fat system, allowing for a faster release of the additional flavor, by infusing or saturating the granulated sugar component of the fat system with the additional flavor. Typically, the granulated sugar component is saturated with an essential oil of a chosen flavor. Apart from the granulated sugar component, the remaining ingredients of the chocolate-based fat system are conched in the usual manner in keeping with chocolate production techniques. A process for production of the edible anhydrous chocolate-based fat system is discussed, and typical machinery for carrying out that process is shown.

Excerpt(s): This invention relates to a new chocolate-based fat system which has improved organoleptic properties. Specifically, the present invention relates to an edible anhydrous chocolate-based fat system having a granulated sugar component which provides the improved organoleptic properties, and which also results in a distinctly different mouth sense. In a particular embodiment of the present invention, the edible anhydrous chocolate-based fat system is flavor infused with an additional sweet flavor, which is brought into the chocolate-based fat system by way of flavor-saturated granulated sugar.... Chocolate has been known in many forms for many years. Traditional forms of chocolate include dark, light, white, and milk chocolates which may be used as a snack item or confection, or for coating other food items. More recently, chocolate has been utilized not only as a flavor but in chip or chunk form as an additive in baked goods and flour confections such as cookies and the like. Finally, chocolate endures almost universal appeal simply for its flavor, its mouth feel--generally, confection chocolates are based on fat systems which melt easily in the mouth, whereas chocolate chips and the like are based on harder fat systems so as to retain their integrity during the baking process--and because of its relatively easy portability. Chocolate may be packaged or wrapped in relatively small portions, for consumption as a snack, for example.... However, until now all chocolate products where chocolate is a principal constituent, and where the chocolate is presented as a stable fat system at room temperature, have been smooth and with a distinct chocolate flavor. That flavor may range from quite sweet to bitter, depending on the sugar content, and whether or not the chocolate is a milk chocolate, light or dark brown chocolate, or white chocolate. Some chocolates may be flavored, typically by the use of mint; but all chocolates are highly conched--that is, they have a high degree of fineness.

Web site: http://appft1.uspto.gov/netahtml/PTO/search-bool.html

- **Cocoa extract compounds and methods for making and using the same**

Inventor(s): Schmitz, Harold H. (Branchburg, NJ), Romanczyk,, Leo J. JR. (Hackettstown, NJ)

Correspondence: CLIFFORD CHANCE US LLP; 200 PARK AVENUE; NEW YORK; NY; 10166; US

Patent Application Number: 20030113290

Date filed: April 22, 2002

Abstract: Disclosed and claimed are cocoa extracts, compounds, combinations thereof and compositions containing the same, such as polyphenols or procyanidins, methods for preparing such extracts, compounds and compositions, as well as uses for them, especially a polymeric compound of the formula A_n, wherein A is a monomer of the formula: 1wherein n is an integer from 2 to 18, such that there is at least one terminal monomeric unit A, and one or a plurality of additional monomeric units;R is 3-(.alpha.)--OH, 3-(.beta.)--OH, 3-(.alpha.)--O-sugar, or 3-(.beta.)--O-sugar;bonding between adjacent monomers takes place at positions 4, 6 or 8;a bond of an additional monomeric unit in position 4 has alpha or beta stereochemistry;X, Y and Z are selected from the group consisting of monomeric unit A, hydrogen, and a sugar, with the provisos that as to the at least one terminal monomeric unit, bonding of the additional monomeric unit thereto (the bonding of the additional monomeric unit adjacent to the terminal monomeric unit) is at position 4 and optionally Y=Z=hydrogen;the sugar is optionally substituted with a phenolic moiety, at any position on the sugar, for instance via an ester bond, andpharmaceutically acceptable salts or derivatives thereof (including oxidation products).

Excerpt(s): Reference is made to copending U.S. application Ser. No. 08/709,406, filed Sep. 6, 1996, Ser. No. 08/631,661, filed Apr. 2, 1996, and Ser. No. 08/317,226, filed Oct. 3, 1994 (now U.S. Pat. No. 5,554,645) and PCT/US96/04497, each of which is incorporated herein by reference.... This invention relates to cocoa extracts and compounds therefrom such as polyphenols preferably polyphenols enriched with procyanidins. This invention also relates to methods for preparing such extracts and compounds, as well as to uses for them; for instance, as antineoplastic agents, antioxidants, DNA topoisomerase II enzyme inhibitors, cyclo-oxygenase and/or lipoxygenase modulators, NO (Nitric Oxide) or NO-synthase modulators, as non-steroidal antiinflammatory agents, apoptosis modulators, platelet aggregation modulators, blood or in vivo glucose modulators, antimicrobials, and inhibitors of oxidative DNA damage.... Documents are cited in this disclosure with a full citation for each appearing thereat or in a References section at the end of the specification, preceding the claims. These documents pertain to the field of this invention; and, each document cited herein is hereby incorporated herein by reference.

Web site: http://appft1.uspto.gov/netahtml/PTO/search-bool.html

- **Cocoa extracts containing solvent-derived cocoa polyphenols from defatted cocoa beans**

Inventor(s): Buck, Margaret M. (Morristown, NJ), Romanczyk, Leo J. JR. (Hackettstown, NJ), Hammerstone, John F. JR. (Nazareth, PA)

Correspondence: CLIFFORD CHANCE US LLP; 200 PARK AVENUE; NEW YORK; NY; 10166; US

Patent Application Number: 20030176493

Date filed: January 15, 2003

Abstract: Disclosed and claimed are cocoa extracts such as polyphenols or procyanidins, methods for preparing such extracts, as well as uses for them, especially as antineoplastic agents and antioxidants. Disclosed and claimed are antineoplastic compositions containing cocoa polyphenols or procyanidins and methods for treating patients employing the compositions. Additionally disclosed and claimed is a kit for treating a patient in need of treatment with an antineoplastic agent containing cocoa polyphenols or procyanidins as well as a lyophilized antineoplastic composition containing cocoa polyphenols or procyanidins. Further, disclosed and claimed is the use of the invention in antioxidant, preservative and topiosomerase-inhibiting compositions and methods.

Excerpt(s): This invention relates to cocoa extracts such as polyphenols preferably polyphenols enriched with procyanidins. This invention also relates to methods for preparing such extracts, as well as to uses for them; for instance, as antineoplastic agents and antioxidants.... Documents are cited in this disclosure with a full citation for each appearing in a References section at the end of the specification, preceding the claims. These documents pertain to the field of this invention; and, each document cited herein is hereby incorporated herein by reference.... Polyphenols are an incredibly diverse group of compounds (Ferreira et al., 1992) which widely occur in a variety of plants, some of which enter into the food chain. In some cases they represent an important class of compounds for the human diet. Although some of the polyphenols are considered to be nonnutrative, interest in these compounds has arisen because of their possible beneficial effects on health. For instance, quercitin (a flavonoid) has been shown to possess anticarcinogenic activity in experimental animal studies (Deshner et al., 1991 and Kato et al., 1983). (+)-Catechin and (-)-epicatechin (flavan-3-ols) have been shown to inhibit Leukemia virus reverse transcriptase activity (Chu et al., 1992). Nobotanin (an oligomeric hydrolyzable tannin) has also been shown to possess anti-tumor activity (Okuda et al., 1992). Statistical reports have also shown that stomach cancer mortality is significantly lower in the tea producing districts of Japan. Epigallocatechin gallate has been reported to be the pharmacologically active material in green tea that inhibits mouse skin tumors (Okuda et al., 1992). Ellagic acid has also been shown to possess anticarcinogen activity in various animal tumor models (Bukharta et al., 1992). Lastly, proanthocyanidin oligomers have been patented by the Kikkoman Corporation for use as antimutageris. Indeed, the area of phenolic compounds in foods and their modulation of tumor development in experimental animal models has been recently presented at the 202nd National Meeting of The American Chemical Society (Ho et al., 1992; Huang et al., 1992).

Web site: http://appft1.uspto.gov/netahtml/PTO/search-bool.html

- **Cocoa sphingolipids, cocoa extracts containing sphingolipids and methods of making and using same**

Inventor(s): Schmitz, Harold H. (Branchburg, NJ), Lazarus, Sheryl; (Centerville, OH), Hammerstone, John F. (Nazareth, PA)

Correspondence: Clifford Chance Rogers & Wells LLP; 200 Park Avenue; New York; NY; 10166-0153; US

Patent Application Number: 20010041683

Date filed: March 8, 2001

Abstract: The invention relates to cocoa sphingolipids, cocoa extracts containing cocoa sphingolipids, and compositions containing cocoa sphingolipids and/or metabolic derivatives thereof. The invention also relates to methods of isolating and purifying sphingolipids and methods of using the cocoa sphingolipids and/or metabolic derivatives thereof.

Excerpt(s): This application claims priority under 35 U.S.C..sctn. 119 from the U.S. Provisional Application Ser. No. 60/187,950, filed Mar. 9, 2000, which application is hereby incorporated herein by reference in its entirety.... The invention relates to cocoa sphingolipids, cocoa extracts containing cocoa sphingolipids, and compositions containing cocoa sphingolipids and/or metabolic derivatives thereof. The invention also relates to methods of isolating and purifying sphingolipids and methods of using the cocoa sphingolipids and/or metabolic derivatives thereof.... In the late nineteenth century, sphingolipids were discovered in the mammalian brain by J. L. W. Thudichum. It is now known that sphingolipids are not limited to the brain; they can be found in all eukaryotic and some prokaryotic organisms (Merrill et al., Symposium: Animal Diets for Nutritional and Toxicological Research, pp. 830S-33S, Am. Soc. Nutr. Sci. 1997, Witaker, Phytochem., 42:627-632, 1996; Ohnishi et al., Biochimica Biophysica Acta, 752: 416-422; 1983; Ohnishi and Fujino, Lipids, 17:803-810 (1982); Laine and Renkonen, Biochem., 13:2837-43; 1974; Walter et al., 36:795-97; 1971)).

Web site: http://appft1.uspto.gov/netahtml/PTO/search-bool.html

- **Composition and process for producing thickened coffee, tea or cocoa beverages**

Inventor(s): O' Connor, Donna Jean; (Maple Grove, MN), Meister, Jeffery D. (Plymouth, MN)

Correspondence: THOMAS HOXIE; NOVARTIS CORPORATION; PATENT AND TRADEMARK DEPT; 564 MORRIS AVENUE; SUMMIT; NJ; 079011027

Patent Application Number: 20020086098

Date filed: December 6, 2001

Abstract: An improved thickened instant coffee beverage mix, comprising a mix of from about 15-90%, preferably 27%, maltodextrin with the rest, to 100%, of an agglomerated starch, and also 0.05-2.0% of mono- and di-glycerides or other wetting agents such as propylene glycol, glycerin, sorbitan monosterate and other emulsifiers, including 0.05-10.0% vegetable oils, together with coffee flavorants, which can be quickly dissolved in water of at least 120.degree. F. water without delay or forming clumps; and an improved thickened instant tea or cocoa beverage mix which can be quickly dissolved in water of at least 120.degree. F. water without delay or forming clumps, comprising 12-50% agglomerated starch as the thickening agent, together with sugar and protein components.

Excerpt(s): This application is a CIP of co-pending U.S. Ser. No. 09/552,373, filed Apr. 19, 2000, now _____, which in turn was a CIP of copending U.S. Ser. No. 09/247,467, filed Feb. 8, 1999, now U.S. Pat. No. 6,217,931, issued Apr. 17, 2001, which was a continuation of U.S. Ser. No. 09/022,195, filed Feb. 11,1998, now abandoned, the latter having been converted to Provisional application USS No. 60/126,422 and also to Provisional application USS No. 60/108,074, filed Nov. 12,1998, both now abandoned.... The present invention relates generally to compositions which when mixed with hot water, yield thickened coffee, tea or cocoa beverages, and to the process for obtaining such compositions.... Thickened beverages are used by patients in long term health care facilities and hospitals to address a swallowing condition known as dysphasia. It has been known that patients with swallowing problems are capable of handling thickened beverages. Because of the nature of this condition, it is important that the patient receive a product that is smooth textured and free of lumps. The degree of thickening needed is determined by the severity of the swallowing condition. Therefore, the beverage must also be consistent in terms of thickness from use to use. In recent years many new products have been introduced to address this need. These have included dry mixes, in which a starch is spooned into a liquid and mixed, as well as ready to serve thickened drinks. While the powered products have worked acceptably well in cold beverages, they have been unsuccessful in hot applications.

Web site: http://appft1.uspto.gov/netahtml/PTO/search-bool.html

- **Composition comprising cocoa**

Inventor(s): Raggers, Rene John; (Amsterdam, NL), Verdegem, Peter Julien Edward; (Zetten, NL), Ter Laak, Wies; (Amsterdam, NL)

Correspondence: YOUNG & THOMPSON; 745 SOUTH 23RD STREET 2ND FLOOR; ARLINGTON; VA; 22202

Patent Application Number: 20020172732

Date filed: March 21, 2001

Abstract: The invention pertains to a composition and a method for the treatment of mood disorders, in particular of treating, preventing or alleviating depression, mood disorders or insufficient mood, obesity, overweight, premenstrual syndrome, craving, carbohydrate craving, chocolate craving, menopausal complaints, erectile dysfunction and/or reduced libido, The composition contains cocoa or one or more of its pharmacologically active components, and a dopamine D2 receptor agonist.

Excerpt(s): The invention concerns nutritional and pharmaceutical compositions containing cocoa components for improving mood.... Cocoa and chocolate comprise several advantageous pharmacologically active components, and have therefore, knowingly or unknowingly, been used to alleviate or treat certain disorders. There remains a vast interest for compositions which induce the pharmacological effects of cocoa or chocolate, however which do not have the adverse side effect induced by chocolate and/or cocoa or one or more of its pharmacological components. Products available within the art, which provide the advantageous effects of the pharmacological compounds within the cocoa/chocolate, appeared insufficient. Many cocoa-containing products have high fat or carbohydrate content, causing obesity and overweight. Alternatives to these products include diet and low fat products, such as low fat cocoa powder, cocoa extracts and the like.... Pharmacological compounds within cocoa or chocolate have been used in products providing appetite suppression and mood improvement.

Web site: http://appft1.uspto.gov/netahtml/PTO/search-bool.html

- **Dry cocoa mix containing a mixture of non-alkalized and alkalized cocoa solids**

Inventor(s): Hammerstone, John F. JR. (Nazareth, PA), Whitacre, Eric J. (Elizabethtown, PA), Nwosu, Chigozie V. (Hackettstown, NJ), Myers, Mary E. (Lititz, PA)

Correspondence: Clifford Chance Rogers & Wells LLP; 200 Park Avenue; New York; NY; 10166-0153; US

Patent Application Number: 20020136819

Date filed: November 9, 2001

Abstract: The invention provides food products, including confectioneries and chocolates, having conserved concentrations of polyphenols, and in particular cocoa polyphenols. The method of this invention avoids the significant and detrimental losses of polyphenols that occur during conventional manufacture by controlling the handling of ingredients in batching processing to provide a product having a significant amount of the cocoa polyphenol concentration present in the raw materials conserved in the finished product. Additionally, the production steps of milling/refining and conching may also be controlled and modified to provide the confectioneries of the present invention having conserved concentrations of cocoa polyphenols relative to the concentration of the polyphenols present in the starting ingredients. The cocoa polyphenol ingredient may be a cocoa ingredient, an extract of a cocoa ingredient (beans, liquor, or powder, etc.) or may be a synthesized derivative thereof, or may be a synthesized polyphenol compound or mixture of polyphenol compounds or derivative thereof.

Excerpt(s): The invention relates to food products having a conserved or enhanced content of cocoa polyphenols and processes for producing the same. The food products prepared by the processes of this invention include edible food products, confectionery products and standard of identity and non-standard of identity chocolate products, and the like, having conserved concentrations of cocoa polyphenols therein.... salts, derivatives and oxidation products thereof.... Advantageously, the saccharide moiety is derived from the group consisting of glucose, galactose, xylose, rhamnose and arabinose. The saccharide moiety and any or all of R, X, Y, and Z may optionally be substituted at any position with a phenolic moiety via an ester bond. The phenolic moiety is selected from the group consisting of caffeic, cinnamic, coumaric, ferulic, gallic, hydroxybenzoic and sinapic acids.

Web site: http://appft1.uspto.gov/netahtml/PTO/search-bool.html

- **Dry drink mix and chocolate flavored drink made therefrom**

Inventor(s): Hammerstone, John F. JR. (Nazareth, PA), Geyer, Hans M. (Hershey, PA), Schmitz, Harold H. (Branchburg, NJ), Myers, Mary E. (Lititz, PA), Romanczyk, Leo J. JR. (Hackettstown, NJ), Snyder, Rodney M. (Elizabethtown, PA), Kealey, Kirk S. (Lancaster, PA), Whitacre, Eric J. (Elizabethtown, PA)

Correspondence: Margaret B. Kelley, Esq. Clifford Chance Rogers & Wells LLP; 200 Park Avenue; New York; NY; 10166-0153; US

Patent Application Number: 20020064584

Date filed: November 5, 2001

Abstract: Cocoa components having enhanced levels of cocoa polyphenols, processes for producing the cocoa components while conserving a significant amount of the cocoa polyphenols, compositions containing the cocoa components or the cocoa polyphenols, and methods of using the cocoa components or the cocoa polyphenols for improving the health of a mammal are described. The cocoa components include partially and fully defatted cocoa solids, cocoa nibs and fractions derived therefrom, cocoa polyphenol extracts, cocoa butter, chocolate liquors, and mixtures thereof. The invention provides processes for extracting fat from cocoa beans and for otherwise processing cocoa beans to yield a cocoa component having conserved concentrations of polyphenols relative to the starting materials.

Excerpt(s): Reference is made to copending U.S. applications Ser. No. 08/317,226, filed Oct. 3, 1994 (allowed, now U.S. Pat. No. 5,554,645), Ser. No. 08/631,661, filed Apr. 2, 1996, Ser. No. 08/709,406, filed Sep. 6, 1996, and Ser. No. 08/831,245, filed Apr. 2, 1997, incorporated herein by reference.... The invention relates to cocoa components having enhanced levels of cocoa polyphenols, processes for producing the same, methods of using the same and compositions containing the same. More specifically, the invention provides a method of producing cocoa components having an enhanced content of cocoa polyphenols, in particular procyanidins. The cocoa components include partially and fully defatted cocoa solids, cocoa nibs and fractions derived therefrom, cocoa polyphenol extracts, cocoa butter, chocolate liquors, and mixtures thereof.... The invention also relates to versatile novel processes for extracting fat from cocoa beans and/or processing cocoa beans to yield a cocoa component having a conserved level of polyphenols, in particular procyanidins. The invention provides a significantly less complex process with respect to total cost of process equipment, maintenance, energy and labor, with the concomitant benefit of obtaining components having conserved concentrations of polyphenols relative to the starting materials.

Web site: http://appft1.uspto.gov/netahtml/PTO/search-bool.html

- **Extraction of sterols from cocoa hulls**

  Inventor(s): Romanczyk, Leo J. JR. (Hackettstown, NJ), McClelland, Craig; (E. Stroudsburg, PA)

  Correspondence: Clifford Chance Rogers & Wells LLP; 200 Park Avenue; New York; NY; 10166-0153; US

  Patent Application Number: 20020048613

  Date filed: April 11, 2001

  Abstract: Cocoa oils containing phytosterols and tocols are prepared by extracting the cocoa hulls from dried unfermented or fermented cocoa beans, micronized cocoa beans, or roasted beans with a solvent such as petroleum ether and then removing the solvent. The cocoa oils are useful in foods, dietary supplements, pharmaceuticals, and cosmetics.

  Excerpt(s): This application claims the benefit of filing date of U.S. provisional application Ser. No. 60/197,134 entitled EXTRACTION OF STEROLS FROM COCOA HULLS which was filed on Apr. 14,2000.... This invention is directed to the extraction of valuable by-products from cocoa hulls.... Cocoa hulls are a waste by-product of the roasting of cocoa beans and have little value in chocolate manufacturing. Generally, the cocoa hulls are used as compost.

  Web site: http://appft1.uspto.gov/netahtml/PTO/search-bool.html

- **Food products having enhanced cocoa polyphenol content and processes for producing the same**

  Inventor(s): Myers, Mary E. (Lititz, PA), Hammerstone, John F. JR. (Nazareth, PA), Nwosu, Chigozie V. (Hackettstown, NJ), Whitacre, Eric J. (Elizabethtown, PA)

  Correspondence: Clifford Chance Rogers & Wells LLP; 200 Park Avenue; New York; NY; 10166-0153; US

  Patent Application Number: 20010007693

  Date filed: January 17, 2001

  Abstract: The invention provides food products, including confectioneries and chocolates, having conserved concentrations of polyphenols, and in particular cocoa polyphenols. The method of this invention avoids the significant and detrimental losses of polyphenols that occur during conventional manufacture by controlling the handling of ingredients in batching processing to provide a product having a significant amount of the cocoa polyphenol concentration present in the raw materials conserved in the finished product. Additionally, the production steps of milling/refining and conching may also be controlled and modified to provide the confectioneries of the present invention having conserved concentrations of cocoa polyphenols relative to the concentration of the polyphenols present in the starting ingredients. The cocoa polyphenol ingredient may be a cocoa ingredient, an extract of a cocoa ingredient (beans, liquor, or powder, etc.) or may be a synthesized derivative thereof, or may be a synthesized polyphenol compound or mixture of polyphenol compounds or derivative thereof.

  Excerpt(s): The invention relates to food products having a conserved or enhanced content of cocoa polyphenols and processes for producing the same. The food products prepared by the processes of this invention include edible food products, confectionery products and standard of identity and non-standard of identity chocolate products, and the like, having conserved concentrations of cocoa polyphenols therein.... salts, derivatives and oxidation products thereof.... Advantageously, the saccharide moiety is derived from the group consisting of glucose, galactose, xylose, rhamnose and arabinose. The saccharide moiety and any or all of R, X, Y, and Z may optionally be substituted at any position with a phenolic moiety via an ester bond. The phenolic moiety is selected from the group consisting of caffeic, cinnamic, coumaric, ferulic, gallic, hydroxybenzoic and sinapic acids.

Web site: http://appft1.uspto.gov/netahtml/PTO/search-bool.html

- **Health of a mammal by administering a composition containing at least one cocoa polyphenol ingredient**

  Inventor(s): Hammerstone, John F. JR. (Nazareth, PA), Geyer, Hans M; (Hershey, PA), Schmitz, Harold H. (Branchburg, NJ), Myers, Mary E. (Lititz, PA), Romanczyk, Leo J. JR. (Hackettstown, NJ), Snyder, Rodney M. (Elizabethtown, PA), Kealey, Kirk S. (Lancaster, PA), Whitacre, Eric J. (Elizabethtown, PA)

  Correspondence: Clifford Chance Rogers & Wells LLP; 200 Park Avenue; New York; NY; 10166-0153; US

  Patent Application Number: 20020045002

  Date filed: October 16, 2001

  Abstract: Cocoa components having enhanced levels of cocoa polyphenols, processes for producing the cocoa components while conserving a significant amount of the cocoa polyphenols, compositions containing the cocoa components or the cocoa polyphenols, and methods of using the cocoa components or the cocoa polyphenols for improving the health of a mammal are described. The cocoa components include partially and fully defatted cocoa solids, cocoa nibs and fractions derived therefrom, cocoa polyphenol extracts, cocoa butter, chocolate liquors, and mixtures thereof. The invention provides processes for extracting fat from cocoa beans and for otherwise processing cocoa beans to yield a cocoa component having conserved concentrations of polyphenols relative to the starting materials.

  Excerpt(s): Reference is made to copending U.S. applications Ser. No. 08/317,226, filed Oct. 3, 1994 (allowed, now U.S. Pat. No. 5,554,645), Ser. No. 08/631,661, filed Apr. 2, 1996, Ser. No. 08/709,406, filed Sep. 6, 1996, and Ser. No. 08/831,245, filed Apr. 2, 1997, incorporated herein by reference.... The invention relates to cocoa components having enhanced levels of cocoa polyphenols, processes for producing the same, methods of using the same and compositions containing the same. More specifically, the invention provides a method of producing cocoa components having an enhanced content of cocoa polyphenols, in particular procyanidins. The cocoa components include partially and fully defatted cocoa solids, cocoa nibs and fractions derived therefrom, cocoa polyphenol extracts, cocoa butter, chocolate liquors, and mixtures thereof.... The invention also relates to versatile novel processes for extracting fat from cocoa beans and/or processing cocoa beans to yield a cocoa component having a conserved level of polyphenols, in particular procyanidins. The invention provides a significantly less complex process with respect to total cost of process equipment, maintenance, energy and labor, with the concomitant benefit of obtaining components having conserved concentrations of polyphenols relative to the starting materials.

  Web site: http://appft1.uspto.gov/netahtml/PTO/search-bool.html

- **Low-flavor cocoa, a method of its production and a use thereof**

  Inventor(s): Lindblom, Marianne Gunilla; (Sollentuna, SE), Biehl, Bole; (Braunschweig, DE)

  Correspondence: FITCH EVEN TABIN AND FLANNERY; 120 SOUTH LA SALLE STREET; SUITE 1600; CHICAGO; IL; 606033406

  Patent Application Number: 20020034579

  Date filed: April 13, 2001

  Abstract: The invention relates to a novel low-flavor cocoa, a method for its production and a use thereof. The novel low-flavor cocoa is obtainable from unfermented cocoa beans by a two step process. In the first step the unfermented beans are treated to destroy the cellular and subcellular structures and then in a second step they are subjected to an oxidation treatment. This method suppresses the formation of flavor and hence low-flavor cocoa is obtained which is e.g. useful as substitute for cocoa butter in the manufacture of chocolate and for the compensation of variations in the flavor intensity of untreated cocoa.

  Excerpt(s): The invention relates to novel low-flavor cocoa, a method of its production and a use thereof.... Cocoa is one of the most important ingredients, it not the most important ingredient, in the production of a variety of cocoa products such as different types of chocolate. Cocoa mass is produced by grinding cocoa nibs. Cocoa nibs are constituents of the seeds of the cocoa tree Theobroma cacao I,. Cocoa seeds are cocoa beans with the surrounding pulp. The cocoa beans consist of the cocoa nibs and a shell that surrounds them.... The cocoa mass consists on the one hand of fatty constituents, the so-called cocoa butter, and on the other hand of non-fatty constituents which will be designated as cocoa powder in the following.

  Web site: http://appft1.uspto.gov/netahtml/PTO/search-bool.html

- **Method and apparatus for producing ice-creams or similar products with stick, covered with chocolate or similar products**

  Inventor(s): Grigoli, Franco Albino Luigi; (Milano, IT)

  Correspondence: NOTARO & MICHALOS P.C. Empire State Building; Suite 6902; 350 Fifth Avenue; New York; NY; 10118-6985; US

  Patent Application Number: 20020146488

  Date filed: January 4, 2002

  Abstract: An apparatus and method for producing ice-creams with sticks includes filling chilled molds with a covering product, for example chocolate. Excess chocolate is suctioned from the molds so that only the desired layer of frozen product adheres to the molds. The molds are then filled with ice-cream or other edible product and insertion of the stick takes place before the starting of the freezing of the product or during or soon afterwards for obtaining the best results. Gas freezing then occurs for obtaining a closing "plug" of the tub followed by brine freezing.

  Excerpt(s): optionally measure such a chocolate layer or other edible product to complete the covering.... Said method according to the invention allows to obtain ice-creams or similar covered products, by accurately giving to the covering layer the desired shape.... In addition, it is also possible to make use of existing apparatuses, without the need to produce ad hoc equipment, but by completing the system with components already in use in the same sector.

Web site: http://appft1.uspto.gov/netahtml/PTO/search-bool.html

- **Method and apparatus for the production of shells of fat-containing, chocolate-like masses under pressure build-up.**

Inventor(s): Aasted, Lars; (Charlottenlund, DK)

Correspondence: JOHN W. FREEMAN, ESQ. Fish & Richardson P.C. 225 Franklin Street; Boston; MA; 02110-2804; US

Patent Application Number: 20030003210

Date filed: August 20, 2002

Abstract: Systems and methods for producing chocolate shells by immersing a core into a liquid filled mold cavity. The temperature of the core member is controlled. A mold-cavity closure extends peripherally around the core member in closing engagement with the mold. The closure is axially movable in relation to the core member. The core member is immersed fully into the liquid mass and pressed in a direction against the mold cavity by a load means to build up pressure in the chocolate mass. Also disclosed is the above mentioned cavity closure which is axially movable in relation to, and connected to, the core.

Excerpt(s): The present invention concerns a method for the production of fat-containing, chocolate-like masses, in particular for chocolate articles, by which an amount of liquid mass is deposited into a mould cavity, whereafter an associated core member is immersed into the mass, the temperature of which core member is being controlled.... Methods of the above mentioned types as well as associated apparatus are to-day well-known within the prior art, and are being used extensively by the chocolate making industry.... EP 0 589 820 A1 (AASTED-MIKROVERK APS) describes the first commercially available method and associated apparatus of the introductory type for industrial use. It relates to a method, where the chocolate-like mass under crystallisation solidifies from the mould cavity and inwardly to form the outer shape of the shell, the temperature of the mould cavity being lower than the temperature of the tempered mass, that a cooling member having a temperature lower than 0.degree. C. is immersed into the mass and kept in the mass in a fully immersed position for a predetermined period of time. The cooling member is furthermore immersed immediately into the mass after this has been filled into the mould cavity. The associated apparatus furthermore comprises means of controlling the up- and down movement of the cooling members, as well as controlling residence times in the fully immersed position. However, by this early teaching within the technical field of the present invention the chocolate-mass is filled into the mould cavity in an amount, which is typically about 10% larger than the volume of the finished chocolate-shell. The early EP-publication teaches no means for enclosing the mould cavity at the rim of the shell, and consequently the mass rises pressureless above the upper surface of the mould plate, when a cooling member is being immersed to the fully immersed position. The teaching describes no means for enclosing the mould cavity fully, nor for building up pressure in the chocolate-mass during moulding.

Web site: http://appft1.uspto.gov/netahtml/PTO/search-bool.html

- **Method and arrangement for processing cocoa mass; resulting products**

  Inventor(s): Gusek, Todd Walter; (Crystal, MN), Purtle, Ian Charles; (Plymouth, MN)

  Correspondence: FOLEY & LARDNER; 777 EAST WISCONSIN AVENUE; MILWAUKEE; WI; 53202; US

  Patent Application Number: 20020176916

  Date filed: November 29, 2001

  Abstract: Techniques for processing cocoa mass are provided. In general, the techniques involve solvent extraction of cocoa fat from cocoa mass, to achieve a desirable cocoa butter and low-fat cocoa powder. In one preferred process, the cocoa mass is the result of grinding cocoa nibs, with absence of a mechanical pressing and heating step, to advantage. Preferred products and uses are characterized.

  Excerpt(s): The present invention relates to processing of cocoa. It particularly concerns processing cocoa mass to generate separated cocoa powder and cocoa butter, both at desirable quality levels and in desirable yields.... Cocoa beans may be processed into cocoa butter and cocoa powder. Cocoa butter represents a portion of the fat content isolated from the cocoa beans. The cocoa powder represents remaining solids, after processing to recover cocoa butter.... Cocoa butters are widely utilized food additives. For example, cocoa butter is used in the production of chocolate. Cocoa powder is also used as a food additive for flavor and color, for example, to produce chocolate flavored milk, cake mixes and brownie mixes.

  Web site: http://appft1.uspto.gov/netahtml/PTO/search-bool.html

- **Method for enhancing post-processing content of beneficial compounds in foodstuffs made with cocoa beans**

  Inventor(s): Zhao, Jifu; (Littleton, CO), Slaga, Thomas J. (Golden, CO), Zapp, Loretta M. (Boulder, CO), Lange, Mark; (Apex, NC)

  Correspondence: DAVID G. HENRY; P.O. Box 1470; 900 Washington Avenue; Waco; TX; 76701; US

  Patent Application Number: 20020081363

  Date filed: November 14, 2001

  Abstract: A new cocoa bean processing technique which, in stark contrast to conventional cocoa processing methods, preserves the beneficial flavanoid compounds of cocoa beans in finished, cocoa bean-based foodstuffs. The present method produces roasted cocoa beans that can be ground and the liquor can be either cooled and allowed to solidify (unsweetened chocolate) or pressed and re-ground to form cocoa powder. The resulting cocoa powder can then be used in a traditional manner to make sweetened chocolate products such as candy and beverages for consumption by humans or animals. The resulting products will be a source of flavanoid compounds, which are known antioxidants.

  Excerpt(s): This is a continuation-in-part with respect to U.S. application, Ser. No. 09/843,543 which was a continuation-in-part of U.S. application Ser. No. 09/481,279 which, in turn, was a continuation-in-part of U.S. application Ser. No. 09/481,279, which, in turn, was a continuation-in-part of U.S. application Ser. No. 09/468,560, from all of which priority is claimed under 35 U.S.C..sctn.120.... The present invention relates to food processing, and in particular to cocoa bean processing and its products.... Test-tube studies by German scientists recently showed that the tetramers found in chocolate were highly beneficial in curbing the type of oxidation damage to blood vessel walls that arise from free-radicals in the blood stream. Chocolate's tetramers and larger procyanidins also help relax the inner surface of blood vessels, according to studies in isolated tissues headed by C. Tissa Kappagoda of the University of California, Davis School of Medicine.

Web site: http://appft1.uspto.gov/netahtml/PTO/search-bool.html

- **Method for extracting cocoa procyanidins**

Inventor(s): Hammerstone, John F. JR. (Nazareth, PA), Chimel, Mark J. (Long Valley, NJ)

Correspondence: Clifford Chance US LLP; 200 Park Avenue; New York; NY; 10166-0153; US

Patent Application Number: 20030157207

Date filed: November 12, 2002

Abstract: A cocoa extract which is rich in procyanidin monomers and oligomers is made by extracting de-fatted, unroasted, unfermented cocoa beans with organic solvents. The yield of procyanidins in an extract varies with type of solvent used, reaction temperature, reaction pH and whether or not the solvent is an aqueous solution. Extraction parameters can be optimized to increase procyanidin yield, and different conditions result in the preferential extraction of the higher or lower oligomers. A preferred extraction method is counter-current extraction method.

Excerpt(s): This invention is directed to improved methods for the extraction of cocoa procyanidin monomers and oligomers from the cocoa solids.... It is known that regular consumption of dietary polyphenols, commonly found in a variety of fruits and vegetables, is beneficial. Red wine, green tea and cocoa have all been identified as being rich in polyphenols, and the regular consumption red wine and green tea have both been shown to be inversely associated with heart disease deaths in industrialized countries.... It is well-known that the polyphenols of cocoa contribute significantly to the development of flavour in the fermented and roasted cocoa bean. Astringent and bitter flavors in cocoa have been traditionally associated with the presence of xanthine alkaloids and polyphenols in the cocoa beans. For this reason, various methods have been developed over the years to extract the cocoa polyphenols to verify their presence, to quantify their amounts, and to identify them. The cocoa polyphenols are primarily cocoa procyanidins. However, no extraction method has thus far been optimized to yield extracts high in cocoa procyanidins.

Web site: http://appft1.uspto.gov/netahtml/PTO/search-bool.html

- **Method for reducing postprandial oxidative stress using cocoa procyanidins**

Inventor(s): Schmitz, Harold H. (Branchburg, NJ), Romanczyk, Leo J. JR. (Hackettstown, NJ)

Correspondence: Clifford Chance US LLP; 200 Park Avenue; New York; NY; 10166-0153; US

Patent Application Number: 20030100601

Date filed: November 27, 2002

Abstract: A method for reducing postprandial oxidative stress and associated pathologies by the dietary intake of cocoa procyanidins, such as epicatechin is disclosed.

Excerpt(s): This invention relates to a method for reducing postprandial oxidative stress.... Studies have linked certain dietary factors with atherosclerosis, a forerunner of coronary heart disease (Addis, P. B., Carr, T. P., Hassel, C. A., Hwang, Z. Z., Warner, G. J., Atherogenic and anti-atherogenic factors in the human diet. Biochem. Soc. Symp. 61, 259-271 (1995)). For example, a diet high in polyunsaturated fatty acids (PUFAS) may render low-density lipoprotein (LDL) more susceptible to peroxidation (Addis et al. 1995). The peroxidation of LDL can cause tissue damage leading to atherosclerosis (Sarkkinen, E. S., Uusitupa, M. I. J., Nyyssonen, K., Parviainen, M., Penttila, I., Salonen, J. T., Effects of two low-fat diets, high and low in polyunsaturated fatty acids, on plasma lipid peroxides and serum vitamin E levels in free-living hypercholesterolaemic men. European Journal of Clinical Nutrition (1993) 47: 623-630). The peroxidation of LDL is a result of the neutrophilic production of a superoxide anion radical or other reactive species (Steinberg, D., Parthasapathy, S., Carew, T. E., Khoo, J. C., Witztum, J. L. (1989) Beyond cholesterol. Modifications of low-density lipoprotein that increases its atherogenicity. New England Journal of Medicine 320: 915-924). The reactive species produced interact with PUFAS to form lipid peroxyl radicals, which subsequently produce lipid hydroperoxides and additional lipid peroxyl radicals (Steinberg et al. 1989). This initiates a peroxidative cascade which may eventually modify an essential part of the lipid's membrane, causing changes in membrane permeability and even cell death (Steinberg et al. 1989). Peroxidative degradation of LDL also leads to the formation of lipid oxidation products such as malondialdehyde (MDA) and other aldehydes which may be potentially toxic to the cell (Steinberg et al. 1989).... Oxidative stress has been implicated in a variety of diseases and pathological conditions, including endothelial cell cytotoxicity, coronary heart diseases (such as thrombosis and hyperlipemia) and cancer. (Addis et al. 1995). Recent studies have shown that elevated lipid peroxidation levels (oxidative stress) may play a role in the pathogenesis of Alzheimer's disease which includes a group of neurodegenerative disorders with diverse etiologies, but the same hallmark brain lesions. Practico D. et al., Increased F2-isoprostanes in Alzheimer's disease: evidence for enhanced lipid peroxidation in vivo. FASEB J. 1998 Dec; 12 (15): 1777-1783.

Web site: http://appft1.uspto.gov/netahtml/PTO/search-bool.html

- **Method of chocolate coating soft confectionery centers**

Inventor(s): Benedict, Shane; (Hackettstown, NJ), Rabinovitch, Kevin; (Hackettstown, NJ)

Correspondence: FITZPATRICK CELLA HARPER & SCINTO; 30 ROCKEFELLER PLAZA; NEW YORK; NY; 10112; US

Patent Application Number: 20030152678

Date filed: January 15, 2003

Abstract: The present invention is directed to a method of coating soft confectionery centers with chocolate. The method comprises the steps of: mixing the soft confectionery centers having a bed temperature of from about 0.degree. C. to about 15.degree. C. applying chocolate onto the soft confectionery centers, wherein the chocolate is at a temperature of from about 36.degree. C. to about 50.degree. C. and cooling the chocolate covered soft confectionery centers.

Excerpt(s): This application claims the benefit of U.S. Provisional Application No. 60/349,143, filed on Jan. 15, 2002.... The present invention relates to a method of coating confectionery centers. More particularly, the present invention relates to a method of coating soft confectionery centers with chocolate by controlling the temperature of the chocolate and the soft confectionery centers.... Confectionery centers are commonly made from a variety of components such as chocolate, peanut butter, raisins, toffee, taffy, fudge and a range of nuts including but not limited to, peanuts and almonds. The centers are often treated further by applying a coating by a panning process. This involves a rotating pan that tumbles the confectionary centers so that they rotate, tumble, and cascade over one another. While this is happening, chocolate or a sugar syrup is applied manually or by one of various spraying methods. The chocolate or sugar syrup is solidified on the confectionery centers by introducing air that cools and/or dries the coating on the centers in the rotating pan.

Web site: http://appft1.uspto.gov/netahtml/PTO/search-bool.html

- **METHOD OF EFFECTING IMPROVED CHOCOLATE PROCESSING USING NOBLE GASES**

Inventor(s): SPENCER, KEVIN C. (HINSDALE, IL)

Correspondence: OBLON SPIVAK MCCLELLAND MAIER & NEUSTADT PC; FOURTH FLOOR; 1755 JEFFERSON DAVIS HIGHWAY; ARLINGTON; VA; 22202; US

Patent Application Number: 20020068120

Date filed: January 25, 1995

Abstract: A method of improving the aromas and/or the flavor of chocolate or a precursor thereof or a chocolate-containing product comprising injecting a gas or gas mixture into the chocolate, precursor thereof or chocolate-containing product in containing means or into the containing means, container, the gas or gas mixture comprising an element selected from the group consisting of argon, krypton, xenon and neon or a mixture thereof substantially saturating the chocolate, precursor thereof or chocolate containing product with the gas or gas mixture; maintaining said saturation substantially throughout the volume of the storage container and during substantially all the time that the chocolate, precursor or chocolate-containing product is stored in said container.

Excerpt(s): The present invention relates to a method of effecting improved chocolate processing using noble gases.... The ability of the noble gases helium (Hi), neon (Ne0< argon (Ar), krypton (Kr), xenon (Xe) and radon (Ra) to enter into chemical combination with other atoms is extremely limited. Generally, only krypton, xenon and radon have been inducted to react with other atoms which are highly reactive, such as fluorine and oxygen, and the compounds thus formed are explosively unstable. See Advanced Inorganic Chemistry, by F. A. Cotton and G. Wilkinson (Wiley, Third Edition). However, while the noble gases are, in general, chemically inert, xenon is known to exhibit certain physiological effects, such as anesthesia. Other physiological effects have also been observed with other inert gases such as nitrogen, which, for example, is known to cause narcosis when used under great pressure in deep-sea diving.... It has been reported in U.S. Pat. No. 3,183,171 to Schreiner that argon and other inert gases can influence the growth rate of fungi and argon is known to improve the preservation of fish or seafood. U.S. Pat. No. 4,946,326 to Schvester, JP 52105232, JP 80002271 and JP 77027699. However, the fundamental lack of understanding of these observations clearly renders such results difficult, if not impossible, to interpret. Moreover, the meaning of such observations is further obscured by the fact that mixtures of many gases, including oxygen, were used in these studies. Further, some of these studies were conducted at hyperbaric pressures and at freezing temperatures. At such high pressures, it is likely that the observed results were caused by pressure damage to cellular components and to the enzymes themselves.

Web site: http://appft1.uspto.gov/netahtml/PTO/search-bool.html

- **Method of making heat-resistant chocolate and chocolate-like compositions with reduced apparent viscosity and products made thereby**

Inventor(s): Finkel, Gilbert; (Morristown, NJ), Davila, Victor R. (Morristown, NJ)

Correspondence: NORMAN E. LEHRER, ESQUIRE; NORMAN E. LEHRER, P.C. 1205 NORTH KINGS HIGHWAY; CHERRY HILL; NJ; 08034; US

Patent Application Number: 20030082291

Date filed: December 3, 2002

Abstract: A heat-resistant chocolate or chocolate-like composition is prepared by mixing a polyol, such as sorbitol or glycerine, with a flowable chocolate or chocolate-like composition through an increased apparent viscosity phase. Upon continued mixing, the mixture returns to a reduced apparent viscosity (fluid) phase. The mixture is subsequently handled in the same manner as an unmodified composition. Upon aging and stabilization, the modified chocolate or chocolate-like composition demonstrates a reduced tendency to deform at elevated temperatures, is less prone to stick to packaging or fingers, and maintains the desired flavor, texture, mouth feel, and other characteristics of ordinary chocolate. The heat-resistant chocolate or chocolate-like composition of the invention is suitable for use in the same manner and for the same purposes for which ordinary chocolate and chocolate-like compositions are used, with the additional benefit of heat-resistance.

Excerpt(s): This application claims the benefit of U.S. Provisional Patent Application Serial No. 60/089,437, filed Jun. 16, 1998.... The present invention is directed toward a method of forming a heat-resistant chocolate or chocolate-like composition and more particularly, toward modified products that demonstrate reduced apparent viscosity in the molten phase. As a result of this reduced apparent viscosity, these products may be handled in the same manner as unmodified compositions. Such products have a reduced tendency to melt or to deform at elevated temperatures and have a tendency to stick to fingers or packing materials.... Chocolate products are typically mixtures of liquid cocoa, cocoa butter, sugar, lecithin, and possibly milk and flavoring substances. Chocolate-like products contain substantially the same ingredients as a chocolate composition and also use any number of vegetable fats, cocoa butter replacers and/or extenders. Since the resulting fat content of these products is relatively high, the corresponding melting point is a function of the melting point of the fat contained therein.

Web site: http://appft1.uspto.gov/netahtml/PTO/search-bool.html

- **Method of shaping chocolate products**

  Inventor(s): Stephens, Steven D. (Greenville, MS), Earis, Frank W. (Maidenhead, GB), Collins, Thomas M. (Nazareth, PA), Lee, Ralph D. (Hampton, NJ), Willcocks, Neil A. (Columbia, NJ), Harding, William; (Gloucester, GB)

  Correspondence: FITZPATRICK CELLA HARPER & SCINTO; 30 ROCKEFELLER PLAZA; NEW YORK; NY; 10112; US

  Patent Application Number: 20020176918

  Date filed: March 29, 2002

  Abstract: Methods of producing shaped, embossed, or decorated confectionery chocolate products by using chilled forming, shaping, or embossing devices.

  Excerpt(s): The present invention relates to methods of forming shaped or embossed chocolate compositions that can include detailed designs and/or planar surfaces.... The unique flavor and mouthfeel of chocolate is a result of the combination of numerous components as well as the process of manufacture. Chocolate contains solid particles dispersed throughout a fat matrix (the term "fat" includes cocoa butter and milk fat).... Similarly, chocolate-like compositions may also contain fats other than cocoa butter or milk fat. Accordingly, melted chocolate and chocolate-like compositions are suspensions of non-fat particles (e.g., sugar, milk powders and cocoa solids) in a continuous liquid fat phase. The fat phase of milk chocolate, for example, is typically a mixture of cocoa butter, a suitable emulsifier, and milk fat. Cocoa butter is typically the predominant fat in the chocolates.

  Web site: http://appft1.uspto.gov/netahtml/PTO/search-bool.html

- **Methods and apparatus for chocolate dispensers**

  Inventor(s): Eckerman, Scott David; (Campbell, CA), Allen, Leslie Earl III; (Riverbank, CA), Small, David; (San Jose, CA)

  Correspondence: BLAKELY SOKOLOFF TAYLOR & ZAFMAN; 12400 WILSHIRE BOULEVARD, SEVENTH FLOOR; LOS ANGELES; CA; 90025; US

  Patent Application Number: 20030129921

  Date filed: January 9, 2002

  Abstract: A system, method and apparatus for dispensing chocolate. Solid chocolate is heated to its melting point within a chamber in order to form a liquid chocolate that is viscous and can flow out an opening in a nozzle at one end when pressure is exerted at another end. The chocolate dispenser is portable and has a housing or case that holds a heating chamber and a heater. The heater heats solid chocolate in the heating chamber into liquid chocolate. A nozzle is snapped or screwed into a dispensing end of the dispenser. A plunger has a piston inserted into the heating chamber to apply pressure to liquid chocolate in order for it to flow out of an opening in the nozzle. A children's playset for use with the chocolate dispenser includes a support structure to support the chocolate dispenser over a dispensing area. One embodiment of the playset includes a turn table and a tapper. A cooling tray may be included in the playset to cool the melted chocolate to its solid form.

Excerpt(s): This invention generally relates to dispensing machines and more particularly to liquid food dispensers.... Chocolate is a food product which is well known throughout the world. Chocolate is typically produced from the seeds of cacao trees. Various types of chocolate can be formed depending upon how it is mixed. The primary ingredient in chocolates, but for white chocolate, is chocolate liquor which is also referred to as unsweetened, bitter, baking, or cooking chocolate. When mixed with certain percentages of milk solids, sugar, vanilla or vanillin, lecithin, and additional cocoa butter, the combinations form extra-bittersweet, bittersweet, semisweet, sweet cooking, dark and milk chocolates. Milk chocolate contains less chocolate liquor than dark chocolate and has some butterfat and a greater percentage of milk solids. White chocolate contains no chocolate liquor but otherwise resembles the composition of milk chocolate.... The melting temperatures of the various types of chocolates can vary depending upon their composition. If chocolate is overheated it can burn easily. For example, dark chocolate should not be heated to temperatures greater than one hundred twenty degrees Fahrenheit (120 F.) while milk and white chocolates should not be heated to temperatures greater than one hundred then degrees Fahrenheit (110 F.). The cooking chocolates can generally handle greater temperatures without burning.

Web site: http://appft1.uspto.gov/netahtml/PTO/search-bool.html

- **Milk chocolate containing water**

  Inventor(s): Windhab, Erich Josef; (Hemishofen, CH), Wang, Junkuan; (Lonay, CH), Hugelshofer, Daniel; (Konolfingen, CH), Beckett, Stephen Thomas; (York, GB)

  Correspondence: WINSTON & STRAWN; PATENT DEPARTMENT; 1400 L STREET, N.W. WASHINGTON; DC; 20005-3502; US

  Patent Application Number: 20030118697

  Date filed: December 13, 2002

  Abstract: A process for manufacturing milk chocolate products containing a higher than normal water content by preparing a dark chocolate containing up to 30% by weight of water, adding a milk powder suspension optionally together with seed crystals of cocoa butter or cocoa butter equivalent, and mixing under low shear. The invention also relates to high water content milk chocolate products, methods of preparing a chocolate coated ice cream article with such products and to the resulting chocolate coated ice cream articles.

  Excerpt(s): This application is a continuation of the US national stage designation of International application PCT/EP01/04767 filed Apr. 26, 2001, the content of which is expressly incorporated herein by reference thereto.... The present invention relates to milk chocolate products containing water and more particularly to a process for manufacturing milk chocolate products containing a higher than normal water content.... Conventional chocolate production and processing methods avoid contact with water since small amounts of added water cause severe rheological changes in the product, usually accompanied by lumping and/or granulation leading to a coarse unacceptable eating texture (Minifie, B. W. Chocolate, Cocoa and Confectionery--Science and Technology, 3 edition, Chapman & Hall (1989)). On the contrary, addition of larger quantities of water, usually in the form of fresh cream or full cream milk, results in the production of "ganache" which is conventionally used as a short shelf-life filling for truffles or as a topping for confections. Ganache is the confectioner's term for a phase-inverted (i.e., oil-in-water) chocolate preparation that has a softer eating texture than normal chocolate and that does not have the snap of traditional chocolate when broken.

Web site: http://appft1.uspto.gov/netahtml/PTO/search-bool.html

- **Nicotine and chocolate compositions**

  Inventor(s): Landh, Thomas; (Lund, SE), Lindberg, Nils-Olof; (Malmo, SE)

  Correspondence: FULBRIGHT & JAWORSKI, LLP; 1301 MCKINNEY; SUITE 5100; HOUSTON; TX; 77010-3095; US

  Patent Application Number: 20030119879

  Date filed: October 15, 2002

  Abstract: The present invention is drawn to nicotine-containing pharmaceutical compositions that comprise chocolate and method of using the compositions in different therapies, such as nicotine replacement therapy.

  Excerpt(s): This application claims priority to U.S. Provisional Application No. 60/329,571, which was filed on Oct. 15, 2001.... This invention relates to novel pharmaceutical compositions of nicotine and use thereof. More particularly, the present invention relates to compositions comprising nicotine and chocolate, methods to prepare the compositions, and to methods for using the compositions in nicotine replacement therapy (NRT), including tobacco substitution and smoking cessation.... Nicotine replacement therapy as a smoking cessation strategy has been successful in the past. Previous nicotine-containing compositions aiming towards the purpose of reducing nicotine craving for subjects wishing to stop their use of tobacco products include i.e., U.S. Pat. No. 3,845,217 disclosing chewable compositions, U.S. Pat. No. 4,579,858 disclosing high-viscous nicotine nose-drop compositions, U.S. Pat. No. 5,525,351 disclosing nicotine-containing saliva-soluble gels, U.S. Pat. No. 5,656,255 disclosing low-viscous nicotine-containing compositions suitable for nasal spray administration, U.S. Pat. No. 4,920,989 and U.S. Pat. No. 4,953,572 disclosing the use of inhalation aerosol, BP 1,528,391 and BP 2,030,862 disclosing liquid aerosol formulations adapted as mouth-sprays, and devices for transdermal delivery of nicotine.

  Web site: http://appft1.uspto.gov/netahtml/PTO/search-bool.html

- **Novel chocolate composition as delivery system for nutrients and medications**

Inventor(s): Hughes, Kerry; (San Rafael, CA), Duberman, Joshua A. (Bellevue, WA), Conn, Alexander R. (Austin, TX), Altaffer, Paulo; (San Francisco, CA), Lytle, David; (Sandy, OR)

Correspondence: CENTRAL COAST PATENT AGENCY; PO BOX 187; AROMAS; CA; 95004; US

Patent Application Number: 20020192316

Date filed: March 26, 2002

Abstract: A novel chocolate product for use in delivering medicaments and/or nutrients to animals, particularly humans, specially formulated so that the craving for such product by animals, particularly humans, is significantly greater than the craving for chocolate conventionally used in pharmaceutical compositions and the concentration, optimization, and the addition of endogenous and exogenous ingredients to increase such craving as well as to treat specific indications. The chocolate product contains: from about 0.5 to about 200 milligrams, more preferably from about 5 to about 20 milligrams, of one or more biogenic amines per 1 gram of the chocolate product; from about 10 to about 500 milligrams, more preferably form about 20 to about 200 milligrams, of one or more amino acids per 1 gram of the chocolate product; (C) from about 1 microgram to about 20 milligrams, more preferably from about 10 micrograms to about 10 milligrams, of one or more of: methyl tetrahydroisoquinoline, N-acylethanolamines, and/or anandamide and/or salsolinol per 1 gram of the chocolate product; (D) from about 0.2 to about 30 milligrams of at least one trace mineral per 1 gram of the chocolate product; and (E) from 0.6 to about 500 milligrams, more preferably from about 35 to about 100 milligrams, of one or more methylxanthine alkaloids per 1 gram of the chocolate product. The chocolate product used in this invention also preferably contains effective amounts of at least one chocolate aroma and at least one vanilla aroma.

Excerpt(s): The present non-provisional patent application claims priority to provisional application Ser. No. 60/279,715, which is incorporated herein in its entirety by reference.... The present invention is in the field of carriers for administering nutrient and/or medicant compositions to animals, particularly to humans, and pertains more particularly to the preparation of such carriers to enhance the probability of consistent use by the animals for which the carrier is intended.... This invention relates to carriers for use in nutrient- and/or medicament-containing compositions designed to treat various ailments health conditions that commonly occur in mammals. More particularly, this invention relates to a novel chocolate composition as a delivery system for nutrients and medications wherein the composition is formulated to increase a patient's desire to consume the nutrients and medications delivered by the composition. In addition, this invention relates to a novel chocolate composition which itself constitutes an effective nutritional product.

Web site: http://appft1.uspto.gov/netahtml/PTO/search-bool.html

- **Partially purified cocoa extracts containing cocoa polyphenols**

Inventor(s): Buck, Margaret M. (Morristown, NJ), Hammerstone, John F. JR. (Nazareth, PA), Romanczyk, Leo J. JR. (Hackettstown, NJ)

Correspondence: Clifford Chance Rogers & Wells LLP; 200 Park Avenue; New York; NY; 10166-0153; US

Patent Application Number: 20020004523

Date filed: January 24, 2001

Abstract: Disclosed and claimed are cocoa extracts such as polyphenols or procyanidins, methods for preparing such extracts, as well as uses for them, especially as antineoplastic agents and antioxidants. Disclosed and claimed are antineoplastic compositions containing cocoa polyphenols or procyanidins and methods for treating patients employing the compositions. Additionally disclosed and claimed is a kit for treating a patient in need of treatment with an antineoplastic agent containing cocoa polyphenols or procyanidins as well as a lyophilized antineoplastic composition containing cocoa polyphenols or procyanidins. Further, disclosed and claimed is the use of the invention in antioxidant, preservative and topiosomerase-inhibiting compositions and methods.

Excerpt(s): This invention relates to cocoa extracts such as polyphenols preferably polyphenols enriched with procyanidins. This invention also relates to methods for preparing such extracts, as well as to uses for them; for instance, as antineoplastic agents and antioxidants.... Documents are cited in this disclosure with a full citation for each appearing in a References section at the end of the specification, preceding the claims. These documents pertain to the field of this invention; and, each document cited herein is hereby incorporated herein by reference.... Polyphenols are an incredibly diverse group of compounds (Ferreira et al., 1992) which widely occur in a variety of plants, some of which enter into the food chain. In some cases they represent an important class of compounds for the human diet. Although some of the polyphenols are considered to be nonnutrative, interest in these compounds has arisen because of their possible beneficial effects on health. For instance, quercitin (a flavonoid) has been shown to possess anticarcinogenic activity in experimental animal studies (Deshner et al., 1991 and Kato et al., 1983). (+)-Catechin and (-)-epicatechin (flavan-3-ols) have been shown to inhibit Leukemia virus reverse transcriptase activity (Chu et al., 1992). Nobotanin (an oligomeric hydrolyzable tannin) has also been shown to possess anti-tumor activity (Okuda et al., 1992). Statistical reports have also shown that stomach cancer mortality is significantly lower in the tea producing districts of Japan. Epigallocatechin gallate has been reported to be the pharmacologically active material in green tea that inhibits mouse skin tumors (Okuda et al., 1992). Ellagic acid has also been shown to possess anticarcinogen activity in various animal tumor models (Bukharta et al., 1992). Lastly, proanthocyanidin oligomers have been patented by the Kikkoman Corporation for use as antimutagens. Indeed, the area of phenolic compounds in foods and their modulation of tumor development in experimental animal models has been recently presented at the 202nd National Meeting of The American Chemical Society (Ho et al., 1992; Huang et al., 1992).

Web site: http://appft1.uspto.gov/netahtml/PTO/search-bool.html

- ## Preparation of crumb products for chocolate production

  Inventor(s): Samuel, Brian; (Wigginton, GB), Gibson, Richard; (Tadcaster, GB), Carli, Sophie; (Heworth, GB), Armstrong, Euan; (St. Andrewgate, GB), Jercher, Loreta; (Heworth, GB)

  Correspondence: ALLAN A. FANUCCI ESQ. WINSTON & STRAWN; 200 PARK AVENUE; NEW YORK; NY; 10166; US

  Patent Application Number: 20010012536

  Date filed: March 30, 2001

  Abstract: A process for the preparation of chocolate crumb which comprises mixing and heating mixing and heating low fat milk solids, sugar, in the absence or presence of cocoa solids and from 1.2 to 8% by weight of water based on the weight of the mixture in a mixer to a temperature of 85.degree. to 120.degree. C., reacting at a temperature of 85.degree. to 180.degree. C. for a period of from 2.5 to 25 minutes followed by drying to a moisture content of less than 3% by weight based on the total weight of the mixture. The present invention also provides a concentrated chocolate crumb comprising low fat milk solids, sugar and optionally cocoa solids wherein the ratio of milk solids to sugar is between 1:1.5 and 1:0.1. When cocoa solids are present, preferably the amount of cocoa solids in the concentrated chocolate crumb is from 10 to 15% by weight based on the total weight of the mixture.

  Excerpt(s): The present invention relates to a chocolate crumb, to a method for its preparation, and to milk chocolate prepared from the chocolate crumb.... Milk chocolate differs from dark or plain chocolate in that it contains milk solids and the essential part of the milk chocolate process is the method used to incorporate the milk solids. Milk chocolate is virtually moisture-free and contains from 0.5-1.5% water while full cream milk contains about 12.5% milk solids including fat, the remainder being about 87.5% water.... One method of removing the 87.5% water from the milk is by evaporation of the liquid milk and drying to a powder and a traditional method of producing milk chocolate is by mixing milk powder together with cocoa liquor or cocoa nibs, sugar, and cocoa butter, followed by refining, conching and tempering.

  Web site: http://appft1.uspto.gov/netahtml/PTO/search-bool.html

- ## Press for separating cocoa mass into cocoa cake and cocoa butter

  Inventor(s): Mantel, Rob Victor; (Wormer, NL)

  Correspondence: KNOBLE & YOSHIDA; EIGHT PENN CENTER; SUITE 1350, 1628 JOHN F KENNEDY BLVD; PHILADELPHIA; PA; 19103; US

  Patent Application Number: 20030161920

  Date filed: December 27, 2002

  Abstract: The invention relates to a press for separating cocoa mass into cocoa cake and cocoa butter, comprising a frame, in which a plurality of pressure elements are disposed, and means for compressing the pressure elements, wherein the pressure elements each comprise a cavity (9) for receiving cocoa mass to be pressed, in which cavity at least one squeezer is present, and wherein a filter (10, 10') is disposed in front of the squeezer and on the side of the cavity opposite said squeezer. In the filling position of the squeezer, the spacing between the said filters (10, 10') is in a range from 40 to 90 mm. This enables a substantial increase in the production capacity of the press.

Excerpt(s): The present invention relates to a press for separating cocoa mass into cocoa cake and cocoa butter, comprising a frame, in which a plurality of pressure elements are disposed, and means for compressing the pressure elements, wherein the pressure elements each comprise a cavity for receiving cocoa mass to be pressed, in which cavity at least one squeezer is present, and wherein a filter is disposed in front of the squeezer and on the side of the cavity opposite said squeezer.... A press of this kind is known from e.g. International patent application WO 92/12853. Such presses are used for separating cocoa mass into cocoa butter (which is liquid at an elevated temperature) on the one hand and solid cakes, which can be processed into cocoa powder, on the other hand. Generally, a hydraulic cylinder is provided, which is formed in a cylinder block which is connected with a retainer by means of two separate tie rods. Present in the cylinder is a plunger, and between said plunger and the retainer there is disposed a series of pressure elements. The pressure elements comprise a so-called pot, which defines a (usually cylindrical) cavity in which a squeezer and for example two filters are present. The space between the filters is intended for receiving an amount of cocoa mass to be pressed.... During a pressure cycle the pots are filled with heated cocoa mass via supply lines, and subsequently they are compressed. The cocoa butter is thereby pressed out through the filters and discharged.

Web site: http://appft1.uspto.gov/netahtml/PTO/search-bool.html

- **Refrigerated product containing pieces of chocolate and a process and an arrangement for its production**

  Inventor(s): Wild, Manfred; (Meitingen, DE), Grassler, Walter; (Polling, DE)

  Correspondence: winston & strawn; 200 park avenue; new york; NY; 10166; US

  Patent Application Number: 20010007692

  Date filed: February 13, 2001

  Abstract: The refrigerated product is based on at least one mousse (2, 3), the mousse containing 2 to 10% by weight of chocolate (4) and the chocolate being sterilized and containing 50 to 70% of fats, 30 to 50% of cocoa powder and 1 to 10% of sugar.

  Excerpt(s): This invention relates to a refrigerated product based on at least one mousse and containing pieces of chocolate. The invention also relates to a process for the production of this product and an installation for carrying out the process.... Refrigerated products containing pieces of chocolate are already available on the market. However, these known products have a storage life in a refrigerator of less than 10 days. This is because, from the moment when pieces of chocolate are dispersed in a mousse treated by UHT, the diffusion of water from the mousse into the chocolate creates microbiological problems because the chocolate is not sterilized. On the other hand, due to the high sugar content of the chocolate, the diffusion of water breaks the crispy texture of the chocolate and the consumer no longer has any sensation of the presence of pieces of chocolate in the mousse.... The problem addressed by the present invention was to provide the consumer with a mousse-based product containing pieces of chocolate which would keep in a refrigerator for 5 to 6 weeks and in which the pieces of chocolate would remain intact over that period.

  Web site: http://appft1.uspto.gov/netahtml/PTO/search-bool.html

- **Solid compositions and liquid preparations for oral administration which contain cocoa polyphenols**

Inventor(s): Buck, Margaret M. (Morristown, NJ), Hammerstone, John F. JR. (Nazareth, PA), Romanczyk, Leo J. JR. (Hackettstown, NJ)

Correspondence: Clifford Chance Rogers & Wells LLP; 200 Park Avenue; New York; NY; 10166-0153; US

Patent Application Number: 20020049166

Date filed: October 11, 2001

Abstract: Disclosed and claimed are cocoa extracts such as polyphenols or procyanidins, methods for preparing such extracts, as well as uses for them, especially as antineoplastic agents and antioxidants. Disclosed and claimed are antineoplastic compositions containing cocoa polyphenols or procyanidins and methods for treating patients employing the compositions. Additionally disclosed and claimed is a kit for treating a patient in need of treatment with an antineoplastic agent containing cocoa polyphenols or procyanidins as well as a lyophilized antineoplastic composition containing cocoa polyphenols or procyanidins. Further, disclosed and claimed is the use of the invention in antioxidant, preservative and topiosomerase-inhibiting compositions and methods.

Excerpt(s): This invention relates to cocoa extracts such as polyphenols preferably polyphenols enriched with procyanidins. This invention also relates to methods for preparing such extracts, as well as to uses for them; for instance, as antineoplastic agents and antioxidants.... Documents are cited in this disclosure with a full citation for each appearing in a References section at the end of the specification, preceding the claims. These documents pertain to the field of this invention; and, each document cited herein is hereby incorporated herein by reference.... Polyphenols are an incredibly diverse group of compounds (Ferreira et al., 1992) which widely occur in a variety of plants, some of which enter into the food chain. In some cases they represent an important class of compounds for the human diet. Although some of the polyphenols are considered to be nonnutrative, interest in these compounds has arisen because of their possible beneficial effects on health. For instance, quercitin (a flavonoid) has been shown to possess anticarcinogenic activity in experimental animal studies (Deshner et al., 1991 and Kato et al., 1983). (+)-Catechin and (-)-epicatechin (flavan-3-ols) have been shown to inhibit Leukemia virus reverse transcriptase activity (Chu et al., 1992). Nobotanin (an oligomeric hydrolyzable tannin) has also been shown to possess anti-tumor activity (Okuda et al., 1992). Statistical reports have also shown that stomach cancer mortality is significantly lower in the tea producing districts of Japan. Epigallocatechin gallate has been reported to be the pharmacologically active material in green tea that inhibits mouse skin tumors (Okuda et al., 1992). Ellagic acid has also been shown to possess anticarcinogen activity in various animal tumor models (Bukharta et al., 1992). Lastly, proanthocyanidin oligomers have been patented by the Kikkoman Corporation for use as antimutagens. Indeed, the area of phenolic compounds in foods and their modulation of tumor development in experimental animal models has been recently presented at the 202nd National Meeting of The American Chemical Society (Ho et al., 1992;Huang et al., 1992).

Web site: http://appft1.uspto.gov/netahtml/PTO/search-bool.html

- **Use of cocoa procyanidins combined with acetylsalicilic acid as an anti-platelet therapy**

Inventor(s): Romanczyk, Leo J. JR. (Hackettstown, NJ), Schmitz, Harold H. (Branchburg, NJ)

Correspondence: Clifford Chance Rogers & Wells LLP; 200 Park Avenue; New York; NY; 10166-0153; US

Patent Application Number: 20020022061

Date filed: March 22, 2001

Abstract: The invention relates to the use of cocoa procyanidins in combination with an aspirin as an anti-platelet therapy and compositions comprising cocoa procyanidins and aspirin (acetylsalicyclic acid).

Excerpt(s): This application claims priority, under 35 U.S.C..sctn. 119, from the U.S. provisional patent application Ser. No. 60/191,203, filed Mar. 22, 2000, the disclosure of which is hereby incorporated herein by reference.... This application is concerned with the use of a combination of cocoa procyanidins and aspirin as an anti-platelet therapy.... A compound consisting of one aromatic ring which contains at least one hydroxyl group is classified as a simple phenol. A polyphenol therefore consists of more than one aromatic ring, each ring containing at least one hydroxyl group. Flavonoids are polyphenols which have a diphenyl propane (C6-C3-C6) skeleton structure, and are found ubiquitously in the plant kingdom. The class of flavonoids called the proanthocyanidins are oligomers of flavan-3-ol monomer units most frequently linked 4.fwdarw.6 or 4.fwdarw.8. One of the most common classes of proanthocyanidins are the procyanidins, which are oligomers of catechin and epicatechin, and their gallic acid esters.

Web site: http://appft1.uspto.gov/netahtml/PTO/search-bool.html

- **Use of non-alkalized cocoa solids in a drink**

Inventor(s): Cipolla, Giovanni G. (Alpha, NJ), Kealey, Kirk S. (Lancaster, PA), Buck, Margaret M. (Morristown, NJ), Hammerstone, John F. JR. (Nazareth, PA), Snyder, Rodney M. (Elizabethtown, PA), Romanczyk, Leo J. JR. (Hackettstown, NJ)

Correspondence: Clifford Chances Rogers & Wells LLP; 200 Park Avenue; New York; NY; 10166-0153; US

Patent Application Number: 20020132018

Date filed: November 8, 2001

Abstract: The present invention is directed to a method of processing a fat-containing bean, e.g., cocoa beans, for producing solids comprising active polyphenols and/or fat-containing products, comprising extracting the fat to produce solids and fat-containing products. Additionally, the inventive method also provides cocoa compositions comprising at least one active polyphenol, wherein the concentration of the polyphenol(s) with respect to the nonfat solids is conserved with respect to the concentration of the active polyphenol(s) in the bean from which the compositions are derived.

Excerpt(s): Reference is made to copending U.S. application Ser. No. 08/317,226, filed Oct. 3, 1994 (allowed, now U.S. Pat. No. 5,554,645), and Ser. No. 08/631,661, filed Apr. 2, 1996, incorporated herein by reference.... The present invention relates to a versatile process for extracting fat from fat-containing beans and/or processing fat-containing beans to yield a solid product having a conserved. level of polyphenols, preferably polyphenols with active procyanidins. More specifically, the invention provides a method of producing cocoa butter and/or cocoa solids having conserved levels of polyphenols from cocoa beans using a unique combination of processing steps which does not require separate bean roasting or liquor milling equipment. The method of the present invention allows for the option of processing cocoa beans without exposure to severe thermal treatment for extended periods of time and/or the use of solvent extraction of fat. The invention provides a significantly less complex process regarding total cost of assets, maintenance, energy and labor, with the concomitant benefit of obtaining solids having conserved concentrations of polyphenols relative to the starting materials.... Documents are cited in this disclosure with a full citation for each appearing thereat. These documents relate to the state-of-the-art to which this invention pertains, and each document cited herein is hereby incorporated by reference.

Web site: http://appft1.uspto.gov/netahtml/PTO/search-bool.html

Keeping Current

In order to stay informed about patents and patent applications dealing with chocolate, you can access the U.S. Patent Office archive via the Internet at the following Web address: **http://www.uspto.gov/patft/index.html**. You will see two broad options: (1) Issued Patent, and (2) Published Applications. To see a list of issued patents, perform the following steps: Under "Issued Patents," click "Quick Search." Then, type "chocolate" (or synonyms) into the "Term 1" box. After clicking on the search button, scroll down to see the various patents which have been granted to date on chocolate.

You can also use this procedure to view pending patent applications concerning chocolate. Simply go back to the following Web address: **http://www.uspto.gov/patft/index.html**. Select "Quick Search" under "Published Applications." Then proceed with the steps listed above.

Chapter 7. Books on Chocolate

Overview

This chapter provides bibliographic book references relating to chocolate. In addition to online booksellers such as **www.amazon.com** and **www.bn.com**, excellent sources for book titles on chocolate include the Combined Health Information Database and the National Library of Medicine. Your local medical library also may have these titles available for loan.

Book Summaries: Federal Agencies

The Combined Health Information Database collects various book abstracts from a variety of healthcare institutions and federal agencies. To access these summaries, go directly to the following hyperlink: **http://chid.nih.gov/detail/detail.html**. You will need to use the "Detailed Search" option. To find book summaries, use the drop boxes at the bottom of the search page where "You may refine your search by." Select the dates and language you prefer. For the format option, select "Monograph/Book." Now type "chocolate" (or synonyms) into the "For these words:" box. You should check back periodically with this database which is updated every three months. The following is a typical result when searching for books on chocolate:

- **Fat Tooth Fat Gram Counter [and] Fat Tooth Restaurant and Fast Food Fat-Gram Counter**

  Source: New York, NY: Workman Publishing. 1993. 592 p.

  Contact: Available from Workman Publishing. 708 Broadway, New York, NY 10003. (212) 254-5900. For multiple copies, call (800) 722-7202, extension 7509 or (212) 614-7509. PRICE: $12.95 for set of 2 books; discounts available for health care providers buying multiple copies. ISBN: 1563051494.

  Summary: These two pocket guides provide information about the fat content in common foods. The Fat Gram Counter consists of general food lists that provide serving size, calories, grams of fat, and percentage fat for foods in the following categories: beverages, candy and **chocolate**, chips and other snacks, dairy products, desserts, eggs, fats, oils and salad dressings, fish and shellfish, fruit, grains and grain products, meats, nuts and seeds, popular ethnic foods, poultry, sauces and gravies, soups, spices, herbs and flavorings, sugar, syrups and spreads, and vegetables. The introductory text enables readers to determine their own 'fat budget' and plan for a healthy diet. The Restaurant and Fast Food Fat Gram Counter is a take-along guide that helps readers make informed choices by providing fat-gram counts for average restaurant servings. The first half of the Restaurant guide lists foods by categories, such as appetizers, breads, desserts, poultry, and vegetables. The second half lists entrees from popular fast food restaurants, including Burger King, Hardee's, Kentucky Fried Chicken, McDonald's, Taco Bell, and Wendy's (and many more).

- **Forbidden Foods: Diabetic Cooking**

  Source: Alexandria, VA: American Diabetes Association. 2000. 230 p.

  Contact: Available from American Diabetes Association (ADA). Order Fulfillment Department, P.O. Box 930850, Atlanta, GA 31193-0850. (800) 232-6733. Fax (770) 442-9742. Website: www.diabetes.org. PRICE: $16.95 plus shipping and handling. ISBN: 1580400450.

  Summary: This cookbook helps people who have diabetes learn how to cook and enjoy their favorite foods. The cookbook includes 150 recipes in the categories of beverages; appetizers and snacks; sauces, gravies, and dressings; faux fried foods; mom's favorites; pizza and pasta; quick breads and muffins; cookies and bars; pies, crumbles, and cobblers; puddings and creamy desserts; and **chocolate** magic. Each recipe includes a nutritional analysis that notes the serving size; the diabetes exchanges; the number of calories; the number of calories from fat; the number of grams of total fat, saturated fat, carbohydrate, protein, and fiber; and number of milligrams of cholesterol and sodium. Preparation, chilling, and cooking times are also provided. In addition, the cookbook teaches readers how to modify their own family recipes to make them healthier without losing the flavor they love. The recipe solution tips focus on ways to replace or reduce fat, sugar, and salt and to increase or change flavorings.

- **Secrets of Fat-Free Baking**

  Source: Garden City Park, NY: Avery, 208 p., 1994.

  Contact: Avery Publishing Group, 120 Old Broadway, Garden City Park, NY 11040. (516) 741-2155, (800) 548-5757. FAX (516) 742-1892.

  Summary: Woodruff has compiled a book of low-fat and non-fat baking recipes. A wide variety of recipes are included, from pies to cookies to breads. Nutritional information is included for each recipe. Sample recipe titles are Strawberry Streusel Muffins, Peach Pizzazz Pie, and Colossal **chocolate** Chippers.

Book Summaries: Online Booksellers

Commercial Internet-based booksellers, such as Amazon.com and Barnes&Noble.com, offer summaries which have been supplied by each title's publisher. Some summaries also include customer reviews. Your local bookseller may have access to in-house and commercial databases that index all published books (e.g. Books in Print®). **IMPORTANT NOTE:** Online booksellers typically produce search results for medical and non-medical books. When searching for "chocolate" at online booksellers' Web sites, you may discover <u>non-medical books</u> that use the generic term "chocolate" (or a synonym) in their titles. The following is indicative of the results you might find when searching for "chocolate" (sorted alphabetically by title; follow the hyperlink to view more details at Amazon.com):

- **"Good Housekeeping" Chocolate: 100 Indulgent Cakes, Cookies, Desserts and Treats;** ISBN: 1855859831;
  http://www.amazon.com/exec/obidos/ASIN/1855859831/icongroupinterna

- **...And on the 28th day God created Chocolate** by Carrie J. Hickman, Patti Williams; ISBN: 0964794918;
  http://www.amazon.com/exec/obidos/ASIN/0964794918/icongroupinterna

- **1001 Chocolate Treats** by Gregg R. Gillespie, Peter Barry (Photographer) (1996); ISBN: 188482286X;
  http://www.amazon.com/exec/obidos/ASIN/188482286X/icongroupinterna

- **101 Chocolate Recipes** by cooking; ISBN: 0785330127;
  http://www.amazon.com/exec/obidos/ASIN/0785330127/icongroupinterna

- **101 Perfect Chocolate Chip Cookies** by Gwen Steege; ISBN: 1580173128;
  http://www.amazon.com/exec/obidos/ASIN/1580173128/icongroupinterna

- **125 Best Chocolate Chip Recipes** by Julie Hasson (2003); ISBN: 0778800725;
  http://www.amazon.com/exec/obidos/ASIN/0778800725/icongroupinterna

- **201 Chocolate Treats: Velvety and Voluptuous Mouthwatering Cakes, Cookies, and Candies** by Gregg R. Gillespie, Peter Barry (Photographer); ISBN: 1579121187;
  http://www.amazon.com/exec/obidos/ASIN/1579121187/icongroupinterna

- **3 Culinary Mysteries: An Audio Book Trilogy of Best Sellers: Dying for Chocolate/Catering to Nobody/the Last Suppers [ABRIDGED]** by Diane Mott Davidson, et al (2002); ISBN: 1578152720;
  http://www.amazon.com/exec/obidos/ASIN/1578152720/icongroupinterna

- **57 More of the Best Chocolate Chip Cookies in the World: The Recipes That Won the Second National Chocolate Chip Cookies Contest** by Honey Zisman (Contributor), Larry Zisman (Editor); ISBN: 031215044X;
  http://www.amazon.com/exec/obidos/ASIN/031215044X/icongroupinterna

- **A Chocolate A Day 2004 Wall Calendar** by Chocolatier Magazine (Author) (2003); ISBN: 0789309181;
  http://www.amazon.com/exec/obidos/ASIN/0789309181/icongroupinterna

- **A Chocolate a Day: Keeps the Doctor Away** by Suzy Ashton, John Dr Ashton (2003); ISBN: 0312307578;
  http://www.amazon.com/exec/obidos/ASIN/0312307578/icongroupinterna

- **A Chocolate Affair** by Sheila Copeland (2003); ISBN: 1583144412;
  http://www.amazon.com/exec/obidos/ASIN/1583144412/icongroupinterna

- **A Chocolate Moose for Dinner** by Fred Gwynne (1988); ISBN: 0671667416;
  http://www.amazon.com/exec/obidos/ASIN/0671667416/icongroupinterna

- **A Chocolate Soldier: A Novel (Contemporary Fiction Series)** by Cyrus Colter; ISBN: 0938410490;
  http://www.amazon.com/exec/obidos/ASIN/0938410490/icongroupinterna

- **A dieta: Con Chocolates !** by Paul Svenson; ISBN: 9686801634;
  http://www.amazon.com/exec/obidos/ASIN/9686801634/icongroupinterna

- **A Guide for Using Charlie & the Chocolate Factory in the Classroom** by Concetta D. Ryan, et al; ISBN: 1557344205;
  http://www.amazon.com/exec/obidos/ASIN/1557344205/icongroupinterna

- **A Guide for Using The Chocolate Touch in the Classroom** by Teacher Created Materials Inc; ISBN: 1576903370;
  http://www.amazon.com/exec/obidos/ASIN/1576903370/icongroupinterna

- **A Passion for Chocolate** by Maurice Bernachon, et al; ISBN: 0688075541;
  http://www.amazon.com/exec/obidos/ASIN/0688075541/icongroupinterna

- **A Passion for Chocolate (Better Homes and Gardens Test Kitchen)** by Kristi Fuller (Editor), et al (2000); ISBN: 0696211742;
  http://www.amazon.com/exec/obidos/ASIN/0696211742/icongroupinterna

- **A Year in Chocolate: Four Seasons of Unforgettable Desserts** by Alice Medrich, et al; ISBN: 0446526649;
  http://www.amazon.com/exec/obidos/ASIN/0446526649/icongroupinterna

- **Alfreda's Reader's Theatre: Black English, Chocolate Slang** by A. Doyle (1998); ISBN: 1568203594;
  http://www.amazon.com/exec/obidos/ASIN/1568203594/icongroupinterna

- **Apples, Brie & Chocolate** by Nell Stehr (1996); ISBN: 0942495543;
  http://www.amazon.com/exec/obidos/ASIN/0942495543/icongroupinterna

- **Baker's Book of Chocolate Riches** (1987); ISBN: 0307492729;
  http://www.amazon.com/exec/obidos/ASIN/0307492729/icongroupinterna

- **Baker's Easiest-Ever Chocolate Recipes** by Outlet; ISBN: 0517056771;
  http://www.amazon.com/exec/obidos/ASIN/0517056771/icongroupinterna

- **Beans to Chocolate (Welcome Books: How Things Are Made)** by Inez Snyder (2003); ISBN: 0516243616;
  http://www.amazon.com/exec/obidos/ASIN/0516243616/icongroupinterna

- **Beat That! Cookbook: The Very, Very Best Recipe for Apple Crisp, Baked Beans, Cheese Souffle, English Muffin Bread, Flank Steak, Hot Chocolate, Key** by Ann Hodgman, et al (1996); ISBN: 1881527921;
  http://www.amazon.com/exec/obidos/ASIN/1881527921/icongroupinterna

- **Best Loved Chocolate** by Caroline Barty, Sourcebooks (2000); ISBN: 1570716072;
  http://www.amazon.com/exec/obidos/ASIN/1570716072/icongroupinterna

- **Best of - Chocolate** (1995); ISBN: 1572150467;
  http://www.amazon.com/exec/obidos/ASIN/1572150467/icongroupinterna

- **Better Homes and Gardens Chocolate**; ISBN: 0696013053;
  http://www.amazon.com/exec/obidos/ASIN/0696013053/icongroupinterna

- **Betty Crocker's Chocolate Cookbook** by Betty Crocker, Betty Crocker; ISBN: 0130849979;
  http://www.amazon.com/exec/obidos/ASIN/0130849979/icongroupinterna

- **Beyond the Chocolate War** by Robert Cormier; ISBN: 044090580X;
  http://www.amazon.com/exec/obidos/ASIN/044090580X/icongroupinterna

- **Bittersweet Journey: A Modestly Erotic Novel of Love, Longing, and Chocolate** by Enid Futterman; ISBN: 0670876941;
  http://www.amazon.com/exec/obidos/ASIN/0670876941/icongroupinterna

- **Bittersweet: Recipes from a Chocolate Life** by Alice Medrich (2003); ISBN: 1579651607;
  http://www.amazon.com/exec/obidos/ASIN/1579651607/icongroupinterna

- **Blood and Chocolate (Laurel-Leaf Books)** by Annette Curtis Klause; ISBN: 0440226686;
  http://www.amazon.com/exec/obidos/ASIN/0440226686/icongroupinterna

- **Blue Corn and Chocolate (Knopf Cooks American)** by Elisabeth Rozin, Elizabeth Rozin (1992); ISBN: 0394583086;
  http://www.amazon.com/exec/obidos/ASIN/0394583086/icongroupinterna

- **Bookmarks: A Companion Text for Like Water for Chocolate** by Janet Giannotti (2000); ISBN: 0472085964;
  http://www.amazon.com/exec/obidos/ASIN/0472085964/icongroupinterna

- **Boxed Chocolates [DOWNLOAD: PDF]** by Mintel International Group Ltd. (Author); ISBN: B00005R9R4;
  http://www.amazon.com/exec/obidos/ASIN/B00005R9R4/icongroupinterna

- **Boxed/ Bagged Chocolates - US [DOWNLOAD: PDF]** by Global Industry Analysts (Author); ISBN: B00005V84O;
  http://www.amazon.com/exec/obidos/ASIN/B00005V84O/icongroupinterna

- **Bread and Chocolate: My Food Life in San Francisco** by Fran Gage (1999); ISBN: 157061153X;
  http://www.amazon.com/exec/obidos/ASIN/157061153X/icongroupinterna

- **Built on Chocolate: The Story of the Hershey Chocolate Company** by James D., Jr. McMahon; ISBN: 1575440334;
  http://www.amazon.com/exec/obidos/ASIN/1575440334/icongroupinterna

- **Celebrate with Chocolate: Totally Over-the-Top Recipes** by Marcel Desaulniers (Author) (2002); ISBN: 0688162983;
  http://www.amazon.com/exec/obidos/ASIN/0688162983/icongroupinterna

- **Chilies to Chocolate: Food the Americas Gave the World** by Nelson Foster (Editor), Linda S. Cordell (Editor) (1992); ISBN: 0816513244;
  http://www.amazon.com/exec/obidos/ASIN/0816513244/icongroupinterna

- **Chocoholic Reasonettes: Little Excuses to Eat Chocolate** by Sherrie Weaver (1998); ISBN: 1562453343;
  http://www.amazon.com/exec/obidos/ASIN/1562453343/icongroupinterna

- **Chocolate** by Elena Maria Costaguta (2003); ISBN: 9502490487;
  http://www.amazon.com/exec/obidos/ASIN/9502490487/icongroupinterna

- **Chocolate** by Sandra Boynton; ISBN: 089480197X;
  http://www.amazon.com/exec/obidos/ASIN/089480197X/icongroupinterna

- **Chocolate** by Aleksandr Tarasov-Rodionov (1973); ISBN: 0883550253;
  http://www.amazon.com/exec/obidos/ASIN/0883550253/icongroupinterna

- **Chocolate** by Southwater Publishing (2000); ISBN: 1842150235;
  http://www.amazon.com/exec/obidos/ASIN/1842150235/icongroupinterna

- **Chocolate** by Christine France (2000); ISBN: 0754802620;
  http://www.amazon.com/exec/obidos/ASIN/0754802620/icongroupinterna

- **Chocolate** by Linda Collister, et al (2002); ISBN: 1841723193;
  http://www.amazon.com/exec/obidos/ASIN/1841723193/icongroupinterna

- **Chocolate** by Gooseberry Patch (2002); ISBN: 1888052929;
  http://www.amazon.com/exec/obidos/ASIN/1888052929/icongroupinterna

- **Chocolate - US [DOWNLOAD: PDF]** by Global Industry Analysts (Author); ISBN:
  B00005UEZR;
  http://www.amazon.com/exec/obidos/ASIN/B00005UEZR/icongroupinterna

- **Chocolate & Baking** (2003); ISBN: 0752575589;
  http://www.amazon.com/exec/obidos/ASIN/0752575589/icongroupinterna

- **Chocolate (From Farm to You)** by Carol Jones; ISBN: 0791070085;
  http://www.amazon.com/exec/obidos/ASIN/0791070085/icongroupinterna

- **Chocolate (Le Cordon Bleu Home Collection , Vol 8)** by Le Cordon Bleu Chefs, Tuttle
  Publishing (1998); ISBN: 9625934316;
  http://www.amazon.com/exec/obidos/ASIN/9625934316/icongroupinterna

- **Chocolate (Starters)** by Saviour Pirotta; ISBN: 1583402640;
  http://www.amazon.com/exec/obidos/ASIN/1583402640/icongroupinterna

- **Chocolate (What's for Lunch)** by Claire Llewellyn, Helaine Cohen (Editor) (1998); ISBN:
  0516262181;
  http://www.amazon.com/exec/obidos/ASIN/0516262181/icongroupinterna

- **Chocolate Ain't Enough No More: Every Woman's Choice** by Arnie Wallace, Adryan
  Russ (1991); ISBN: 0962534129;
  http://www.amazon.com/exec/obidos/ASIN/0962534129/icongroupinterna

- **Chocolate and Cocoa: Health and Nutrition** by Ian Knight (Editor) (1999); ISBN:
  0632054158;
  http://www.amazon.com/exec/obidos/ASIN/0632054158/icongroupinterna

- **Chocolate and Confectionery Manufacturing in Indonesia [DOWNLOAD: PDF]** by
  IBISWorld (Author); ISBN: B000096C3Q;
  http://www.amazon.com/exec/obidos/ASIN/B000096C3Q/icongroupinterna

- **Chocolate and French Fries** by Carlos Trillo (2003); ISBN: 1593960034;
  http://www.amazon.com/exec/obidos/ASIN/1593960034/icongroupinterna

- **Chocolate Artistry**; ISBN: 0809255448;
  http://www.amazon.com/exec/obidos/ASIN/0809255448/icongroupinterna

- **Chocolate Artistry: Techniques for Molding, Decorating, and Designing With
  Chocolate** by Elaine Gonzalez; ISBN: 0809252740;
  http://www.amazon.com/exec/obidos/ASIN/0809252740/icongroupinterna

- **Chocolate Astrology: Delectable Recipes and Readings for Every Sign of the Zodiac**
  by Joy Nagy (2003); ISBN: 0609609416;
  http://www.amazon.com/exec/obidos/ASIN/0609609416/icongroupinterna

- **Chocolate Burnout: The Road to Freedom** by Vicki L. Hubbard, Vicky L. Hubbard
  (2001); ISBN: 0595148743;
  http://www.amazon.com/exec/obidos/ASIN/0595148743/icongroupinterna

- **Chocolate by Hershey: A Story About Milton S. Hershey (A Carolrhoda Creative
  Minds Book)** by Betty Burford, Loren Chantland (Illustrator) (1994); ISBN: 0876146418;
  http://www.amazon.com/exec/obidos/ASIN/0876146418/icongroupinterna

- **Chocolate Cake: From the Simple to the Sublime** by Michele Urvater (2001); ISBN:
  0767906071;
  http://www.amazon.com/exec/obidos/ASIN/0767906071/icongroupinterna

- **Chocolate Cake: The MIND Method of Weight Control** by Jakki Wendt; ISBN: 0930306120;
  http://www.amazon.com/exec/obidos/ASIN/0930306120/icongroupinterna

- **Chocolate Cakes for Weddings and Celebrations** by John Slattery (2002); ISBN: 1853918792;
  http://www.amazon.com/exec/obidos/ASIN/1853918792/icongroupinterna

- **Chocolate Caliente Para El Alma de Quien Ha..** by Jack Canfield, et al (1998); ISBN: 9580440832;
  http://www.amazon.com/exec/obidos/ASIN/9580440832/icongroupinterna

- **Chocolate Candies - US [DOWNLOAD: PDF]** by Global Industry Analysts (Author); ISBN: B00005RC30;
  http://www.amazon.com/exec/obidos/ASIN/B00005RC30/icongroupinterna

- **Chocolate Candy: 80 Recipes for Chocolate Treats from Fudge to Truffles** by Anita Prichard; ISBN: 0517559382;
  http://www.amazon.com/exec/obidos/ASIN/0517559382/icongroupinterna

- **Chocolate Chili Pepper Love: Stories That Prove Opposites Attract** by Becky Freeman (2000); ISBN: 0736902376;
  http://www.amazon.com/exec/obidos/ASIN/0736902376/icongroupinterna

- **Chocolate Chip Challah and Other Twists on the Jewish Holiday Table: An Interactive Family Cookbook** by Lisa Rauchwerger (Illustrator) (1999); ISBN: 0807407003;
  http://www.amazon.com/exec/obidos/ASIN/0807407003/icongroupinterna

- **Chocolate Chip Cookie Murder** by Joanne Fluke; ISBN: 075820230X;
  http://www.amazon.com/exec/obidos/ASIN/075820230X/icongroupinterna

- **Chocolate Chip Cookies** by Karen Wagner, Leah P. Preiss (Illustrator); ISBN: 0805012680;
  http://www.amazon.com/exec/obidos/ASIN/0805012680/icongroupinterna

- **Chocolate Chipmunks and Canoes: An American Indian Words Coloring Book** by Juan Alvarez (1992); ISBN: 1878610031;
  http://www.amazon.com/exec/obidos/ASIN/1878610031/icongroupinterna

- **Chocolate Chips - Contemporary Haiku** by Michael Moore, Windy Barker (Editor) (1995); ISBN: 0961070242;
  http://www.amazon.com/exec/obidos/ASIN/0961070242/icongroupinterna

- **Chocolate Chips and Trumpet Tricks (Alex Devotions)** by Nancy Simpson Levene, et al; ISBN: 0781401038;
  http://www.amazon.com/exec/obidos/ASIN/0781401038/icongroupinterna

- **Chocolate Companion** by Cynthia Shade Rogers, Lisa Adams (Illustrator) (1994); ISBN: 1883283027;
  http://www.amazon.com/exec/obidos/ASIN/1883283027/icongroupinterna

- **Chocolate Confectionery - US [DOWNLOAD: PDF]** by Global Industry Analysts (Author); ISBN: B00005UEZQ;
  http://www.amazon.com/exec/obidos/ASIN/B00005UEZQ/icongroupinterna

- **Chocolate Confectionery [DOWNLOAD: PDF]** by Mintel International Group Ltd. (Author); ISBN: B00005R9S6;
  http://www.amazon.com/exec/obidos/ASIN/B00005R9S6/icongroupinterna

- **Chocolate Confectionery Industry Guide [DOWNLOAD: PDF]** by Datamonitor (Author); ISBN: B00008R3RI;
  http://www.amazon.com/exec/obidos/ASIN/B00008R3RI/icongroupinterna

- **Chocolate Confectionery Market - US Report [DOWNLOAD: PDF]** by Mintel International Group Ltd. (Author); ISBN: B00005U85A;
  http://www.amazon.com/exec/obidos/ASIN/B00005U85A/icongroupinterna

- **Chocolate Cookies : The Taste of Sweet Seduction** by Vincent Tyler; ISBN: 0967027217;
  http://www.amazon.com/exec/obidos/ASIN/0967027217/icongroupinterna

- **Chocolate Covered Ants** by Stephen Manes; ISBN: 0590409611;
  http://www.amazon.com/exec/obidos/ASIN/0590409611/icongroupinterna

- **Chocolate Covered Clue (New Bobbsey Twins, No 10)** by Laura Lee Hope; ISBN: 0671630733;
  http://www.amazon.com/exec/obidos/ASIN/0671630733/icongroupinterna

- **Chocolate covered raisins** by Detrick Oliver Hughes; ISBN: 0964898004;
  http://www.amazon.com/exec/obidos/ASIN/0964898004/icongroupinterna

- **Chocolate Crazy** by Sylvia Balser Hirsch; ISBN: 0452257298;
  http://www.amazon.com/exec/obidos/ASIN/0452257298/icongroupinterna

- **Chocolate Creams and Dollars** by Mohammed Mrabet, et al (1993); ISBN: 096251196X;
  http://www.amazon.com/exec/obidos/ASIN/096251196X/icongroupinterna

- **Chocolate days, popsicle weeks** by Edward Hannibal (Author); ISBN: B00005VL8G;
  http://www.amazon.com/exec/obidos/ASIN/B00005VL8G/icongroupinterna

- **Chocolate Desserts by Pierre Herme** by Pierre Herme, et al; ISBN: 0316357413;
  http://www.amazon.com/exec/obidos/ASIN/0316357413/icongroupinterna

- **Chocolate Everything** by Jean Pare (2000); ISBN: 1895455642;
  http://www.amazon.com/exec/obidos/ASIN/1895455642/icongroupinterna

- **Chocolate Fads, Folklore, & Fantasies: 1,000+ Chunks of Chocolate Information** by Linda K., Phd Fuller (1996); ISBN: 1560230274;
  http://www.amazon.com/exec/obidos/ASIN/1560230274/icongroupinterna

- **Chocolate fantasies**; ISBN: 0848708164;
  http://www.amazon.com/exec/obidos/ASIN/0848708164/icongroupinterna

- **Chocolate Fantasies: 70 Irresistible Recipes to Die for** by Christine France; ISBN: 1859678211;
  http://www.amazon.com/exec/obidos/ASIN/1859678211/icongroupinterna

- **Chocolate for a Lover's Heart: Soul-Soothing Stories That Celebrate the Power of Love** by Kay Allenbaugh (Editor); ISBN: 0684862980;
  http://www.amazon.com/exec/obidos/ASIN/0684862980/icongroupinterna

- **Chocolate for a Mother's Heart: Inspiring Stories That Celebrate the Spirit of Motherhood** by Kay Allenbaugh (Editor); ISBN: 0684862999;
  http://www.amazon.com/exec/obidos/ASIN/0684862999/icongroupinterna

- **Chocolate for a Teen's Dreams : Heartwarming Stories About Making Your Wishes Come True** by Kay Allenbaugh (Editor); ISBN: 074323703X;
  http://www.amazon.com/exec/obidos/ASIN/074323703X/icongroupinterna

- **Chocolate for a Teen's Heart: Unforgettable Stories for Young Women About Love, Hope, and Happiness** by Kay Allenbaugh (Editor); ISBN: 0743213807; http://www.amazon.com/exec/obidos/ASIN/0743213807/icongroupinterna

- **Chocolate for a Teen's Soul: Life-Changing Stories for Young Women About Growing Wise and Growing Strong** by Kay Allenbaugh (Editor); ISBN: 0684870819; http://www.amazon.com/exec/obidos/ASIN/0684870819/icongroupinterna

- **Chocolate for a Teen's Spirit: Inspiring Stories for Young Women About Hope, Strength, and Wisdom** by Kay Allenbaugh (Editor); ISBN: 074322289X; http://www.amazon.com/exec/obidos/ASIN/074322289X/icongroupinterna

- **Chocolate For A Woman's Blessings : 77 Heartwarming Tales Of Gratitude That Celebrate The Good Things In Life** by Kay Allenbaugh (Editor); ISBN: 0743203089; http://www.amazon.com/exec/obidos/ASIN/0743203089/icongroupinterna

- **Chocolate for a Woman's Courage : 77 Stories That Honor Your Strength and Wisdom** by Kay Allenbaugh (Compiler); ISBN: 0743236998; http://www.amazon.com/exec/obidos/ASIN/0743236998/icongroupinterna

- **Chocolate for a Woman's Dreams : 77 Stories to Treasure as You Make Your Wishes Come True** by Kay Allenbaugh (Editor); ISBN: 0743217772; http://www.amazon.com/exec/obidos/ASIN/0743217772/icongroupinterna

- **Chocolate for a Woman's Heart & Soul** by Kay Allenbaugh (Editor) (1998); ISBN: 0684857855; http://www.amazon.com/exec/obidos/ASIN/0684857855/icongroupinterna

- **Chocolate For A Womans Heart : 77 Stories Of Love Kindness And Compassion To Nourish Your Soul And Sweeten Yo** by Kay Allenbaugh (Editor); ISBN: 0684848961; http://www.amazon.com/exec/obidos/ASIN/0684848961/icongroupinterna

- **Chocolate for Breakfast and Tea: B&B Innkeepers Share Their Finest Recipes** by Laura Zahn (Editor), Laura Zohn; ISBN: 0939301970; http://www.amazon.com/exec/obidos/ASIN/0939301970/icongroupinterna

- **Chocolate for the Poor: A Story of Rape in 1805** by David Beasley (1999); ISBN: 0915317044; http://www.amazon.com/exec/obidos/ASIN/0915317044/icongroupinterna

- **Chocolate from the Cake Mix Doctor** by Anne Byrn; ISBN: 0761122710; http://www.amazon.com/exec/obidos/ASIN/0761122710/icongroupinterna

- **Chocolate Girls** by Annie Murray; ISBN: 0330492136; http://www.amazon.com/cxcc/obidos/ASIN/0330492136/icongroupinterna

- **Chocolate Horse (Bryant, Bonnie. Saddle Club, No. 32.)** by Bonnie Bryant (1994); ISBN: 0553481460; http://www.amazon.com/exec/obidos/ASIN/0553481460/icongroupinterna

- **Chocolate Icing on Vanilla Prose** by Sandra Glassman (2002); ISBN: 140106065X; http://www.amazon.com/exec/obidos/ASIN/140106065X/icongroupinterna

- **Chocolate Island (Usborne Young Puzzle Adventures)** by Karen Dolby, Caroline Church (Illustrator) (1995); ISBN: 0746014589; http://www.amazon.com/exec/obidos/ASIN/0746014589/icongroupinterna

- **Chocolate Lover's Cookbook for Dummies** by Carole Bloom (Author) (2002); ISBN: 0764554662; http://www.amazon.com/exec/obidos/ASIN/0764554662/icongroupinterna

- **Chocolate Lover's Cookies and Brownies** (1993); ISBN: 0881768510;
  http://www.amazon.com/exec/obidos/ASIN/0881768510/icongroupinterna

- **Chocolate Lovers Diet: Enjoy Chocolate and Say Goodbye to Fat** by Robert F. MD Joseph; ISBN: 0963414712;
  http://www.amazon.com/exec/obidos/ASIN/0963414712/icongroupinterna

- **Chocolate Magnetic 2004 Calendar** by Sandra Boynton (2003); ISBN: 0761130748;
  http://www.amazon.com/exec/obidos/ASIN/0761130748/icongroupinterna

- **Chocolate Malts and Nickel Sodas** by Margaret. Johnson; ISBN: 0310266610;
  http://www.amazon.com/exec/obidos/ASIN/0310266610/icongroupinterna

- **Chocolate Memorabilia (Schiffer Book for Collectors)** by Donna S. Baker (2001); ISBN: 0764311530;
  http://www.amazon.com/exec/obidos/ASIN/0764311530/icongroupinterna

- **Chocolate Moulds: A History & Encyclopedia** by Judene Divone (1987); ISBN: 0939047020;
  http://www.amazon.com/exec/obidos/ASIN/0939047020/icongroupinterna

- **Chocolate Mousse and Other Fabulous Chocolate Creations** by Betty M. Potter (1986); ISBN: 0913703117;
  http://www.amazon.com/exec/obidos/ASIN/0913703117/icongroupinterna

- **Chocolate Mud Cake** by Harriet Ziefert; ISBN: 0060268921;
  http://www.amazon.com/exec/obidos/ASIN/0060268921/icongroupinterna

- **Chocolate On The Brain : Foolproof Recipes for Unrepentant Chocoholics** by Kevin Mills (Author), Nancy Mills (Author); ISBN: 0395983584;
  http://www.amazon.com/exec/obidos/ASIN/0395983584/icongroupinterna

- **Chocolate Passion: Recipes and Inspiration from the Kitchens of Chocolatier Magazine** by Tish Boyle (Author), Timothy Moriarty (Author); ISBN: 0471293172;
  http://www.amazon.com/exec/obidos/ASIN/0471293172/icongroupinterna

- **Chocolate Products - US [DOWNLOAD: PDF]** by Global Industry Analysts (Author); ISBN: B00005UEZS;
  http://www.amazon.com/exec/obidos/ASIN/B00005UEZS/icongroupinterna

- **Chocolate Pudding, and Other Approaches to Intensive Multiple-Family Therapy** by Ruth McClendon; ISBN: 0831400668;
  http://www.amazon.com/exec/obidos/ASIN/0831400668/icongroupinterna

- **Chocolate Quake** by Nancy Fairbanks; ISBN: 0425189465;
  http://www.amazon.com/exec/obidos/ASIN/0425189465/icongroupinterna

- **Chocolate Quick Fix** by Milton Zelman, Jeannine Winquist (Editor) (1985); ISBN: 0942320182;
  http://www.amazon.com/exec/obidos/ASIN/0942320182/icongroupinterna

- **Chocolate Sangria** by Tracy Price-Thompson (2003); ISBN: 0375506519;
  http://www.amazon.com/exec/obidos/ASIN/0375506519/icongroupinterna

- **Chocolate Sauce and Malice** by Arline Potter (2000); ISBN: 1583488499;
  http://www.amazon.com/exec/obidos/ASIN/1583488499/icongroupinterna

- **Chocolate Temptations** by Linda Collister, Patrice De Villiers (Photographer); ISBN: 1841720909;
  http://www.amazon.com/exec/obidos/ASIN/1841720909/icongroupinterna

- **Chocolate Temptations** by Christine Lacey (2000); ISBN: 1562454102;
  http://www.amazon.com/exec/obidos/ASIN/1562454102/icongroupinterna

- **Chocolate Thematic Unit** by Janna Reed, Kathee Gosnell; ISBN: 1557342393;
  http://www.amazon.com/exec/obidos/ASIN/1557342393/icongroupinterna

- **Chocolate Therapy: Dare to Discover Your Inner Center!** by Murray Langham (2003);
  ISBN: 1580081088;
  http://www.amazon.com/exec/obidos/ASIN/1580081088/icongroupinterna

- **Chocolate Thunder: The In-Your-Face, All-Over-The-Place, Death-Defyin',
  Mesmerizin', Slam-Jam Adventures of Double-D** by Darryl Dawkins, George Wirt;
  ISBN: 0809248867;
  http://www.amazon.com/exec/obidos/ASIN/0809248867/icongroupinterna

- **Chocolate Thunder: The Uncensored Life and Time of Darryl Dawkins** by Darryl
  Dawkins, Charley Rosen (2003); ISBN: 0973144327;
  http://www.amazon.com/exec/obidos/ASIN/0973144327/icongroupinterna

- **Chocolate to Morphine: Understanding Mind-Active Drugs** by Andrew Weil,
  Winifred Rosen; ISBN: 0395331900;
  http://www.amazon.com/exec/obidos/ASIN/0395331900/icongroupinterna

- **Chocolate Touch** by Patrick Skene Catling, Margot Apple (Illustrator) (1996); ISBN:
  0440412897;
  http://www.amazon.com/exec/obidos/ASIN/0440412897/icongroupinterna

- **Chocolate Truffles** by Carrie Huber; ISBN: 0942320158;
  http://www.amazon.com/exec/obidos/ASIN/0942320158/icongroupinterna

- **Chocolate Unwrapped: The Surprising Health Benefits of America's Favorite Passion**
  by Rowan Jacobsen; ISBN: 1931229317;
  http://www.amazon.com/exec/obidos/ASIN/1931229317/icongroupinterna

- **Chocolate! [CLV]** by Carin Kuoni (Author), et al; ISBN: 1884692036;
  http://www.amazon.com/exec/obidos/ASIN/1884692036/icongroupinterna

- **Chocolate, a Glacier Grizzly** by Peggy Christian, Carol Cottone-Kolthoff (Illustrator)
  (1997); ISBN: 1882728637;
  http://www.amazon.com/exec/obidos/ASIN/1882728637/icongroupinterna

- **Chocolate, Chocolate, Chocolate** by Barbara Myers; ISBN: 0892562196;
  http://www.amazon.com/exec/obidos/ASIN/0892562196/icongroupinterna

- **Chocolate, Cocoa, and Confectionery : Science and Technology** by Bernard W. Minifie
  (1995); ISBN: 083421301X;
  http://www.amazon.com/exec/obidos/ASIN/083421301X/icongroupinterna

- **Chocolate: An Exquisite Indulgence (Miniature Edition)** by Brian Perrin (Editor), et al
  (1995); ISBN: 1561386219;
  http://www.amazon.com/exec/obidos/ASIN/1561386219/icongroupinterna

- **Chocolate: From Simple Cookies to Extravagant Showstoppers** by Nick Malgieri
  (Author) (1998); ISBN: 0060187115;
  http://www.amazon.com/exec/obidos/ASIN/0060187115/icongroupinterna

- **Chocolate: From Start to Finish (Made in the U.S.A)** by Samuel G. Woods, Gale Zucker
  (Photographer) (1999); ISBN: 1567113915;
  http://www.amazon.com/exec/obidos/ASIN/1567113915/icongroupinterna

- **Chocolate: Over 250 Recipes for Cakes and Bakes, Desserts, Party Food, and Drinks** by Katherine Edelson (Editor), Jo Richardson (2003); ISBN: 1571459561; http://www.amazon.com/exec/obidos/ASIN/1571459561/icongroupinterna

- **Chocolate: Savor the Flavor (Landau, Elaine. Tasty Treats.)** by Elaine Landau (2001); ISBN: 157103336X; http://www.amazon.com/exec/obidos/ASIN/157103336X/icongroupinterna

- **Chocolate: The Consuming Passion** by Sandra Boynton (1982); ISBN: 0894801996; http://www.amazon.com/exec/obidos/ASIN/0894801996/icongroupinterna

- **Chocolate: The Nature of Indulgence** by Ruth Lopez (2002); ISBN: 0810904039; http://www.amazon.com/exec/obidos/ASIN/0810904039/icongroupinterna

- **Chocolates (Heavenly Recipes)**; ISBN: 1840721928; http://www.amazon.com/exec/obidos/ASIN/1840721928/icongroupinterna

- **Chocolates and Candies (Chocolates and Candies)** by Rebecca Gilpin, et al (2002); ISBN: 0794501591; http://www.amazon.com/exec/obidos/ASIN/0794501591/icongroupinterna

- **Chocolates for the Pillows Nightmares for the Guests: The Failure of the Hotel Industry to Protect the Traveling Public from Violent Crime** by Kenneth Lane Prestia (1993); ISBN: 0910155259; http://www.amazon.com/exec/obidos/ASIN/0910155259/icongroupinterna

- **Chocolates on the Pillow** by Gail Greco (Author), Tom Bagley (Author) (1996); ISBN: 1558534547; http://www.amazon.com/exec/obidos/ASIN/1558534547/icongroupinterna

- **Chocolates, Sweets & Candies: Hand-Made Temptations to Give for Every Season** by Sarah Ainley (2000); ISBN: 0754803481; http://www.amazon.com/exec/obidos/ASIN/0754803481/icongroupinterna

- **Chocolates, Sweets and Candies (Gifts from Nature Series)** by Southwater (Editor) (2003); ISBN: 1842157868; http://www.amazon.com/exec/obidos/ASIN/1842157868/icongroupinterna

- **Cholesterol Cures: More Than 325 Natural Ways to Lower Cholesterol and Live Longer from Almonds and Chocolate to Garlic and Wine** by William P. Castelli (Editor), Prevention Health Books (Editor) (2002); ISBN: 1579544819; http://www.amazon.com/exec/obidos/ASIN/1579544819/icongroupinterna

- **Cockadoodle Moo (Twinkle, Twinkle, Chocolate Bar)** by John Foster (Editor); ISBN: 0192762656; http://www.amazon.com/exec/obidos/ASIN/0192762656/icongroupinterna

- **Cocoa and Chocolate Painting** by Marsha Winbeckler, Roland A. Winbeckler (Illustrator) (1987); ISBN: 093011308X; http://www.amazon.com/exec/obidos/ASIN/093011308X/icongroupinterna

- **Cocoa and Chocolate, 1765-1914** by William Gervase Clarence-Smith; ISBN: 0415215765; http://www.amazon.com/exec/obidos/ASIN/0415215765/icongroupinterna

- **Collector's Guide to Antique Chocolate Molds With Values** by Wendy Mullen (2002); ISBN: 0875886183; http://www.amazon.com/exec/obidos/ASIN/0875886183/icongroupinterna

- **Cooking class chocolate cookies & brownies cookbook**; ISBN: 0785306676; http://www.amazon.com/exec/obidos/ASIN/0785306676/icongroupinterna

- **Cooks, Cakes, and Chocolate Shakes (Sanders, Nancy I. Parables in Action.)** by Nancy I. Sanders, et al (2000); ISBN: 0570071127;
  http://www.amazon.com/exec/obidos/ASIN/0570071127/icongroupinterna

- **Crafting the Culture and History of French Chocolate** by Susan J. Terrio; ISBN: 0520221265;
  http://www.amazon.com/exec/obidos/ASIN/0520221265/icongroupinterna

- **Crazy As Chocolate** by Elisabeth Hyde, Elizabeth Hyde (2003); ISBN: 0425192466;
  http://www.amazon.com/exec/obidos/ASIN/0425192466/icongroupinterna

- **Crisis in Candyland: Melting the Chocolate Shell of the Mars Family Empire** by Jan Pottker (1995); ISBN: 0788199870;
  http://www.amazon.com/exec/obidos/ASIN/0788199870/icongroupinterna

- **Curious George Goes to a Chocolate Factory** by Margaret Rey, et al; ISBN: 061311454X;
  http://www.amazon.com/exec/obidos/ASIN/061311454X/icongroupinterna

- **Dancin in Chocolate Heaven & Silence Cries out: How the Djembe got it's Voice** by DeBorah Devonne Ahmed (1999); ISBN: 0741400871;
  http://www.amazon.com/exec/obidos/ASIN/0741400871/icongroupinterna

- **Death by Chocolate** by Marcel Desavlniers (1993); ISBN: 0394223527;
  http://www.amazon.com/exec/obidos/ASIN/0394223527/icongroupinterna

- **Death by Chocolate : Revised and Expanded** by Marcel Desaulniers (Author) (2004); ISBN: 0847825574;
  http://www.amazon.com/exec/obidos/ASIN/0847825574/icongroupinterna

- **Death by Chocolate : What You Must Know Before Taking a Cruise** by Ross Klein; ISBN: 155081172X;
  http://www.amazon.com/exec/obidos/ASIN/155081172X/icongroupinterna

- **Death by Chocolate Cakes : An Astonishing Array of Chocolate Enchantments** by Marcel Desaulniers (Author) (2000); ISBN: 0688162975;
  http://www.amazon.com/exec/obidos/ASIN/0688162975/icongroupinterna

- **Death by Chocolate Cookies** by Marcel Desaulniers (1997); ISBN: 068483197X;
  http://www.amazon.com/exec/obidos/ASIN/068483197X/icongroupinterna

- **Death by Chocolate: A Savannah Reid Mystery** by G. A. McKevett (2003); ISBN: 1575667126;
  http://www.amazon.com/exec/obidos/ASIN/1575667126/icongroupinterna

- **Death by Chocolate: The Last Word on a Consuming Passion** by Marcel Desaulniers, Michael Grand (Photographer) (1992); ISBN: 0847815641;
  http://www.amazon.com/exec/obidos/ASIN/0847815641/icongroupinterna

- **Delicious Holiday Chocolate & Cookies** by Evelyn L. Beilenson, Joanna Roy (Illustrator) (1998); ISBN: 0880884088;
  http://www.amazon.com/exec/obidos/ASIN/0880884088/icongroupinterna

- **Dying for Chocolate** by Diane Mott Davidson; ISBN: 0553560247;
  http://www.amazon.com/exec/obidos/ASIN/0553560247/icongroupinterna

- **Eat Chocolate Naked** by Cam Johnson (2003); ISBN: 1402200978;
  http://www.amazon.com/exec/obidos/ASIN/1402200978/icongroupinterna

- **Eating Chocolates and Dancing in the Kitchen** by Tom Plummer, Louise Plummer (Introduction); ISBN: 1573453056;
  http://www.amazon.com/exec/obidos/ASIN/1573453056/icongroupinterna

- **Eating the Chocolate Elephant: Take Charge of Change Through Total Process Management** by Mark Youngblood; ISBN: 1571870024;
http://www.amazon.com/exec/obidos/ASIN/1571870024/icongroupinterna

- **Ebony Bitter-Sweet, a Chocolate Girl in a Vanilla World: Poetry and Prose for the Soul** by Rita Hall (1999); ISBN: 1881524310;
http://www.amazon.com/exec/obidos/ASIN/1881524310/icongroupinterna

- **El chocolate (La dolce vita series)** by Blume Staff, Edimat Libros; ISBN: 848403285X;
http://www.amazon.com/exec/obidos/ASIN/848403285X/icongroupinterna

- **El Libro De Contar De Los Chocolates ""M&M'S"" Brand** by Barbara Barbieri McGrath, et al (2003); ISBN: 1570913706;
http://www.amazon.com/exec/obidos/ASIN/1570913706/icongroupinterna

- **Everything Kids' Cookbook: From Mac ' N Cheese to Double Chocolate Chip Cookies-All You Need to Have Some Finger Lickin' Fun (Everything Kids Series)** by Sandra, M.S., R.D. Nissenberg, Sandra K. Nissenberg (2002); ISBN: 1580626580;
http://www.amazon.com/exec/obidos/ASIN/1580626580/icongroupinterna

- **Fabulous No-Guilt Desserts: From Sorbet to Chocolate Cake, Sin-Free Desserts for Every Occasion (Prevention Magazine's Quick & Healthy Low-Fat Cooking)** by The Food Editors of Prevention Magazine (Editor), Prevention Magazine; ISBN: 0875963285;
http://www.amazon.com/exec/obidos/ASIN/0875963285/icongroupinterna

- **Farm Journals Choice Chocolate Recipes** by Farm Journ, Farm Journal; ISBN: 0345301846;
http://www.amazon.com/exec/obidos/ASIN/0345301846/icongroupinterna

- **Farm Journal's Choice Chocolate Recipes** by Manning; ISBN: 0385147775;
http://www.amazon.com/exec/obidos/ASIN/0385147775/icongroupinterna

- **Favorite brand name best-loved chocolate recipes**; ISBN: 0785317910;
http://www.amazon.com/exec/obidos/ASIN/0785317910/icongroupinterna

- **Favorite Chocolate Recipes** by Christie Katona, et al (2003); ISBN: 1558671544;
http://www.amazon.com/exec/obidos/ASIN/1558671544/icongroupinterna

- **Favourite Chocolate Recipes**; ISBN: 1902842030;
http://www.amazon.com/exec/obidos/ASIN/1902842030/icongroupinterna

- **Faye Levy's Sensational Chocolate** by Faye Levy; ISBN: 1557880492;
http://www.amazon.com/exec/obidos/ASIN/1557880492/icongroupinterna

- **For the Love of Chocolate** by Margaret Brownley (Contributor), et al (2000); ISBN: 0312957912;
http://www.amazon.com/exec/obidos/ASIN/0312957912/icongroupinterna

- **For the Love of Chocolate Labrador Retrievers Deluxe 2004 Calendar** (2003); ISBN: 0763163139;
http://www.amazon.com/exec/obidos/ASIN/0763163139/icongroupinterna

- **Forrest Gump: My Favorite Chocolate Recipes: Mama's Fudge, Cookies, Cakes, and Candies** by Winston Groom, Leisure Arts; ISBN: 0848714873;
http://www.amazon.com/exec/obidos/ASIN/0848714873/icongroupinterna

- **French Toast & Dutch Chocolate** by Karen O'Connor; ISBN: 0570047714;
http://www.amazon.com/exec/obidos/ASIN/0570047714/icongroupinterna

- **Fresa y Chocolate** by Alea T. Gutierrez, J. C. Tabio (2002); ISBN: 844931254X;
http://www.amazon.com/exec/obidos/ASIN/844931254X/icongroupinterna

- **From Chocolate to Morphine : Everything You Need to Know About Mind-Altering Drugs** by Winifred Rosen (Author), Andrew T. Weil (Author); ISBN: 0395911524;
  http://www.amazon.com/exec/obidos/ASIN/0395911524/icongroupinterna

- **From Cocoa Bean to Chocolate (Start to Finish (Minneapolis, Minn.).)** by Robin Nelson; ISBN: 0822546655;
  http://www.amazon.com/exec/obidos/ASIN/0822546655/icongroupinterna

- **Germany Chocolate Confectionery 2003 [DOWNLOAD: PDF]** by Snapshots International Ltd (Author); ISBN: B0000ANM93;
  http://www.amazon.com/exec/obidos/ASIN/B0000ANM93/icongroupinterna

- **Germany Chocolate Tablets Report 2002 [DOWNLOAD: PDF]** by Snapshots International Ltd (Author); ISBN: B00006CRZ3;
  http://www.amazon.com/exec/obidos/ASIN/B00006CRZ3/icongroupinterna

- **Ghirardelli Original Chocolate Cookbook** by Phyllis Larsen, et al; ISBN: 0961021802;
  http://www.amazon.com/exec/obidos/ASIN/0961021802/icongroupinterna

- **Gourmet Coffee, Tea and Chocolate Drinks: Creating Your Favorite Recipes at Home** by Mathew Tekulsky (2002); ISBN: 0517221187;
  http://www.amazon.com/exec/obidos/ASIN/0517221187/icongroupinterna

- **Great Chefs Great Chocolate: Spectacular Desserts from America's Great Chefs** by Julia M. Pitkin (Editor) (1998); ISBN: 1888952830;
  http://www.amazon.com/exec/obidos/ASIN/1888952830/icongroupinterna

- **Great Movie Songs: Selections from: Hook, Home Alone, Victor/Victoria, the Last Emperor, Superman: The Movie, Doctor Dolittle, Willy Wonka & the Chocolate Factory scro** by Leslie Bricusse, Milton Okun (Editor); ISBN: 0895247003;
  http://www.amazon.com/exec/obidos/ASIN/0895247003/icongroupinterna

- **Growing Up on the Chocolate Diet** by Lora Brody; ISBN: 0805001190;
  http://www.amazon.com/exec/obidos/ASIN/0805001190/icongroupinterna

- **Growing Up on the Chocolate Diet: A Memoir With Recipes** by Lora Brody; ISBN: 0316108979;
  http://www.amazon.com/exec/obidos/ASIN/0316108979/icongroupinterna

- **Heavenly Chocolate** by Linda Collister, Debi Treloar (Photographer) (2002); ISBN: 1841722111;
  http://www.amazon.com/exec/obidos/ASIN/1841722111/icongroupinterna

- **Heavenly Chocolate: Divinely Decadent: The Ultimate Cookbook** by Christine France (2003); ISBN: 1842158155;
  http://www.amazon.com/exec/obidos/ASIN/1842158155/icongroupinterna

- **Hershey Milk Chocolate Weights and Measures** by Jerry Pallotta, Rob Bolster (Illustrator) (2003); ISBN: 0439388767;
  http://www.amazon.com/exec/obidos/ASIN/0439388767/icongroupinterna

- **Hershey's Chocolate and Cocoa Cookbook** by Ideals Publications Inc, Hershey Foods Corporation; ISBN: 082493007X;
  http://www.amazon.com/exec/obidos/ASIN/082493007X/icongroupinterna

- **Hershey's Chocolate Cookbook** by Hershey Food Corporation; ISBN: 0517675587;
  http://www.amazon.com/exec/obidos/ASIN/0517675587/icongroupinterna

- **Hershey's Chocolate for Every Season: 81 Luscious Creations** by Meredith Books (2001); ISBN: 0696213389;
http://www.amazon.com/exec/obidos/ASIN/0696213389/icongroupinterna

- **Hersheys Chocolate Lovers Cookbook** by Hersheys (Author); ISBN: 0887057624;
http://www.amazon.com/exec/obidos/ASIN/0887057624/icongroupinterna

- **Hershey's Chocolate Lovers Cookbook** by Wishing Well; ISBN: 0887057616;
http://www.amazon.com/exec/obidos/ASIN/0887057616/icongroupinterna

- **Hershey's Chocolate Memories: Sweets and Treats Since 1895, Through the Years Cookbook** by Nao Hauser; ISBN: 0943296005;
http://www.amazon.com/exec/obidos/ASIN/0943296005/icongroupinterna

- **Hershey's Chocolate Treasury**; ISBN: 0307492745;
http://www.amazon.com/exec/obidos/ASIN/0307492745/icongroupinterna

- **Hot Chocolate** by Suzanne Forster (Editor), et al (1999); ISBN: 0515124524;
http://www.amazon.com/exec/obidos/ASIN/0515124524/icongroupinterna

- **Hot Chocolate at Hanselmann's (European Women Writers Series)** by Rosetta Loy, Gregory Conti (Introduction) (2003); ISBN: 0803280068;
http://www.amazon.com/exec/obidos/ASIN/0803280068/icongroupinterna

- **Hot Chocolate for the Mystical Lover: 101 True Stories of Soul Mates Brought Together by Divine Intervention** by Arielle Ford (Editor), Deepak Chopra (Introduction) (2001); ISBN: 0452282179;
http://www.amazon.com/exec/obidos/ASIN/0452282179/icongroupinterna

- **Hot Chocolate for the Mystical Soul: 101 True Stories of Angels, Miracles, and Healings** by Arielle Ford, Mark Victor Hansen (1998); ISBN: 0452279259;
http://www.amazon.com/exec/obidos/ASIN/0452279259/icongroupinterna

- **Hot Chocolate for the Mystical Teenage Soul: 101 True Stories of Angels, Miracles, and Healings** by Arielle Ford (Editor), Gotham Chopra (2000); ISBN: 0452280702;
http://www.amazon.com/exec/obidos/ASIN/0452280702/icongroupinterna

- **Hot Chocolate Friendship (Alex Series 3)** by Nancy S. Levene, et al (1999); ISBN: 078143257X;
http://www.amazon.com/exec/obidos/ASIN/078143257X/icongroupinterna

- **Hot Chocolate Honeymoon (Harlequin American Romance, No 717)** by Cathy Gillen Thacker (1998); ISBN: 0373167172;
http://www.amazon.com/exec/obidos/ASIN/0373167172/icongroupinterna

- **How God Gives Us Chocolate** by Henrietta Gambill; ISBN: 0874038626;
http://www.amazon.com/exec/obidos/ASIN/0874038626/icongroupinterna

- **How Monkeys Make Chocolate: Foods and Medicines from the Rainforests** by Adrian Forsyth (1995); ISBN: 1895688329;
http://www.amazon.com/exec/obidos/ASIN/1895688329/icongroupinterna

- **How to Turn Exercise Into Chocolate: The Mother and Son Chocoholics' Guide to Making Exercise Delicious!** by Ken Rutkowski, Anne Rutkowski (Contributor) (2003); ISBN: 0966293347;
http://www.amazon.com/exec/obidos/ASIN/0966293347/icongroupinterna

- **I Like Chocolate (Welcome Books)** by Robin Pickering (2000); ISBN: 0516230085;
http://www.amazon.com/exec/obidos/ASIN/0516230085/icongroupinterna

- **I Love You More Than Chocolate!** by Marcia Tabram Philips (2002); ISBN: 0972434003;
  http://www.amazon.com/exec/obidos/ASIN/0972434003/icongroupinterna

- **I Want Chocolate!** by Trish Deseine, Marie-Pierre Morel (Photographer) (2003); ISBN: 1592230083;
  http://www.amazon.com/exec/obidos/ASIN/1592230083/icongroupinterna

- **Ice Cool: An Enticing Guide to Making Ice Cream and Ice Desserts With over 55 Irresistible Recipes - From Creamy Vanilla to Rich Chocolate Ripple** by Sara Lewis (2001); ISBN: 1842153684;
  http://www.amazon.com/exec/obidos/ASIN/1842153684/icongroupinterna

- **I'm Chocolate, You're Vanilla : Raising Healthy Black and Biracial Children in a Race-Conscious World** by Marguerite Wright (Author); ISBN: 0787952346;
  http://www.amazon.com/exec/obidos/ASIN/0787952346/icongroupinterna

- **Indulgence: Around the World in Search of Chocolate** by Paul Richardson (2003); ISBN: 0316860956;
  http://www.amazon.com/exec/obidos/ASIN/0316860956/icongroupinterna

- **Is It a Sin to Eat a Chocolate Bar?** by Mary Hoffman Wolf (2000); ISBN: 0595097367;
  http://www.amazon.com/exec/obidos/ASIN/0595097367/icongroupinterna

- **Italy Chocolate Confectionery Report 2002 [DOWNLOAD: PDF]** by Snapshots International Ltd (Author); ISBN: B00006CS6M;
  http://www.amazon.com/exec/obidos/ASIN/B00006CS6M/icongroupinterna

- **Just Hand over the Chocolate and No One Will Get Hurt** by Karen Scalf Linamen (1999); ISBN: 0800756940;
  http://www.amazon.com/exec/obidos/ASIN/0800756940/icongroupinterna

- **Knocking Chocolate Off the Trees: The Chronicle of a Serial Entrepreneur** by Kaliel Tuzman, Kristin Kimball (2003); ISBN: 1578518245;
  http://www.amazon.com/exec/obidos/ASIN/1578518245/icongroupinterna

- **La Dolce Vita: Chocolate** by New Holland (2001); ISBN: 1859748856;
  http://www.amazon.com/exec/obidos/ASIN/1859748856/icongroupinterna

- **Land Without Chocolate: A Memoir** by Faizal Deen (1999); ISBN: 0919897673;
  http://www.amazon.com/exec/obidos/ASIN/0919897673/icongroupinterna

- **Like Chocolate for Women: Indulge and Recharge with Everyday Aromatherapy** by Kim Morrison, et al (2002); ISBN: 1877178861;
  http://www.amazon.com/exec/obidos/ASIN/1877178861/icongroupinterna

- **Lilly's Chocolate Heart** by Kevin Henkes (Author) (2003); ISBN: 0060560665;
  http://www.amazon.com/exec/obidos/ASIN/0060560665/icongroupinterna

- **Little Black Book of Chocolate** by Barbara Bloch Benjamin (2003); ISBN: 0880883618;
  http://www.amazon.com/exec/obidos/ASIN/0880883618/icongroupinterna

- **Llams, Weavings, and Organic Chocolate: Multicultural Grassroots Development in the Andes and Amazon of Bolivia (From the Helen Kellogg Institue for International Studies)** by Kevin Healy (2001); ISBN: 0268013268;
  http://www.amazon.com/exec/obidos/ASIN/0268013268/icongroupinterna

- **Look & Cook: Chocolate** by Anne Willan; ISBN: 1564580318;
  http://www.amazon.com/exec/obidos/ASIN/1564580318/icongroupinterna

- **Louis Simpson's "Chocolates": A Study Guide from Gale's "Poetry for Students"** [DOWNLOAD: PDF]; ISBN: B000096BGC;
  http://www.amazon.com/exec/obidos/ASIN/B000096BGC/icongroupinterna

- **Love Adds a Little Chocolate: 100 Stories to Brighten Your Day and Sweeten Your Life** by Medard Laz (Introduction) (1998); ISBN: 0446524247;
  http://www.amazon.com/exec/obidos/ASIN/0446524247/icongroupinterna

- **Love Adds the Chocolate** by Linda Andersen, Vicki Wehrman (Illustrator) (2000); ISBN: 1578563259;
  http://www.amazon.com/exec/obidos/ASIN/1578563259/icongroupinterna

- **Love by Chocolate** by Rosanne Bittner, et al; ISBN: 0515120146;
  http://www.amazon.com/exec/obidos/ASIN/0515120146/icongroupinterna

- **Low-Fat Living for Real People: The Fat-Free Chocolate-Covered Creme-Filled Mini-Cakes Diet and Other Confusions of Low-Fat Eating Explained** by Linda Levy, Francine Grabowski (1998); ISBN: 096274039X;
  http://www.amazon.com/exec/obidos/ASIN/096274039X/icongroupinterna

- **Lucky Pennies and Hot Chocolate (Picture Puffins)** by Carol Diggory Shields, Hiroe Nakata (Illustrator) (2002); ISBN: 0142301906;
  http://www.amazon.com/exec/obidos/ASIN/0142301906/icongroupinterna

- **Luxury Chocolates [DOWNLOAD: PDF]** by Mintel International Group Ltd. (Author); ISBN: B00005R9TT;
  http://www.amazon.com/exec/obidos/ASIN/B00005R9TT/icongroupinterna

- **Mable Hoffman's Chocolate Cookery** by Mable Hoffman; ISBN: 0895860163;
  http://www.amazon.com/exec/obidos/ASIN/0895860163/icongroupinterna

- **Maida Heatter's Book of Great Chocolate Desserts** by Maida Heatter, Toni Evins (Illustrator) (1995); ISBN: 0679765336;
  http://www.amazon.com/exec/obidos/ASIN/0679765336/icongroupinterna

- **Making Chocolates** by Alec Leaver (Author); ISBN: 051721637X;
  http://www.amazon.com/exec/obidos/ASIN/051721637X/icongroupinterna

- **Making Your Own Gourmet Chocolate Drinks: Hot Drinks, Cold Drinks, Sodas, Floats, Shakes, and More!** by Mathew Tekulsky, et al; ISBN: 0517702657;
  http://www.amazon.com/exec/obidos/ASIN/0517702657/icongroupinterna

- **Marketlooks: The U.S. Market for Chocolate Candy [DOWNLOAD: PDF]** by MarketLooks - Packaged Facts (Author); ISBN: B000083FNC;
  http://www.amazon.com/exec/obidos/ASIN/B000083FNC/icongroupinterna

- **Marshall Field's Frango Chocolate Cookbook** by Marshall Field; ISBN: 0809244357;
  http://www.amazon.com/exec/obidos/ASIN/0809244357/icongroupinterna

- **Mary Marony and the Chocolate Surprise** by Suzy Kline, Blanche Sims (Illustrator) (1995); ISBN: 0399228292;
  http://www.amazon.com/exec/obidos/ASIN/0399228292/icongroupinterna

- **Mas Matematicas Con Los Chocolates De M&M's** by Barbara Barbieri McGrath, et al (2001); ISBN: 1570914818;
  http://www.amazon.com/exec/obidos/ASIN/1570914818/icongroupinterna

- **Max's Chocolate Chicken (Max and Ruby)** by Rosemary Wells (Illustrator) (2000); ISBN: 0140566724;
  http://www.amazon.com/exec/obidos/ASIN/0140566724/icongroupinterna

- **Meat & Potatoes: Home-Cooked Favorites from Perfect Pot Roast to Chocolate Cream Pie (American Kitchen Classics)** by Judith Choate; ISBN: 0671735489;
  http://www.amazon.com/exec/obidos/ASIN/0671735489/icongroupinterna

- **Men Love Chocolates But They Don't Say** by Mildred Kiconco Barya (2002); ISBN: 9970988808;
  http://www.amazon.com/exec/obidos/ASIN/9970988808/icongroupinterna

- **Mercedes and the Chocolate Pilot: A True Story of the Berlin Airlift and the Candy That Dropped from the Sky** by Margot Theis Raven, Gijsbert Van Frankenhuyzen (Illustrator) (2002); ISBN: 1585360694;
  http://www.amazon.com/exec/obidos/ASIN/1585360694/icongroupinterna

- **Milk Chocolate Naked Moon** by Joe Okonkwo (2002); ISBN: 0595248993;
  http://www.amazon.com/exec/obidos/ASIN/0595248993/icongroupinterna

- **Mocha, the Chocolate Puppy** by Peggy Simpson; ISBN: 1585970778;
  http://www.amazon.com/exec/obidos/ASIN/1585970778/icongroupinterna

- **Modeling Chocolate Made Easy: A Decorating Guide** by Peggy Alter (1995); ISBN: 0964800403;
  http://www.amazon.com/exec/obidos/ASIN/0964800403/icongroupinterna

- **More Hot Chocolate for the Mystical Soul: 101 True Stories of Angels, Miracles, and Healings** by Arielle Ford (1999); ISBN: 0452280699;
  http://www.amazon.com/exec/obidos/ASIN/0452280699/icongroupinterna

- **More M&M's Brand Chocolate Candies Math** by Barbara Barbieri McGrath, Roger Glass (Illustrator) (1998); ISBN: 0881069949;
  http://www.amazon.com/exec/obidos/ASIN/0881069949/icongroupinterna

- **Mr. Food Simply Chocolate** by Art Ginsburg; ISBN: 0688144195;
  http://www.amazon.com/exec/obidos/ASIN/0688144195/icongroupinterna

- **Mr. Pin: The Chocolate Files** by Mary Elise Monsell, et al (1992); ISBN: 0671740857;
  http://www.amazon.com/exec/obidos/ASIN/0671740857/icongroupinterna

- **Mr. Roopratna's Chocolates: The Winning Stories from the Rhys Davies Competition** by Cary Archard (Editor) (2000); ISBN: 1854112678;
  http://www.amazon.com/exec/obidos/ASIN/1854112678/icongroupinterna

- **Mrs. Fields I Love Chocolate! Cookbook: 100 Easy & Irresistible Recipes** by Debbi Fields, Robert A. Doyle (Editor) (1999); ISBN: 0809478080;
  http://www.amazon.com/exec/obidos/ASIN/0809478080/icongroupinterna

- **Multipack Chocolate Confectionery [DOWNLOAD: PDF]** by Mintel International Group Ltd. (Author); ISBN: B00005U84A;
  http://www.amazon.com/exec/obidos/ASIN/B00005U84A/icongroupinterna

- **Music from Cuba: Mongo Santamaria, Chocolate Armenteros, and Other Stateside Cuban Musicians** by Charley Gerard (Author); ISBN: 0275966828;
  http://www.amazon.com/exec/obidos/ASIN/0275966828/icongroupinterna

- **Mystery Cat and the Chocolate Trap** by Susan Saunders; ISBN: 055315415X;
  http://www.amazon.com/exec/obidos/ASIN/055315415X/icongroupinterna

- **Netherlands Chocolate Confectionery Report 2002 [DOWNLOAD: PDF]** by Snapshots International Ltd (Author); ISBN: B00006CS7K;
  http://www.amazon.com/exec/obidos/ASIN/B00006CS7K/icongroupinterna

- **New Chocolate Classics: Over 100 of Your Favorite Recipes Now Irresistibly in Chocolate** by Diana Dalsass (1999); ISBN: 0393318818;
  http://www.amazon.com/exec/obidos/ASIN/0393318818/icongroupinterna

- **New Cuisine Alternatives: Cream Puff Volcanoes & Chocolate Roller Blades** by Pam Moroso; ISBN: 0967880408;
  http://www.amazon.com/exec/obidos/ASIN/0967880408/icongroupinterna

- **New York Chocolate Lovers Guide: The Best Candy, Cakes and Chocolate Treats in Town** by William Gillen, et al (1996); ISBN: 1885492367;
  http://www.amazon.com/exec/obidos/ASIN/1885492367/icongroupinterna

- **Non-Chocolate Candy - US [DOWNLOAD: PDF]** by Global Industry Analysts (Author); ISBN: B00005UEZP;
  http://www.amazon.com/exec/obidos/ASIN/B00005UEZP/icongroupinterna

- **Of Course You Know That Chocolate Is a Vegetable and Other Stories (Five Star First Edition Mystery Series.)** by Barbara D'Amato; ISBN: 0786225394;
  http://www.amazon.com/exec/obidos/ASIN/0786225394/icongroupinterna

- **Once upon a Chocolate Kiss** by Cheryl Wolverton (2003); ISBN: 0373872364;
  http://www.amazon.com/exec/obidos/ASIN/0373872364/icongroupinterna

- **One Smart Cookie: How a Housewife's Chocolate Chip Recipe Turned into a Multimillion-Dollar Business: The Story of Mrs. Fields Cookies** by Debbi Fields, Alan Furst (Contributor); ISBN: 0671618385;
  http://www.amazon.com/exec/obidos/ASIN/0671618385/icongroupinterna

- **Patisserie: An Encyclopedia of Cakes, Pastries, Cookies, Biscuits, Chocolate, Confectionery & Desserts** by Aaron Maree; ISBN: 020718478X;
  http://www.amazon.com/exec/obidos/ASIN/020718478X/icongroupinterna

- **Peace, Love and Chocolate: Spiritual Humor and Other Stuff** by Benny Aabamadamabaa (2001); ISBN: 0595190650;
  http://www.amazon.com/exec/obidos/ASIN/0595190650/icongroupinterna

- **Percy's Chocolate Crunch** by W. Awdry (2004); ISBN: 0375827242;
  http://www.amazon.com/exec/obidos/ASIN/0375827242/icongroupinterna

- **Petits Fours, Chocolate, Frozen Desserts, and Sugar Work** by Roland Bilheux (Author), Alain Escoffier (Author) (1997); ISBN: 0470244100;
  http://www.amazon.com/exec/obidos/ASIN/0470244100/icongroupinterna

- **Plays 2: Cigarettes and Chocolate/Hang Up/What If It's Raining?/Truly, Madly, Deeply/Mosiac/Days Like These** by Anthony Minghella (1997); ISBN: 0413715205;
  http://www.amazon.com/exec/obidos/ASIN/0413715205/icongroupinterna

- **Pocket Book of Sex and Chocolate: What More Could a Body Want?** by Richard Craze; ISBN: 0897933206;
  http://www.amazon.com/exec/obidos/ASIN/0897933206/icongroupinterna

- **Poland Chocolate Confectionery Report 2002 [DOWNLOAD: PDF]** by Snapshots International Ltd (Author); ISBN: B000083FHE;
  http://www.amazon.com/exec/obidos/ASIN/B000083FHE/icongroupinterna

- **Poland Chocolate Tablets Report 2002 [DOWNLOAD: PDF]** by Snapshots International Ltd (Author); ISBN: B000083FHF;
  http://www.amazon.com/exec/obidos/ASIN/B000083FHF/icongroupinterna

- **Psyche Delicacies: Coffee, Chocolate, Chiles, Kava, and Cannabis, and Why They're Good for You** by Christopher Kilham, Chris Kilham (2001); ISBN: 1579543472;
  http://www.amazon.com/exec/obidos/ASIN/1579543472/icongroupinterna

- **Pure Imagination: The Making of Willy Wonka and the Chocolate Factory** by Mel Stuart, Josh Young (Contributor); ISBN: 0312287771;
  http://www.amazon.com/exec/obidos/ASIN/0312287771/icongroupinterna

- **Quick & Easy Chocolate: 70 Imaginative Recipes for the Busy Cook** by Gina Steer (1995); ISBN: 0943231744;
  http://www.amazon.com/exec/obidos/ASIN/0943231744/icongroupinterna

- **Quilts for Chocolate Lovers** by Janet Jones Worley, Janet Jones Worley (2001); ISBN: 1574327607;
  http://www.amazon.com/exec/obidos/ASIN/1574327607/icongroupinterna

- **Real Chocolate** by Chantal Coady (2003); ISBN: 0847825159;
  http://www.amazon.com/exec/obidos/ASIN/0847825159/icongroupinterna

- **Rinkle-Ronkle the Rhinocerwurst & the Big Chocolate Milk Spill** by Dr Paul, VI Paul (1997); ISBN: 0965968103;
  http://www.amazon.com/exec/obidos/ASIN/0965968103/icongroupinterna

- **Rosie's Bakery Chocolate-Packed Jam-Filled Butter-Rich No-Holds-Barred Cookie Book** by Judy Rosenberg, Sara Love (1996); ISBN: 1563055066;
  http://www.amazon.com/exec/obidos/ASIN/1563055066/icongroupinterna

- **Russia Chocolate Confectionery Report 2002 [DOWNLOAD: PDF]** by Snapshots International Ltd (Author); ISBN: B000083FJR;
  http://www.amazon.com/exec/obidos/ASIN/B000083FJR/icongroupinterna

- **Seasonal Chocolate Confectionery [DOWNLOAD: PDF]** by Mintel International Group Ltd. (Author); ISBN: B00005RC4U;
  http://www.amazon.com/exec/obidos/ASIN/B00005RC4U/icongroupinterna

- **Seduction by Chocolate** by Nina Bangs, et al; ISBN: 0843946679;
  http://www.amazon.com/exec/obidos/ASIN/0843946679/icongroupinterna

- **Sex, Drugs, Gambling, & Chocolate : A Workbook for Overcoming Addictions** by A. Thomas Horvath, Reid K. Hester (1998); ISBN: 1886230153;
  http://www.amazon.com/exec/obidos/ASIN/1886230153/icongroupinterna

- **Shoes: Chocolate For The Feet - A Cathy Collection** by Cathy Guisewite; ISBN: 0740705555;
  http://www.amazon.com/excc/obidos/ASIN/0740705555/icongroupinterna

- **Simple Chocolate Step-By-Step** by Gina Steer (Editor) (2002); ISBN: 1571457496;
  http://www.amazon.com/exec/obidos/ASIN/1571457496/icongroupinterna

- **Sin-Free Chocolate Smoothies: A Chocolate Lover's Guide to 70 Nutritious Blended Drinks** by Gabriel Constans (2002); ISBN: 1583331220;
  http://www.amazon.com/exec/obidos/ASIN/1583331220/icongroupinterna

- **Situation Desperate: Send Chocolate** by Polly Craig (2002); ISBN: 1403346275;
  http://www.amazon.com/exec/obidos/ASIN/1403346275/icongroupinterna

- **Slices of Chocolate Lives** by Linda F. Waters; ISBN: 096308870X;
  http://www.amazon.com/exec/obidos/ASIN/096308870X/icongroupinterna

- **Slow Chocolate Autopsy : Incidents from the Notorious Career of Norton, Prisoner of London** by Iain Sinclair, David McKean (1997); ISBN: 1861590881;
  http://www.amazon.com/exec/obidos/ASIN/1861590881/icongroupinterna

- **Smack, A.K.A. Plum Wine Dark Chocolate: A Love Story-The Shadow's Journey, Where Man Is Not Truly One, but Truly Two** by Renaldo, MD Fischer, Renaldo Fischer MD (2002); ISBN: 059522217X;
  http://www.amazon.com/exec/obidos/ASIN/059522217X/icongroupinterna

- **Sorcery and Cecelia or The Enchanted Chocolate Pot: Being the Correspondence of Two Young Ladies of Quality Regarding Various Magical Scandals in London and the Country** by Caroline Stevermer (Author), Patricia C. Wrede (Author); ISBN: 0152046151;
  http://www.amazon.com/exec/obidos/ASIN/0152046151/icongroupinterna

- **Spago Chocolate** by Mary Bergin (Introduction), et al (1999); ISBN: 0679448330;
  http://www.amazon.com/exec/obidos/ASIN/0679448330/icongroupinterna

- **Spiritual Chocolate for the Christmas Season** by Glenn Mollette (2002); ISBN: 0972070508;
  http://www.amazon.com/exec/obidos/ASIN/0972070508/icongroupinterna

- **Spiritual Chocolate Sweet Delights for Friends and Special People** by Glenn Mollette (2002); ISBN: 1592680038;
  http://www.amazon.com/exec/obidos/ASIN/1592680038/icongroupinterna

- **Spiritual Chocolate: Inspirational Delights for the Heart** by Glenn Mollette (2001); ISBN: 0970465025;
  http://www.amazon.com/exec/obidos/ASIN/0970465025/icongroupinterna

- **Spiritual Chocolate: Prayer-Filled Delights** by Glenn Mollette (2002); ISBN: 0970465084;
  http://www.amazon.com/exec/obidos/ASIN/0970465084/icongroupinterna

- **Sunset Over Chocolate Mountains** by Susan Elderkin; ISBN: 0802137997;
  http://www.amazon.com/exec/obidos/ASIN/0802137997/icongroupinterna

- **Sweet Seduction: Chocolate Truffles** by Adrienne Welch; ISBN: 0060911875;
  http://www.amazon.com/exec/obidos/ASIN/0060911875/icongroupinterna

- **Swimming in Chocolate: Poems and Drawings** by Mr. Mike, Mr Mike (1998); ISBN: 0965836541;
  http://www.amazon.com/exec/obidos/ASIN/0965836541/icongroupinterna

- **The 2003-2008 World Outlook for Chocolate Biscuit Countlines [DOWNLOAD: PDF]**; ISBN: B00009KFO5;
  http://www.amazon.com/exec/obidos/ASIN/B00009KFO5/icongroupinterna

- **The 2003-2008 World Outlook for Chocolate Countlines [DOWNLOAD: PDF]**; ISBN: B00009KFO6;
  http://www.amazon.com/exec/obidos/ASIN/B00009KFO6/icongroupinterna

- **The 2003-2008 World Outlook for Multipack Chocolate and Ice Cream Sticks [DOWNLOAD: PDF]**; ISBN: B00009KFAR;
  http://www.amazon.com/exec/obidos/ASIN/B00009KFAR/icongroupinterna

- **The 2003-2008 World Outlook for Seasonal Chocolate Confectionery [DOWNLOAD: PDF]**; ISBN: B00009KFEB;
  http://www.amazon.com/exec/obidos/ASIN/B00009KFEB/icongroupinterna

- **The 2003-2008 World Outlook for Seasonal Easter Chocolates [DOWNLOAD: PDF]**;
  ISBN: B00009KFEC;
  http://www.amazon.com/exec/obidos/ASIN/B00009KFEC/icongroupinterna

- **The 37 best chocolate chip cookies in America : the winning recipes in American Reflections' national cookie contest**; ISBN: 0936136006;
  http://www.amazon.com/exec/obidos/ASIN/0936136006/icongroupinterna

- **The 47 Best Chocolate Chip Cookies in the World** by Larry Zisman, Honey Zisman (1983); ISBN: 0312299834;
  http://www.amazon.com/exec/obidos/ASIN/0312299834/icongroupinterna

- **The Adventures of Sunny & The Chocolate Dog: Sunny & The Chocolate Dog Go to the Beach** by Susie Neimark, Kent Hammerstrom (Illustrator); ISBN: 0972594515;
  http://www.amazon.com/exec/obidos/ASIN/0972594515/icongroupinterna

- **The Adventures of Sunny & The Chocolate Dog: Sunny & The Chocolate Dog Go to the Doctor** by Susie Neimark; ISBN: 0972594523;
  http://www.amazon.com/exec/obidos/ASIN/0972594523/icongroupinterna

- **The Adventures of Sunny & The Chocolate Dog: Sunny Meets Her Baby Sister** by Susie Neimark, Kent Hammerstrom (Illustrator); ISBN: 0972594507;
  http://www.amazon.com/exec/obidos/ASIN/0972594507/icongroupinterna

- **The Art of Chocolate: Techniques & Recipes for Simply Spectacular Desserts & Confections** by Elaine Gonzalez, Frankie Frankeny (Photographer) (1998); ISBN: 081181811X;
  http://www.amazon.com/exec/obidos/ASIN/081181811X/icongroupinterna

- **The Best Chocolate Desserts: Cakes, Cookies, Brownies, and Other Sinful Sweets** by Gregg R. Gillespie (2003); ISBN: 1579122922;
  http://www.amazon.com/exec/obidos/ASIN/1579122922/icongroupinterna

- **The Big Chocolate Cookbook** by Gertrude Parke; ISBN: 0883656094;
  http://www.amazon.com/exec/obidos/ASIN/0883656094/icongroupinterna

- **The Book of Chocolate (Haworth Popular Culture)** by Nathalie Bailleux (Editor), et al (1996); ISBN: 2080135880;
  http://www.amazon.com/exec/obidos/ASIN/2080135880/icongroupinterna

- **The Book of Chocolates and Petit Fours** by Beverley Sutherland Smith, Beverly Sutherland Smith (1989); ISBN: 0895864819;
  http://www.amazon.com/exec/obidos/ASIN/0895864819/icongroupinterna

- **The Boy With Chocolate Mumps: With the Ultimate Lesson Plan** by Ernest R. Hurtado (2003); ISBN: 0533142334;
  http://www.amazon.com/exec/obidos/ASIN/0533142334/icongroupinterna

- **The Carob Way to Health: All-Natural Recipes for Cooking With Nature's Healthful Chocolate Alternative** by Frances Goulart; ISBN: 0446373028;
  http://www.amazon.com/exec/obidos/ASIN/0446373028/icongroupinterna

- **The Chocolate Bear Burglary: A Chocoholic Mystery** by Joanna Carl; ISBN: 0451207475;
  http://www.amazon.com/exec/obidos/ASIN/0451207475/icongroupinterna

- **The Chocolate Bible** by Christian Teubner, et al (2003); ISBN: 1552855007;
  http://www.amazon.com/exec/obidos/ASIN/1552855007/icongroupinterna

- **The Chocolate Book** by Sara Perry, Ben Garvie (Illustrator) (1992); ISBN: 0811802469;
  http://www.amazon.com/exec/obidos/ASIN/0811802469/icongroupinterna

- **The Chocolate Cat Caper** by Joanna Carl; ISBN: 0451205561;
  http://www.amazon.com/exec/obidos/ASIN/0451205561/icongroupinterna

- **The Chocolate Cookbook** by Elizabeth Wolf Cohen; ISBN: 0517073153;
  http://www.amazon.com/exec/obidos/ASIN/0517073153/icongroupinterna

- **The Chocolate Cookbook** by Christine France (2003); ISBN: 0754811026;
  http://www.amazon.com/exec/obidos/ASIN/0754811026/icongroupinterna

- **The Chocolate Cream Society: A Novel** by Leonard Barras; ISBN: 0906228581;
  http://www.amazon.com/exec/obidos/ASIN/0906228581/icongroupinterna

- **The Chocolate Deal: A Novel** by Haim Gouri, et al (1999); ISBN: 0814328008;
  http://www.amazon.com/exec/obidos/ASIN/0814328008/icongroupinterna

- **The Chocolate Debutante** by Marion Chesney; ISBN: 0449222594;
  http://www.amazon.com/exec/obidos/ASIN/0449222594/icongroupinterna

- **The Chocolate Diet** by Sally Ann Voak (2001); ISBN: 1857824377;
  http://www.amazon.com/exec/obidos/ASIN/1857824377/icongroupinterna

- **The Chocolate Frog Frame-Up** by Joanna Carl; ISBN: 0451209850;
  http://www.amazon.com/exec/obidos/ASIN/0451209850/icongroupinterna

- **The Chocolate Korndog** by Jonathan Pearce; ISBN: 074141127X;
  http://www.amazon.com/exec/obidos/ASIN/074141127X/icongroupinterna

- **The Chocolate Lover** (2004); ISBN: 0142500429;
  http://www.amazon.com/exec/obidos/ASIN/0142500429/icongroupinterna

- **The Chocolate Lovers' Companion** by Norman. Kolpas; ISBN: 0825631262;
  http://www.amazon.com/exec/obidos/ASIN/0825631262/icongroupinterna

- **The Chocolate Lover's Guide to the Pacific Northwest** by Bobbie Hasselbring, Bobbie J. Hasselbring; ISBN: 0966561902;
  http://www.amazon.com/exec/obidos/ASIN/0966561902/icongroupinterna

- **The Chocolate Lovers: A Children's Story and Cookbook** by Joan Van Loon, et al (2001); ISBN: 1552852334;
  http://www.amazon.com/exec/obidos/ASIN/1552852334/icongroupinterna

- **The Chocolate Man** by Randy Ross; ISBN: 0966267508;
  http://www.amazon.com/exec/obidos/ASIN/0966267508/icongroupinterna

- **The Chocolate Man** by Jeremy Fox (1996); ISBN: 0920953891;
  http://www.amazon.com/exec/obidos/ASIN/0920953891/icongroupinterna

- **The Chocolate Market [DOWNLOAD: PDF]** by Packaged Facts (Author); ISBN: B00005R94K;
  http://www.amazon.com/exec/obidos/ASIN/B00005R94K/icongroupinterna

- **The Chocolate Seduction (Sex & Candy)** by Carrie Alexander (2003); ISBN: 0373691254;
  http://www.amazon.com/exec/obidos/ASIN/0373691254/icongroupinterna

- **The Chocolate Ship** by Marissa Monteilh (Author) (2003); ISBN: 0060011483;
  http://www.amazon.com/exec/obidos/ASIN/0060011483/icongroupinterna

- **The Chocolate Side of Life** by Cindy Sigler Dagnan (2003); ISBN: 1892435284;
  http://www.amazon.com/exec/obidos/ASIN/1892435284/icongroupinterna

- **The Chocolate Snowball: and Other Fabulous Pastries from Deer Valley Bakery** by Letty Flatt Halloran (Author) (1999); ISBN: 1560448288;
  http://www.amazon.com/exec/obidos/ASIN/1560448288/icongroupinterna

- **The Chocolate Sundae Mystery (Boxcar Children Mysteries, 46)** by Gertrude Chandler Warner, Charles Tang (Illustrator) (1995); ISBN: 0807511455;
  http://www.amazon.com/exec/obidos/ASIN/0807511455/icongroupinterna

- **The Chocolate Train** by Joanne Kornfeld; ISBN: 097046293X;
  http://www.amazon.com/exec/obidos/ASIN/097046293X/icongroupinterna

- **The Chocolate War** by Robert Cormier; ISBN: 0440944597;
  http://www.amazon.com/exec/obidos/ASIN/0440944597/icongroupinterna

- **The Chocolate War: A Unit Plan** by Janine H. Sherman, Barbara M. Linde; ISBN: 1583372288;
  http://www.amazon.com/exec/obidos/ASIN/1583372288/icongroupinterna

- **The Chocolate-Covered Contest** by Carolyn Keene (Author); ISBN: 067103443X;
  http://www.amazon.com/exec/obidos/ASIN/067103443X/icongroupinterna

- **The Chocolate-Covered-Cookie Tantrum** by Harvey Stevenson (Illustrator), Deborah Blumenthal (Author) (1999); ISBN: 0395700280;
  http://www.amazon.com/exec/obidos/ASIN/0395700280/icongroupinterna

- **The Diabetic Chocolate Cookbook** by Mary Jane Finsand, James D. Healy (1990); ISBN: 0806979003;
  http://www.amazon.com/exec/obidos/ASIN/0806979003/icongroupinterna

- **The Dilettante Book of Chocolate and Confections** by Ruth Reed, Dana Taylor Davenport; ISBN: 0060912235;
  http://www.amazon.com/exec/obidos/ASIN/0060912235/icongroupinterna

- **The Discovery of Chocolate** by James Runcie (Author) (2002); ISBN: 0060959436;
  http://www.amazon.com/exec/obidos/ASIN/0060959436/icongroupinterna

- **The East India Company Book of Chocolate** by Antony Wild, Anthony Wild; ISBN: 0004127749;
  http://www.amazon.com/exec/obidos/ASIN/0004127749/icongroupinterna

- **The Emperors of Chocolate: Inside the Secret World of Hershey and Mars** by Joel Glenn Brenner; ISBN: 0767904575;
  http://www.amazon.com/exec/obidos/ASIN/0767904575/icongroupinterna

- **The European Market for Chocolate to 2006 [DOWNLOAD: PDF]** by Datamonitor (Author); ISBN: B00008R3QV;
  http://www.amazon.com/exec/obidos/ASIN/B00008R3QV/icongroupinterna

- **The Everything Chocolate Cookbook: A Chocolate-Lover's Dream Collection of Cookies, Cakes, Brownies, Candies, and Confections (Everything Series)** by Laura Tyler Samuels (2000); ISBN: 1580624057;
  http://www.amazon.com/exec/obidos/ASIN/1580624057/icongroupinterna

- **The Food Lover's Guide to Chocolate and Vanilla** by Sharon Tyler Herbst; ISBN: 0688137709;
  http://www.amazon.com/exec/obidos/ASIN/0688137709/icongroupinterna

- **The Ghirardelli Chocolate Cookbook** by Neva Beach, Ghirardelli Company (1995); ISBN: 0898157692;
  http://www.amazon.com/exec/obidos/ASIN/0898157692/icongroupinterna

- **The Ghost Who Ate Chocolate (Black Cat Club, No. 1)** by Susan Saunders, Jane K. Manning (Illustrator) (1996); ISBN: 0064420353;
  http://www.amazon.com/exec/obidos/ASIN/0064420353/icongroupinterna

- **The Good Web Guide to Chocolate**; ISBN: 1903282349;
  http://www.amazon.com/exec/obidos/ASIN/1903282349/icongroupinterna

- **The Great American Chocolate Cookbook**; ISBN: 0871972301;
  http://www.amazon.com/exec/obidos/ASIN/0871972301/icongroupinterna

- **The Haigh's Book of Chocolate** by Cath Kerry; ISBN: 1862544603;
  http://www.amazon.com/exec/obidos/ASIN/1862544603/icongroupinterna

- **The Hershey's Milk Chocolate Bar Fractions Book** by Jerry Pallotta, et al (1999); ISBN: 0439135192;
  http://www.amazon.com/exec/obidos/ASIN/0439135192/icongroupinterna

- **The Hershey's Milk Chocolate Multiplication Book** by Jerry Pallotta, Rob Bolster (Illustrator) (2002); ISBN: 0439236231;
  http://www.amazon.com/exec/obidos/ASIN/0439236231/icongroupinterna

- **The Hollow Chocolate Bunnies of the Apocalypse (Gollancz S.F.)** by Robert Rankin; ISBN: 0575073136;
  http://www.amazon.com/exec/obidos/ASIN/0575073136/icongroupinterna

- **The International Chocolate Cookbook** by Nancy Baggett, Martin Jacobs (Photographer); ISBN: 1556703635;
  http://www.amazon.com/exec/obidos/ASIN/1556703635/icongroupinterna

- **The Joy of Chocolate** by Judith Olney; ISBN: 0812054350;
  http://www.amazon.com/exec/obidos/ASIN/0812054350/icongroupinterna

- **The Kid's Book of Chocolate** by Richard Ammon; ISBN: 068931292X;
  http://www.amazon.com/exec/obidos/ASIN/068931292X/icongroupinterna

- **The Legend of Frango Chocolate** by Robert Spector (1993); ISBN: 0935503145;
  http://www.amazon.com/exec/obidos/ASIN/0935503145/icongroupinterna

- **The Little Book of Chocolate** by Katherine Khodorowsky, Herve Robert (2001); ISBN: 2080105434;
  http://www.amazon.com/exec/obidos/ASIN/2080105434/icongroupinterna

- **The M&M's Brand Chocolate Candies Counting Board Book** by Barbara Barbieri McGrath, Barbara Barbieri McGarth (1997); ISBN: 0881069485;
  http://www.amazon.com/exec/obidos/ASIN/0881069485/icongroupinterna

- **The New Taste of Chocolate: A Cultural and Natural History of Cacao with Recipes** by Maricel E. Presilla (2001); ISBN: 1580081436;
  http://www.amazon.com/exec/obidos/ASIN/1580081436/icongroupinterna

- **The Official M&M's Brand History of Chocolate** by Karen Pellaton (Illustrator), Red Yellow Green and Blue (2001); ISBN: 1570914494;
  http://www.amazon.com/exec/obidos/ASIN/1570914494/icongroupinterna

- **The Only Thing Better Than Chocolate** by Janet Dailey, et al; ISBN: 0821772937;
  http://www.amazon.com/exec/obidos/ASIN/0821772937/icongroupinterna

- **The Passion of Chocolate** by Patrick Caton (1996); ISBN: 156245272X;
  http://www.amazon.com/exec/obidos/ASIN/156245272X/icongroupinterna

- **The Perfect Chocolate Desert** by Outlet (1988); ISBN: 0517363313;
  http://www.amazon.com/exec/obidos/ASIN/0517363313/icongroupinterna

- **The Pillsbury Chocolate Lover's Cookbook** by Pillsbury Company; ISBN: 038523869X;
  http://www.amazon.com/exec/obidos/ASIN/038523869X/icongroupinterna

- **The Poisoned Chocolates Case** by Anthony Berkeley (2003); ISBN: 184262217X;
  http://www.amazon.com/exec/obidos/ASIN/184262217X/icongroupinterna

- **The Pond Vol. 2: Chocolate For Life Cassette 6 Pack : [ABRIDGED]** by Charlie Richards (Author); ISBN: 140030220X;
  http://www.amazon.com/exec/obidos/ASIN/140030220X/icongroupinterna

- **The Pursuit of Romance: A Husband's Guide to Thinking Beyond Chocolate, Roses and Candlelight** by David J. Frahm, Anne Frahm (Contributor) (1997); ISBN: 1562922572;
  http://www.amazon.com/exec/obidos/ASIN/1562922572/icongroupinterna

- **The Science of Chocolate** by Stephen T. Beckett (2000); ISBN: 0854046003;
  http://www.amazon.com/exec/obidos/ASIN/0854046003/icongroupinterna

- **The Search for the Perfect Chocolate Chip Cookie** by Gwen Steege; ISBN: 0882664786;
  http://www.amazon.com/exec/obidos/ASIN/0882664786/icongroupinterna

- **The Totally Chocolate Cookbook** by Helene Siegel, Karen Gillingham (1996); ISBN: 0890878056;
  http://www.amazon.com/exec/obidos/ASIN/0890878056/icongroupinterna

- **The True History of Chocolate** by Sophie D. Coe, Michael D. Coe (2000); ISBN: 0500282293;
  http://www.amazon.com/exec/obidos/ASIN/0500282293/icongroupinterna

- **The U.S. Gourmet Chocolate Market [DOWNLOAD: PDF]** by Packaged Facts (Author); ISBN: B00005R8VE;
  http://www.amazon.com/exec/obidos/ASIN/B00005R8VE/icongroupinterna

- **The U.S. Market for Chocolate Candy: Volume 1 in the Series [DOWNLOAD: PDF]** by Packaged Facts (Author); ISBN: B00007EIEB;
  http://www.amazon.com/exec/obidos/ASIN/B00007EIEB/icongroupinterna

- **The U.S. Market for Non-Chocolate Candy: Volume 2 in the series [DOWNLOAD: PDF]** by Packaged Facts (Author); ISBN: B000087GJ4;
  http://www.amazon.com/exec/obidos/ASIN/B000087GJ4/icongroupinterna

- **The Ultimate Encyclopedia of Chocolate: With over 200 Recipes** by Christine McFadden, Christine France (Contributor); ISBN: 0765194767;
  http://www.amazon.com/exec/obidos/ASIN/0765194767/icongroupinterna

- **The Ultimate Healthy Eating Plan: That Still Leaves Room for Chocolate** by Mairlyn Smith, Liz Pearson (2002); ISBN: 1552853349;
  http://www.amazon.com/exec/obidos/ASIN/1552853349/icongroupinterna

- **The Unsolved Chocolate Pudding Files** by Alex Gabbard (1994); ISBN: 0962260851;
  http://www.amazon.com/exec/obidos/ASIN/0962260851/icongroupinterna

- **The Usborne Book of Young Puzzle Adventures: Lucy and the Sea Monster, Chocolate Island, Dragon in the Cupboard (Young Puzzles Adventures Series)** by Karen Dolby, Caroline Church (Illustrator) (1996); ISBN: 0746022905;
  http://www.amazon.com/exec/obidos/ASIN/0746022905/icongroupinterna

- **Theodoras Wedding: Faith, Love, and Chocolate** by Penny Culliford (2003); ISBN: 0310250390;
  http://www.amazon.com/exec/obidos/ASIN/0310250390/icongroupinterna

- **There Are No Bad Chocolate Chip Cookies** by Nathan P. Boyd (2003); ISBN: 1412004004;
  http://www.amazon.com/exec/obidos/ASIN/1412004004/icongroupinterna
- **Thomas and Friends: Percy's Chocolate Crunch and Other Thomas the Tank Enginestories** by Random House (2003); ISBN: 0375813926;
  http://www.amazon.com/exec/obidos/ASIN/0375813926/icongroupinterna
- **Three Hundred and Sixty-Five Great Chocolate Desserts** by Natalie Haughton; ISBN: 0060165375;
  http://www.amazon.com/exec/obidos/ASIN/0060165375/icongroupinterna
- **Travel Tips for the Sophisticated Woman: Over 1,000 Practical Tips on Enjoying Museums, Shopping, Performances, Dining, Chocolate, Looking Great, and More While Traveling in Europe and North** by Laura Vestanen (2001); ISBN: 1401033792;
  http://www.amazon.com/exec/obidos/ASIN/1401033792/icongroupinterna
- **Treasury of Chocolate Recipes**; ISBN: 1561736597;
  http://www.amazon.com/exec/obidos/ASIN/1561736597/icongroupinterna
- **Truffles and Other Chocolate Confections** by Pamella Asquith, Laura Hartman (Illustrator); ISBN: 0030633567;
  http://www.amazon.com/exec/obidos/ASIN/0030633567/icongroupinterna
- **UK Chocolate Confectionery 2001 [DOWNLOAD: PDF]** by Snapshots International Ltd (Author); ISBN: B00006CSOU;
  http://www.amazon.com/exec/obidos/ASIN/B00006CSOU/icongroupinterna
- **UK Chocolate Confectionery 2003 [DOWNLOAD: PDF]** by Snapshots International Ltd (Author); ISBN: B0000ANM96;
  http://www.amazon.com/exec/obidos/ASIN/B0000ANM96/icongroupinterna
- **Ultimate Chocolate (DK Living)** by Patricia Lousada, et al; ISBN: 0789448386;
  http://www.amazon.com/exec/obidos/ASIN/0789448386/icongroupinterna
- **Ultimate Cook Book : Chocolate Sensations** by Stephane Souvlis (Editor), et al; ISBN: 158279118X;
  http://www.amazon.com/exec/obidos/ASIN/158279118X/icongroupinterna
- **Una Casa De Chocolate/a House Out of Chocolate (How 2 Series)** by Silver Dolphin (2002); ISBN: 9685308543;
  http://www.amazon.com/exec/obidos/ASIN/9685308543/icongroupinterna
- **US CHOCOLATE CONFECTIONERY REPORT 2002 [DOWNLOAD: PDF]** by Snapshots International Ltd (Author); ISBN: B00006SLLZ;
  http://www.amazon.com/exec/obidos/ASIN/B00006SLLZ/icongroupinterna
- **Western Europe Chocolate Confectionery 2001 [DOWNLOAD: PDF]** by Snapshots International Ltd (Author); ISBN: B00006CSTE;
  http://www.amazon.com/exec/obidos/ASIN/B00006CSTE/icongroupinterna
- **What's Cooking Chocolate (What's Cooking Series)** by Jacqueline Bellefontaine (1998); ISBN: 157145151X;
  http://www.amazon.com/exec/obidos/ASIN/157145151X/icongroupinterna
- **When Chocolate Milk Moved In** by Ken Harvey, Marysue Hermes (Illustrator); ISBN: 1930093160;
  http://www.amazon.com/exec/obidos/ASIN/1930093160/icongroupinterna
- **White Chocolate** by Janice Wald Henderson; ISBN: 0809247836;
  http://www.amazon.com/exec/obidos/ASIN/0809247836/icongroupinterna

- **White Chocolate** by Elizabeth Atkins Bowman, Elizabeth Atkins Bowman; ISBN: 0812571819;
  http://www.amazon.com/exec/obidos/ASIN/0812571819/icongroupinterna

- **White Chocolate** by Dr. Michael Helzner, Michael Helzner (Preface) (1999); ISBN: 0887391605;
  http://www.amazon.com/exec/obidos/ASIN/0887391605/icongroupinterna

- **Why Women Need Chocolate: Eat What You Crave to Look Good & Feel Great** by Debra Waterhouse (1995); ISBN: 0788192507;
  http://www.amazon.com/exec/obidos/ASIN/0788192507/icongroupinterna

- **Yummy Chocolate Bunny** by Jocelyn Jamison, Jui Ishida (Illustrator) (2003); ISBN: 0843102594;
  http://www.amazon.com/exec/obidos/ASIN/0843102594/icongroupinterna

- **Zingerman's Guide to Good Eating : How to Choose the Best Bread, Cheeses, Olive Oil, Pasta, Chocolate, and Much More** by Ari Weinzweig (Author) (2003); ISBN: 0395926165;
  http://www.amazon.com/exec/obidos/ASIN/0395926165/icongroupinterna

The National Library of Medicine Book Index

The National Library of Medicine at the National Institutes of Health has a massive database of books published on healthcare and biomedicine. Go to the following Internet site, **http://locatorplus.gov/**, and then select "Search LOCATORplus." Once you are in the search area, simply type "chocolate" (or synonyms) into the search box, and select "books only." From there, results can be sorted by publication date, author, or relevance. The following was recently catalogued by the National Library of Medicine:[11]

- **A treatise on tobacco, tea, coffee, and chocolate:... the whole illustrated with copper plates, exhibiting the tea utensils of the Chinese and Perians** Author: Paulli, Simon,; Year: 1746; London: Printed for T. Osborne..., J. Hildyard, at York, M. Bryson, at Newcastle, and J. Leake, at Bath, 1746

- **Chocolate and cocoa: health and nutrition.** Author: edited by Ian Knight; Year: 1999

- **Coffee, tea, and chocolate: their influence upon the health, the intellect, and the moral nature of man. Tr. from the French of A. Saint-Arroman...** Author: Saint-Arroman, Auguste.; Year: 1846; Philadelphia, T. Ward, 1846

- **Coffee, tea, chocolate, and the brain** Author: Nehlig, Astrid.; Year: 1717; London; New York: Taylor; Francis, 2004; ISBN: 0415306914
  http://www.amazon.com/exec/obidos/ASIN/0415306914/icongroupinterna

- **Coffee, tea, chocolate, and the brain.** Author: edited by Astrid Nehlig; Year: 2004

- **Natural history of coffee, chocolate, thee, tobacco, in four several sections: with a tract of elder and juniper-berries, shewing how useful they may be in our coffee-houses;**

---

[11] In addition to LOCATORPlus, in collaboration with authors and publishers, the National Center for Biotechnology Information (NCBI) is currently adapting biomedical books for the Web. The books may be accessed in two ways: (1) by searching directly using any search term or phrase (in the same way as the bibliographic database PubMed), or (2) by following the links to PubMed abstracts. Each PubMed abstract has a "Books" button that displays a facsimile of the abstract in which some phrases are hypertext links. These phrases are also found in the books available at NCBI. Click on hyperlinked results in the list of books in which the phrase is found. Currently, the majority of the links are between the books and PubMed. In the future, more links will be created between the books and other types of information, such as gene and protein sequences and macromolecular structures. See **http://www.ncbi.nlm.nih.gov/entrez/query.fcgi?db=Books**.

and also the way of making mum, with some remarks upon that liquor. Author: collected; Year: 1682

- Psyche delicacies: coffee, chocolate, chiles, kava, and cannabis, and why they're good for you. Author: by Chris Kilham; Year: 2001

- Tablet triturates, hypodermic and compressed tablets, chocolate coated tablets, physicians' private formulas, and vial cases. Author: Fraser Tablet Triturate Mfg. Company.; Year: 1693; New York: The Fraser Tablet Triturate Mfg. Company..., 1899

- Tablet triturates, hypodermic and compressed tablets, chocolate coated tablets, physicians' private formulas, and vial cases. Author: Fraser Tablet Triturate Mfg. Company; Year: 1899

- The natural history of chocolate. Being a distinct and particular account of the cocao-tree, its growth and culture, and the preparation, excellent properties, and medicinal vertues of its fruit... Translated from the last edition of the French, by a physician. Author: Quélus, D. de.; Year: 1796; London, J. Roberts, 1724

Chapters on Chocolate

In order to find chapters that specifically relate to chocolate, an excellent source of abstracts is the Combined Health Information Database. You will need to limit your search to book chapters and chocolate using the "Detailed Search" option. Go to the following hyperlink: http://chid.nih.gov/detail/detail.html. To find book chapters, use the drop boxes at the bottom of the search page where "You may refine your search by." Select the dates and language you prefer, and the format option "Book Chapter." Type "chocolate" (or synonyms) into the "For these words:" box. The following is a typical result when searching for book chapters on chocolate:

- Hyperoxaluria and Nephrolithiasis

  Source: in Bayless, T.M. and Hanauer, S.B. Advanced Therapy of Inflammatory Bowel Disease. Hamilton, Ontario: B.C. Decker Inc. 2001. p. 475-478.

  Contact: Available from B.C. Decker Inc. 20 Hughson Street South, P.O. Box 620, L.C.D. 1 Hamilton, Ontario L8N 3K7. (905) 522-7017 or (800) 568-7281. Fax (905) 522-7839. Email: info@bcdecker.com. Website: www.bcdecker.com. PRICE: $129.00 plus shipping and handling. ISBN: 1550091220.

  Summary: This chapter on hyperoxaluria (excessive amounts of oxalate in the urine) and nephrolithiasis (kidney stones) is from the second edition of a book devoted to the details of medical, surgical, and supportive management of patients with Crohn's disease (CD) and Ulcerative Colitis (UC), together known as inflammatory bowel disease (IBD). The finding of kidney stones in association with IBD occurs with a frequency ranging from 1 percent to 5 percent. The author cautions that not all kidney stones found in patients with IBD are oxalate stones. Chemical analysis of a passed stone or of the urine must be made before enteric hyperoxaluria (the urologic term for IBD associated hyperoxaluria) can be assumed to be the cause of the nephrolithiasis. Kidney stones classically present as renal colic (pain in the area of the kidneys). Unfortunately, in patients with IBD a high index of suspicion is necessary, because the pain associated with the kidney stone may easily (and erroneously) be attributed to the underlying IBD. Microscopic hematuria (blood in the urine) is suggestive of the diagnosis. The treatment for acute, symptomatic kidney stones is initially narcotic analgesia (pain medication) with copious hydration in an attempt to help the patient pass the stone spontaneously. If this is unsuccessful, a urologist is consulted, and the stone can be removed transureterally, surgically, or by using extracorporeal shock wave lithotripsy (ESWL). Once alleviation of the stone is accomplished, preventing stone recurrence becomes important. Prevention strategies include restriction of dietary oxalate (common sources include rhubarb, spinach, beets, peanuts, **chocolate**, parsley, celery, tea, and coffee) and protein reduction (protein is an indirect dietary source of oxalate). 3 tables. 9 references.

- **Everything You Ever Wanted to Ask Your Dietitian About IBS**

  Source: in Magee, E. Tell Me What to Eat If I Have Irritable Bowel Syndrome. Franklin Lakes, NJ: Career Press, Inc. 2000. p. 30-46.

  Contact: Available from Career Press, Inc. 3 Tice Road, P.O. Box 687, Franklin Lakes, NJ 07417. (800) 227-3371. Website: www.careerpress.com or www.newpagebooks.com. PRICE: $10.99 plus shipping and handling.

  Summary: This chapter is from a book that offers eating and nutrition guidelines for people who have been diagnosed with irritable bowel syndrome (IBS). People with IBS have bowels that tend to overreact in certain situations. Whatever affects the bowels of the population at large, such as diet, hormones, or stress, affects those of people with IS even more, resulting in the symptoms of the disorder. This chapter notes that a big part of treating and managing IBS involves what the patient eats, how and how much they eat, and where they eat. Certain foods and nutrients can help the condition, and others can make symptoms worse. The author emphasizes that IBS is a very individual disorder and that it may take some time for each patient to determine his or her own food triggers. And even for those patients whose IS is particularly affected by stress, limiting personal food triggers during stressful times will contribute to minimizing the resulting symptoms. For readers who are not sure what foods trigger their symptoms, the author recommends the use of an F's (food, feelings, symptoms) journal to help find the links between foods, eating patterns, and symptoms. In addition, the simple act of eating normally causes the muscles in the colon to contract. In people with IBS, the resulting need to defecate may be urgent and occur soon after eating, with accompanying cramps and diarrhea. The author recommends eating smaller meals more often to reduce this post-meal challenge. The author then considers specific food items, including potential problems such as fructose (the natural sugar found in fruits and berries), soft drinks, sorbitol, olestra (a calorie free fat substitute), and **chocolate**; and vegetables and fruits that tend to be well tolerated by the bowels. The chapter concludes with a lengthy discussion of lactose intolerance and the role it may play in people with IBS. 2 tables.

- **Food-Related Illnesses and Allergies**

  Source: in Townsend, C.E. and Roth, R.A. Nutrition and Diet Therapy. 7th ed. Albany, NY: Delmar Publishers. 1999. 171-187 p.

  Contact: Available from Delmar Publishers. 3 Columbia Circle, Albany, NY 12212. (800) 865-5840. E-mail: info@delmar.com. PRICE: $44.95 plus shipping and handling. ISBN: 0766802965.

  Summary: This chapter on food related illnesses and allergies is from an undergraduate textbook on nutrition and diet therapy. The chapter identifies the diseases caused by contaminated food, along with their signs and the means by which they are spread; lists the signs of food contamination; reviews precautions for protecting food from contamination; and covers allergies and elimination diets and their uses. Foodborne illnesses covered include Campylobacter jejuni, Clostridium botulinum, Clostridium perfringens, Cyclospora, Escherichia coli (O157:H7), Listeria monocytogenes, Salmonella, Shigella, and Staphylococcus aureas. The authors stress that infection or poisoning traced to food is usually caused by human ignorance or carelessness. Food should not be prepared by anyone who has or carries a contagious disease. All fresh fruits and vegetables should be washed before being eaten. Meats, poultry, fish, eggs, and dairy products should be refrigerated. Food should be covered to prevent contamination by dust, insects, or animals. Food allergies can cause many different and unpleasant symptoms, and elimination diets are used to determine their causes. Some of the most common food allergens are milk, **chocolate**, eggs, tomatoes, fish, citrus fruit, legumes, strawberries, and wheat. The chapter includes lists of key terms to learn, recommended discussion topics, and suggested supplemental activities, and a section of review questions so readers can test their comprehension of the material. Two illustrative case studies are appended. 1 figure. 4 tables.

- **Sweet Talk: Sugar and Other Sweeteners**

Source: in Duyff, R.L. American Dietetic Association's Complete Food and Nutrition Guide. Minneapolis, MN: Chronimed Publishing. 1996. p. 119-137.

Contact: Available from Chronimed Publishing. P.O. Box 59032, Minneapolis, MN 55459. (800) 848-2793 or (612) 541-0239. Fax (800) 395-3344 or (612) 541-0210. PRICE: $29.95; bulk orders available. ISBN: 1565610989.

Summary: This chapter on sugar and other sweeteners is from a food and nutrition guide that focuses on healthful eating for all stages of life. Traditional sweeteners (sugars and sugar alcohols) are nutritive sweeteners, which nourish the body by supplying energy. Intense sweeteners, such as aspartame and saccharin, are many times sweeter than sugar. However, because they supply few, if any, calories, they're considered nonnutritive. The author defines sugar, then discusses sugar and oral health, sugar myths, the recommended amounts of carbohydrate to include in one's diet, where sugars come from, the role of sugars in a healthful diet, myths about **chocolate**, the types of intense sweeteners (aspartame, saccharin, and acesulfame K), and cooking with intense sweeteners. The chapter concludes with a self assessment, with which readers can measure their own eating styles and sugar habits.

- **Early Movement Center: West Shore YMCA, Camp Hill, Pennsylvania**

Source: in Health and Fitness Programs. YMCA of the USA. Champaign, IL, National Council of Young Men's Christian Associations of the United States of America, YMCA Program Discovery Series, Volume 2, Number 4, pp. 5-18, 1992.

Contact: YMCA Program Store, P.O. Box 5077, Champaign, IL 61825. (217) 351-5077.

Summary: Early Movement Center: West Shore YMCA, a book chapter in Health and Fitness Programs, discusses a physical activity program established by a Harrisburg, Pennsylvania, area Young Men's Christian Association (YMCA). The Early Movement Center expanded on an earlier program called Kids Klub, which offered gymnastics and swimming to a limited number of preschoolers 1 day a week for 5-week sessions. The Early Movement Center provides learning opportunities and motor activities, including gymnastics and swimming, for 3-year-olds 2 days a week and for 4- and 5-year-olds 3 days a week throughout the school year. Initially, a single staff person, who had responsibility for directing all of the West Shore YMCA's preschool programs, administered the program. Later, the program developed its own staff, which includes a full-time director and a part-time assistant director. For the movement education, gymnastics, and swimming components of the program, the YMCA relies on part-time instructors, all of whom have had special training. Program staff incorporate field trips and special events into the lesson plans whenever possible. Trips have included a sheep farm, a cavern, and Hershey's **chocolate** World. Twice a year, the staff observes each child's motor abilities and rates those abilities against a checklist of movement skills children should be able to accomplish at certain ages. Skills include walking, standing, balancing, climbing, catching, jumping, and throwing. Program staff also periodically rate children on their progress in swimming and gymnastics. The Center's director meets with parents twice a year to review all of the skills checklists and to review their child's progress. The YMCA has used newspaper advertisements and mailed brochures to YMCA members to publicize the program. Parents can visit the center at any time during the program, as long as they do not interfere with the activities. At the end of each session, parents complete a questionnaire that asks for input on such topics as program content and structure, leadership, facilities, and suggested improvements.

CHAPTER 8. MULTIMEDIA ON CHOCOLATE

Overview

In this chapter, we show you how to keep current on multimedia sources of information on chocolate. We start with sources that have been summarized by federal agencies, and then show you how to find bibliographic information catalogued by the National Library of Medicine.

Video Recordings

An excellent source of multimedia information on chocolate is the Combined Health Information Database. You will need to limit your search to "Videorecording" and "chocolate" using the "Detailed Search" option. Go directly to the following hyperlink: **http://chid.nih.gov/detail/detail.html**. To find video productions, use the drop boxes at the bottom of the search page where "You may refine your search by." Select the dates and language you prefer, and the format option "Videorecording (videotape, videocassette, etc.)." Type "chocolate" (or synonyms) into the "For these words:" box. The following is a typical result when searching for video recordings on chocolate:

- **Movement, Music, and Memories**

  Source: Salt Lake City, UT: Innovative Caregiving Resources. 1995.

  Contact: Available from Innovative Caregiving Resources, Inc. PO Box 17809, Salt Lake City, UT 84117-1809. (800) 249-5600; (801) 272-9806; FAX: 801-272-9805. Internet: http://www.videorespite.com. PRICE: $57.75.

  Summary: This videotape is designed to capture and hold the attention of people with dementia and provide respite for caregivers. Cathy, the facilitator, evokes childhood memories by singing songs, telling stories, and playing games from her youth. She shares songs such as "Mary had a Little Lamb," "Ring Around the Rosie," "Let Me Call You Sweetheart," "I'm Forever Blowing Bubbles," and "Grandfather's Clock," and recalls events including attending school, picking apples, eating **chocolate** chip cookies, and playing kickball. A visit from a young child sparks memories of what it is like to be young. Cathy engages the memory-impaired individual using conversation, sing-a-longs, and light stretching and arm and leg movements.

CHAPTER 9. PERIODICALS AND NEWS ON CHOCOLATE

Overview

In this chapter, we suggest a number of news sources and present various periodicals that cover chocolate.

News Services and Press Releases

One of the simplest ways of tracking press releases on chocolate is to search the news wires. In the following sample of sources, we will briefly describe how to access each service. These services only post recent news intended for public viewing.

PR Newswire

To access the PR Newswire archive, simply go to **http://www.prnewswire.com/**. Select your country. Type "chocolate" (or synonyms) into the search box. You will automatically receive information on relevant news releases posted within the last 30 days. The search results are shown by order of relevance.

Reuters Health

The Reuters' Medical News and Health eLine databases can be very useful in exploring news archives relating to chocolate. While some of the listed articles are free to view, others are available for purchase for a nominal fee. To access this archive, go to **http://www.reutershealth.com/en/index.html** and search by "chocolate" (or synonyms). The following was recently listed in this archive for chocolate:

- **Skip the milk chocolate, dark is better for you**
  Source: Reuters Health eLine
  Date: August 27, 2003
  http://www.reutershealth.com/archive/2003/08/27/eline/links/20030827elin013.html

- **Eating dark chocolate raises antioxidant levels**
  Source: Reuters Medical News
  Date: August 27, 2003

- **Scans show why we always have room for chocolate**
  Source: Reuters Health eLine
  Date: August 21, 2003

- **Chocolate-derived chemical could suppress cough**
  Source: Reuters Health eLine
  Date: December 18, 2002

- **Chemical in chocolate could prevent coughs**
  Source: Reuters Medical News
  Date: December 18, 2002

- **Coffee, chocolate compounds potential cancer drugs**
  Source: Reuters Health eLine
  Date: August 21, 2002

- **Same health benefits from less chocolate: report**
  Source: Reuters Health eLine
  Date: May 01, 2002

- **Doctors say a chocolate a day keeps them away**
  Source: Reuters Health eLine
  Date: September 04, 2001

- **Tea, chocolate may be heart-healthy snacks**
  Source: Reuters Health eLine
  Date: August 06, 2001

- **Consumption of tea, chocolate may reduce risk of death from heart disease**
  Source: Reuters Medical News
  Date: August 06, 2001

- **Drinkers, chocolate lovers may share same craving**
  Source: Reuters Health eLine
  Date: November 02, 2000

- **Evidence for cardiovascular benefits of chocolate continues to grow**
  Source: Reuters Industry Breifing
  Date: August 30, 2000

- **Chocolate-flavored cereal lowers cholesterol**
  Source: Reuters Health eLine
  Date: August 22, 2000

- **Skin patch could reduce chocolate cravings**
  Source: Reuters Health eLine
  Date: July 24, 2000

- **Cocoa may help fight cholesterol**
  Source: Reuters Health eLine
  Date: April 17, 2000

- **Chocolate may benefit the physical heart, too**
  Source: Reuters Health eLine
  Date: February 21, 2000

- **Cardiovascular benefits claimed for cocoa flavonoids**
  Source: Reuters Medical News
  Date: February 21, 2000

- **Chocolate craving is real**
  Source: Reuters Health eLine
  Date: October 06, 1999

- **Fat-free chocolate ice cream worth screaming for**
  Source: Reuters Health eLine
  Date: August 25, 1999

- **A chocolate a day might keep the doctor away**
  Source: Reuters Health eLine
  Date: August 06, 1999

- **Chocolate may lengthen your life**
  Source: Reuters Health eLine
  Date: December 18, 1998

- **Chocolate "addiction" a fiction?**
  Source: Reuters Health eLine
  Date: December 16, 1998

- **Chocolate Doesn't Trigger Migraines**
  Source: Reuters Health eLine
  Date: January 08, 1998

- **Salmonella in Chocolate and Pepper**
  Source: Reuters Health eLine
  Date: May 12, 1997

- **Chocolate Contains Antioxidants**
  Source: Reuters Health eLine
  Date: September 20, 1996

- **Substances In Chocolate Mimic Effects Of Cannabis**
  Source: Reuters Medical News
  Date: August 22, 1996

- **Chocolate, Marijuana Separated At Birth**
  Source: Reuters Health eLine
  Date: August 22, 1996

The NIH

Within MEDLINEplus, the NIH has made an agreement with the New York Times Syndicate, the AP News Service, and Reuters to deliver news that can be browsed by the public. Search news releases at **http://www.nlm.nih.gov/medlineplus/alphanews_a.html**. MEDLINEplus allows you to browse across an alphabetical index. Or you can search by date at the following Web page: **http://www.nlm.nih.gov/medlineplus/newsbydate.html**. Often, news items are indexed by MEDLINEplus within its search engine.

Business Wire

Business Wire is similar to PR Newswire. To access this archive, simply go to **http://www.businesswire.com/**. You can scan the news by industry category or company name.

Market Wire

Market Wire is more focused on technology than the other wires. To browse the latest press releases by topic, such as alternative medicine, biotechnology, fitness, healthcare, legal, nutrition, and pharmaceuticals, access Market Wire's Medical/Health channel at **http://www.marketwire.com/mw/release_index?channel=MedicalHealth**. Or simply go to Market Wire's home page at **http://www.marketwire.com/mw/home**, type "chocolate" (or synonyms) into the search box, and click on "Search News." As this service is technology oriented, you may wish to use it when searching for press releases covering diagnostic procedures or tests.

Search Engines

Medical news is also available in the news sections of commercial Internet search engines. See the health news page at Yahoo (**http://dir.yahoo.com/Health/News_and_Media/**), or you can use this Web site's general news search page at **http://news.yahoo.com/**. Type in "chocolate" (or synonyms). If you know the name of a company that is relevant to chocolate, you can go to any stock trading Web site (such as **http://www.etrade.com/**) and search for the company name there. News items across various news sources are reported on indicated hyperlinks. Google offers a similar service at **http://news.google.com/**.

BBC

Covering news from a more European perspective, the British Broadcasting Corporation (BBC) allows the public free access to their news archive located at **http://www.bbc.co.uk/**. Search by "chocolate" (or synonyms).

Newsletter Articles

Use the Combined Health Information Database, and limit your search criteria to "newsletter articles." Again, you will need to use the "Detailed Search" option. Go directly to the following hyperlink: **http://chid.nih.gov/detail/detail.html**. Go to the bottom of the search page where "You may refine your search by." Select the dates and language that you prefer. For the format option, select "Newsletter Article." Type "chocolate" (or synonyms) into the "For these words:" box. You should check back periodically with this database as it is updated every three months. The following is a typical result when searching for newsletter articles on chocolate:

- **What Causes Kidney Stones**

  Source: Columbia-Presbyterian Urology. p. 4. Fall 1996.

  Contact: Available from Columbia-Presbyterian Urology. Dana W. Atchley Pavilion, 11 Floor, 161 Fort Washington Avenue, New York, NY 10032-3784. (212) 305-0111.

  Summary: This brief newsletter article describes the causes of kidney stones. There are four factors that lead to stone formation: urine saturation, crystallization, particle retention, and matrix foundation. The author first describes who is at risk for forming kidney stones and briefly outlines the different types of stones: calcium oxalate (75 percent of patients develop these), uric acid, and struvite stones. Urine saturation occurs when urine has excessive amounts of calcium, uric acid, and oxalate crystals, which are all stone-forming substances. This saturation may occur during the day but frequently occurs after meals or during the sleeping hours or hot weather because of the lack of fluids consumed. Stone inhibiting substances include pyrophosphate, citrate, magnesium, and nephrocalcin. Freshly voided urine from most healthy individuals contains small crystals, which are flushed out of the urinary tract. However, some people have anatomic abnormalities in the kidney and or ureter, making the crystals stick to the lining of these structures. In addition to being composed of crystals, stones are also formed from an organic material called matrix. Matrix acts as the foundation for stone formation by controlling crystallization. The matrix is composed of a carbohydrate and protein. The article concludes with a section on preventing kidney stones, offering the following suggestions: increase fluid intake to lower saturation; make sure one half the fluid intake is water; produce two and a half quarts of urine in 24 hours; avoid eating grapes, berries, plums and citrus fruits; limit intake of coffee, tea and **chocolate**; avoid eating sardines, shrimp, and oysters; and, to prevent uric acid stones, avoid eating liver, sweet breads, and brains. Some people may require medication because they form calcium and uric acid stones even though they have adequate fluid intake and do not consume an excessive amount of dairy products. 1 figure.

Academic Periodicals covering Chocolate

Numerous periodicals are currently indexed within the National Library of Medicine's PubMed database that are known to publish articles relating to chocolate. In addition to these sources, you can search for articles covering chocolate that have been published by any of the periodicals listed in previous chapters. To find the latest studies published, go to **http://www.ncbi.nlm.nih.gov/pubmed**, type the name of the periodical into the search box, and click "Go."

If you want complete details about the historical contents of a journal, you can also visit the following Web site: **http://www.ncbi.nlm.nih.gov/entrez/jrbrowser.cgi**. Here, type in the name of the journal or its abbreviation, and you will receive an index of published articles. At **http://locatorplus.gov/**, you can retrieve more indexing information on medical periodicals (e.g. the name of the publisher). Select the button "Search LOCATORplus." Then type in the name of the journal and select the advanced search option "Journal Title Search."

APPENDICES

APPENDIX A. PHYSICIAN RESOURCES

Overview

In this chapter, we focus on databases and Internet-based guidelines and information resources created or written for a professional audience.

NIH Guidelines

Commonly referred to as "clinical" or "professional" guidelines, the National Institutes of Health publish physician guidelines for the most common diseases. Publications are available at the following by relevant Institute[12]:

- Office of the Director (OD); guidelines consolidated across agencies available at **http://www.nih.gov/health/consumer/conkey.htm**

- National Institute of General Medical Sciences (NIGMS); fact sheets available at **http://www.nigms.nih.gov/news/facts/**

- National Library of Medicine (NLM); extensive encyclopedia (A.D.A.M., Inc.) with guidelines: **http://www.nlm.nih.gov/medlineplus/healthtopics.html**

- National Cancer Institute (NCI); guidelines available at **http://www.cancer.gov/cancerinfo/list.aspx?viewid=5f35036e-5497-4d86-8c2c-714a9f7c8d25**

- National Eye Institute (NEI); guidelines available at **http://www.nei.nih.gov/order/index.htm**

- National Heart, Lung, and Blood Institute (NHLBI); guidelines available at **http://www.nhlbi.nih.gov/guidelines/index.htm**

- National Human Genome Research Institute (NHGRI); research available at **http://www.genome.gov/page.cfm?pageID=10000375**

- National Institute on Aging (NIA); guidelines available at **http://www.nia.nih.gov/health/**

---

[12] These publications are typically written by one or more of the various NIH Institutes.

- National Institute on Alcohol Abuse and Alcoholism (NIAAA); guidelines available at http://www.niaaa.nih.gov/publications/publications.htm

- National Institute of Allergy and Infectious Diseases (NIAID); guidelines available at http://www.niaid.nih.gov/publications/

- National Institute of Arthritis and Musculoskeletal and Skin Diseases (NIAMS); fact sheets and guidelines available at http://www.niams.nih.gov/hi/index.htm

- National Institute of Child Health and Human Development (NICHD); guidelines available at http://www.nichd.nih.gov/publications/pubskey.cfm

- National Institute on Deafness and Other Communication Disorders (NIDCD); fact sheets and guidelines at http://www.nidcd.nih.gov/health/

- National Institute of Dental and Craniofacial Research (NIDCR); guidelines available at http://www.nidr.nih.gov/health/

- National Institute of Diabetes and Digestive and Kidney Diseases (NIDDK); guidelines available at http://www.niddk.nih.gov/health/health.htm

- National Institute on Drug Abuse (NIDA); guidelines available at http://www.nida.nih.gov/DrugAbuse.html

- National Institute of Environmental Health Sciences (NIEHS); environmental health information available at http://www.niehs.nih.gov/external/facts.htm

- National Institute of Mental Health (NIMH); guidelines available at http://www.nimh.nih.gov/practitioners/index.cfm

- National Institute of Neurological Disorders and Stroke (NINDS); neurological disorder information pages available at http://www.ninds.nih.gov/health_and_medical/disorder_index.htm

- National Institute of Nursing Research (NINR); publications on selected illnesses at http://www.nih.gov/ninr/news-info/publications.html

- National Institute of Biomedical Imaging and Bioengineering; general information at http://grants.nih.gov/grants/becon/becon_info.htm

- Center for Information Technology (CIT); referrals to other agencies based on keyword searches available at http://kb.nih.gov/www_query_main.asp

- National Center for Complementary and Alternative Medicine (NCCAM); health information available at http://nccam.nih.gov/health/

- National Center for Research Resources (NCRR); various information directories available at http://www.ncrr.nih.gov/publications.asp

- Office of Rare Diseases; various fact sheets available at http://rarediseases.info.nih.gov/html/resources/rep_pubs.html

- Centers for Disease Control and Prevention; various fact sheets on infectious diseases available at http://www.cdc.gov/publications.htm

NIH Databases

In addition to the various Institutes of Health that publish professional guidelines, the NIH has designed a number of databases for professionals.[13] Physician-oriented resources provide a wide variety of information related to the biomedical and health sciences, both past and present. The format of these resources varies. Searchable databases, bibliographic citations, full-text articles (when available), archival collections, and images are all available. The following are referenced by the National Library of Medicine:[14]

- **Bioethics:** Access to published literature on the ethical, legal, and public policy issues surrounding healthcare and biomedical research. This information is provided in conjunction with the Kennedy Institute of Ethics located at Georgetown University, Washington, D.C.: **http://www.nlm.nih.gov/databases/databases_bioethics.html**

- **HIV/AIDS Resources:** Describes various links and databases dedicated to HIV/AIDS research: **http://www.nlm.nih.gov/pubs/factsheets/aidsinfs.html**

- **NLM Online Exhibitions:** Describes "Exhibitions in the History of Medicine": **http://www.nlm.nih.gov/exhibition/exhibition.html**. Additional resources for historical scholarship in medicine: **http://www.nlm.nih.gov/hmd/hmd.html**

- **Biotechnology Information:** Access to public databases. The National Center for Biotechnology Information conducts research in computational biology, develops software tools for analyzing genome data, and disseminates biomedical information for the better understanding of molecular processes affecting human health and disease: **http://www.ncbi.nlm.nih.gov/**

- **Population Information:** The National Library of Medicine provides access to worldwide coverage of population, family planning, and related health issues, including family planning technology and programs, fertility, and population law and policy: **http://www.nlm.nih.gov/databases/databases_population.html**

- **Cancer Information:** Access to cancer-oriented databases: **http://www.nlm.nih.gov/databases/databases_cancer.html**

- **Profiles in Science:** Offering the archival collections of prominent twentieth-century biomedical scientists to the public through modern digital technology: **http://www.profiles.nlm.nih.gov/**

- **Chemical Information:** Provides links to various chemical databases and references: **http://sis.nlm.nih.gov/Chem/ChemMain.html**

- **Clinical Alerts:** Reports the release of findings from the NIH-funded clinical trials where such release could significantly affect morbidity and mortality: **http://www.nlm.nih.gov/databases/alerts/clinical_alerts.html**

- **Space Life Sciences:** Provides links and information to space-based research (including NASA): **http://www.nlm.nih.gov/databases/databases_space.html**

- **MEDLINE:** Bibliographic database covering the fields of medicine, nursing, dentistry, veterinary medicine, the healthcare system, and the pre-clinical sciences: **http://www.nlm.nih.gov/databases/databases_medline.html**

---

[13] Remember, for the general public, the National Library of Medicine recommends the databases referenced in MEDLINE*plus* (**http://medlineplus.gov/** or **http://www.nlm.nih.gov/medlineplus/databases.html**).

[14] See **http://www.nlm.nih.gov/databases/databases.html**.

- **Toxicology and Environmental Health Information (TOXNET):** Databases covering toxicology and environmental health: **http://sis.nlm.nih.gov/Tox/ToxMain.html**

- **Visible Human Interface:** Anatomically detailed, three-dimensional representations of normal male and female human bodies: **http://www.nlm.nih.gov/research/visible/visible_human.html**

The Combined Health Information Database

A comprehensive source of information on clinical guidelines written for professionals is the Combined Health Information Database. You will need to limit your search to one of the following: Brochure/Pamphlet, Fact Sheet, or Information Package, and "chocolate" using the "Detailed Search" option. Go directly to the following hyperlink: **http://chid.nih.gov/detail/detail.html**. To find associations, use the drop boxes at the bottom of the search page where "You may refine your search by." For the publication date, select "All Years." Select your preferred language and the format option "Fact Sheet." Type "chocolate" (or synonyms) into the "For these words:" box. The following is a sample result:

- **La Nutricion y el Virus HIV: Normas Dieteticas Practicas Para la Gente Infectada con el Virus HIV o el SIDA... [Nutrition and HIV: Practical Dietary Guidelines for People With HIV Infection or AIDS.]**

  Contact: Abbott Laboratories/US, Ross Laboratories, 625 Cleveland Ave, Columbus, OH, 43215, (614) 227-3333.

  Summary: This manual is provided to health care professionals as an aid in counseling HIV/AIDS patients on nutrition. It discusses the benefits of good nutrition, offers guidelines on building a nutritious diet, and suggests ways of increasing the calorie and protein content of a diet without serving larger portions. Directions for proper food handling are provided, as are tips for managing nutrition and alleviating symptoms in the event of fatigue, nausea, diarrhea, sore mouth or throat, and changing sense of taste. The manual promotes the use of the nutritional product Advera, designed to meet the nutritional needs of people with HIV and AIDS. Patents are pending on the low-fat, high-fiber product, meant to be used as an oral supplement or meal replacement. Several recipes are included using **chocolate** and orange cream flavors of Advera.

The NLM Gateway[15]

The NLM (National Library of Medicine) Gateway is a Web-based system that lets users search simultaneously in multiple retrieval systems at the U.S. National Library of Medicine (NLM). It allows users of NLM services to initiate searches from one Web interface, providing one-stop searching for many of NLM's information resources or databases.[16] To use the NLM Gateway, simply go to the search site at **http://gateway.nlm.nih.gov/gw/Cmd**. Type "chocolate" (or synonyms) into the search box and click "Search." The results will be presented in a tabular form, indicating the number of references in each database category.

---

[15] Adapted from NLM: **http://gateway.nlm.nih.gov/gw/Cmd?Overview.x**

[16] The NLM Gateway is currently being developed by the Lister Hill National Center for Biomedical Communications (LHNCBC) at the National Library of Medicine (NLM) of the National Institutes of Health (NIH).

Results Summary

Category	Items Found
Journal Articles	1377
Books / Periodicals / Audio Visual	45
Consumer Health	76
Meeting Abstracts	23
Other Collections	0
Total	1521

HSTAT[17]

HSTAT is a free, Web-based resource that provides access to full-text documents used in healthcare decision-making.[18] These documents include clinical practice guidelines, quick-reference guides for clinicians, consumer health brochures, evidence reports and technology assessments from the Agency for Healthcare Research and Quality (AHRQ), as well as AHRQ's Put Prevention Into Practice.[19] Simply search by "chocolate" (or synonyms) at the following Web site: **http://text.nlm.nih.gov.**

Coffee Break: Tutorials for Biologists[20]

Coffee Break is a general healthcare site that takes a scientific view of the news and covers recent breakthroughs in biology that may one day assist physicians in developing treatments. Here you will find a collection of short reports on recent biological discoveries. Each report incorporates interactive tutorials that demonstrate how bioinformatics tools are used as a part of the research process. Currently, all Coffee Breaks are written by NCBI staff.[21] Each report is about 400 words and is usually based on a discovery reported in one or more articles from recently published, peer-reviewed literature.[22] This site has new articles every few weeks, so it can be considered an online magazine of sorts. It is intended for general background information. You can access the Coffee Break Web site at the following hyperlink: **http://www.ncbi.nlm.nih.gov/Coffeebreak/.**

---

[17] Adapted from HSTAT: **http://www.nlm.nih.gov/pubs/factsheets/hstat.html.**

[18] The HSTAT URL is **http://hstat.nlm.nih.gov/.**

[19] Other important documents in HSTAT include: the National Institutes of Health (NIH) Consensus Conference Reports and Technology Assessment Reports; the HIV/AIDS Treatment Information Service (ATIS) resource documents; the Substance Abuse and Mental Health Services Administration's Center for Substance Abuse Treatment (SAMHSA/CSAT) Treatment Improvement Protocols (TIP) and Center for Substance Abuse Prevention (SAMHSA/CSAP) Prevention Enhancement Protocols System (PEPS); the Public Health Service (PHS) Preventive Services Task Force's *Guide to Clinical Preventive Services*; the independent, nonfederal Task Force on Community Services' *Guide to Community Preventive Services*; and the Health Technology Advisory Committee (HTAC) of the Minnesota Health Care Commission (MHCC) health technology evaluations.

[20] Adapted from **http://www.ncbi.nlm.nih.gov/Coffeebreak/Archive/FAQ.html.**

[21] The figure that accompanies each article is frequently supplied by an expert external to NCBI, in which case the source of the figure is cited. The result is an interactive tutorial that tells a biological story.

[22] After a brief introduction that sets the work described into a broader context, the report focuses on how a molecular understanding can provide explanations of observed biology and lead to therapies for diseases. Each vignette is accompanied by a figure and hypertext links that lead to a series of pages that interactively show how NCBI tools and resources are used in the research process.

Other Commercial Databases

In addition to resources maintained by official agencies, other databases exist that are commercial ventures addressing medical professionals. Here are some examples that may interest you:

- **CliniWeb International:** Index and table of contents to selected clinical information on the Internet; see **http://www.ohsu.edu/cliniweb/**.

- **Medical World Search:** Searches full text from thousands of selected medical sites on the Internet; see **http://www.mwsearch.com/**.

Appendix B. Patient Resources

Overview

Official agencies, as well as federally funded institutions supported by national grants, frequently publish a variety of guidelines written with the patient in mind. These are typically called "Fact Sheets" or "Guidelines." They can take the form of a brochure, information kit, pamphlet, or flyer. Often they are only a few pages in length. Since new guidelines on chocolate can appear at any moment and be published by a number of sources, the best approach to finding guidelines is to systematically scan the Internet-based services that post them.

Patient Guideline Sources

The remainder of this chapter directs you to sources which either publish or can help you find additional guidelines on topics related to chocolate. Due to space limitations, these sources are listed in a concise manner. Do not hesitate to consult the following sources by either using the Internet hyperlink provided, or, in cases where the contact information is provided, contacting the publisher or author directly.

The National Institutes of Health

The NIH gateway to patients is located at **http://health.nih.gov/**. From this site, you can search across various sources and institutes, a number of which are summarized below.

Topic Pages: MEDLINEplus

The National Library of Medicine has created a vast and patient-oriented healthcare information portal called MEDLINEplus. Within this Internet-based system are "health topic pages" which list links to available materials relevant to chocolate. To access this system, log on to **http://www.nlm.nih.gov/medlineplus/healthtopics.html**. From there you can either search using the alphabetical index or browse by broad topic areas. Recently, MEDLINEplus listed the following when searched for "chocolate":

- Other Guides

  Amphetamine Abuse
  http://www.nlm.nih.gov/medlineplus/amphetamineabuse.html

  Diabetic Diet
  http://www.nlm.nih.gov/medlineplus/diabeticdiet.html

  Heart Failure
  http://www.nlm.nih.gov/medlineplus/heartfailure.html

  Osteoporosis
  http://www.nlm.nih.gov/medlineplus/osteoporosis.html

  Taste and Smell Disorders
  http://www.nlm.nih.gov/medlineplus/tasteandsmelldisorders.html

You may also choose to use the search utility provided by MEDLINEplus at the following Web address: **http://www.nlm.nih.gov/medlineplus/**. Simply type a keyword into the search box and click "Search." This utility is similar to the NIH search utility, with the exception that it only includes materials that are linked within the MEDLINEplus system (mostly patient-oriented information). It also has the disadvantage of generating unstructured results. We recommend, therefore, that you use this method only if you have a very targeted search.

The Combined Health Information Database (CHID)

CHID Online is a reference tool that maintains a database directory of thousands of journal articles and patient education guidelines on chocolate. CHID offers summaries that describe the guidelines available, including contact information and pricing. CHID's general Web site is **http://chid.nih.gov/**. To search this database, go to **http://chid.nih.gov/detail/detail.html**. In particular, you can use the advanced search options to look up pamphlets, reports, brochures, and information kits. The following was recently posted in this archive:

- **Taking Care of Irritable Bowel Syndrome**

  Source: Santa Cruz, CA: ETR Associates. 1997. 4 p.

  Contact: Available from ETR Associates. P.O. Box 1830, Santa Cruz, CA 95061-1830. (800) 321-4407. PRICE: $16.00 for 50 copies.

  Summary: This patient education brochure explains the basics of living with irritable bowel syndrome (IBS). The brochure encourages readers to check with their health care provider for assistance in dealing with the discomfort and inconvenience of recurrent and chronic cramps, gas, bloating, diarrhea, or constipation. The brochure discusses causes of IBS, the physiology of normal digestion, how to discover individual triggers of symptoms, common dietary triggers of IBS symptoms (caffeine; dairy products; **chocolate**; alcohol; and acidic, fatty, or spicy foods), how to manage symptoms, the role of medications, and how to learn to manage stress (a common trigger of IBS symptoms). The brochure emphasizes the role of exercise and nutrition in managing IBS. The brochure also lists symptoms for which a health care provider should be consulted, including blood in the stool, continuous abdominal pain and fever, and when symptoms interfere with normal activities. The brochure concludes with a brief list of references and the contact information for the National Digestive Diseases Information Clearinghouse. 1 figure. 3 references. (AA-M).

- **FAN Flashbacks: Milk**

  Source: Fairfax, VA: Food Allergy and Anaphylaxis Network (FAAN). 1996. 11 p.

  Contact: Available from Food Allergy and Anaphylaxis Network (FAAN). 10400 Eaton Place, Suite 107, Fairfax, VA 22030. (800) 929-4040 or (703) 691-3179. Fax (703) 691-2713. E-mail: faan@foodallergy.org. Web site: http://www.foodallergy.org/. Price: $2.00 each.

  Summary: This brochure reprints relevant information on specific topics from previous issues of Food Allergy News, the newsletter of the Food Allergy and Anaphylaxis Network. This brochure focuses on milk allergy, particularly in children. Articles are reprinted on topics including altering a child's diet to accommodate a milk allergy; protein hydrolysate formulas to substitute for cow milk or soy formulas; determining the need for vitamin or other supplements; calcium compounds, including calcium citrate, calcium carbonate, and calcium gluconate; kosher foods and allergies, including understanding kosher rules and markings; new products, including Simplesse, and Vitamite nondairy beverage; consumer guidelines for specific brand name products; calcium-fortified products; milk-free products; the different types of **chocolate** products, including cocoa powder, cocoa butter, **chocolate** liquor, baking **chocolate**, milk **chocolate**, semisweet and sweet chocolates, and unsweetened **chocolate**; finding desserts and dessert substitutes for children who are allergic to milk; goat milk as a substitute for cow milk; and kosher processing and food allergies. The brochure includes the address, telephone numbers, and email addresses for the Food Allergy and Anaphylaxis Network, a national nonprofit organization established to help families living with food allergies and to increase public awareness about food allergies and anaphylaxis. (AA-M).

- **Milk-Free General Foods Products**

  Source: White Plains, NY: Kraft General Foods Consumer Center. March 1993. 5 p.

  Contact: Available from Kraft General Foods Consumer Center. 250 North Street, White Plains, NY 10625. (800) 431-1003. PRICE: Free.

  Summary: An informational flier lists foods for patients who must use milk-free foods. Included are beverage products and ready-to-drink beverages; breakfast cereals; dessert ingredients including baking powder, **chocolate**, and coconut; dessert products including dietetic gelatin and pudding, gelatin desserts, pectin, cooked pudding, tapioca, and frozen novelty desserts; and main meal products including coating mixes for poultry and meat, rice, rice mixes, salad dressings, and syrups.

- **Lactose-Free General Foods Products**

  Source: White Plains, NY: Kraft General Foods Consumer Center. March 1993. 5 p.

  Contact: Available from Kraft General Foods Consumer Center. 250 North Street, White Plains, NY 10625. (800) 431-1003. PRICE: Free.

  Summary: An informational flier lists foods for patients who must use lactose-free foods. Included are beverage powders and ready-to-drink beverages; breakfast cereals; dessert ingredients including baking powder, **chocolate**, and coconut; desserts including dietetic gelatin and pudding mixes, gelatin desserts, pectin, cooked pudding, tapioca, and frozen novelty desserts; and main meal products including coating mixes for pultry and meat, rice, rice mixes, salad dressing, and syrup.

- **Flexible Meal Planning with Diabetes**

  Source: Washington, D.C.: Sugar Association, Inc. 1994. 4 p.

  Contact: Available from Sugar Association, Inc. 1101 15th Street, N.W., Suite 600, Washington, D.C. 20005. (202) 785-1122. PRICE: Up to 50 copies free.

  Summary: This brochure is designed to help readers with diabetes follow the new dietary guidelines, which allow the limited use of sugar in a diabetic diet. The guidelines also address proportions of carbohydrates, fats, and protein in the diet. Topics include weight loss; the use of sugar in moderation; and meal planning and optimal nutrition. Three meal plans are provided; as are recipes for **chocolate** Dunking Biscotti; Blackberry Tea Bars; Watermelon Ice; and Cinnamon Apple-Nut Muffins.

- **Recipes for Calorie Watchers**

  Source: Parsipanny, NJ: Estee Corporation. 1992. 5 p.

  Contact: Available from Estee Corporation, Professional Services Department. 169 Lackawanna Avenue, Parsipanny, NJ 07054. (800) 523-1734, ext. 200, or (201) 335-1000. PRICE: Single copy free.

  Summary: This booklet was developed to help readers plan and enjoy meals while following a weight reduction or weight conscious diet. The recipes in the booklet are lower in calories, fat, and sodium and contain no table sugar (sucrose). The introductory section reminds readers with noninsulin-dependent diabetes (NIDDM) about the importance of weight control in their diabetes management program. Recipes included are Pasta with Broccoli and Shrimp; Curried Turkey Salad; Chicken Sate; **chocolate** Crumb Pie; Sesame Slaw; Little Lemon Cakes; Strawberry Pineapple Trifle; and Fajita Salad. The recipes feature products available from the Estee Corporation. Complete nutritional information and diabetic exchange information follow each recipe. (AA-M).

- **Pierogi, Pasta and Pastry**

  Source: Carlisle, PA: Patricia Amadure. 1991. 29 p.

  Contact: Available from Patricia Amadure. Cookbook, 243 West Baltimore Street, Carlisle, PA 17013. (717) 243-6846. PRICE: $4 plus $0.50 shipping and handling. Make checks payable to the Juvenile Diabetes Foundation (JDF).

  Summary: This cookbook, designed by the mother of a teenager with diabetes, brings family recipes up-to-date for people with diabetes. Recipes are divided into two main categories, main dishes and sweets, and include such favorites as Hungarian goulash, macaroni and cheese, crab cakes, pasta dishes, apple pie, and **chocolate** chip cookies. Each recipes includes exchange list information and caloric values. The author also includes a table of sweeteners and a few cooking hints.

- **Questions and Answers on Urinary Tract Infections**

  Source: Alexandria, VA: American Medical Women's Association. 1997. 4 p.

  Contact: Available from American Medical Women's Association. 801 North Fairfax Street, Alexandria, VA 22314. (781) 585-8220. PRICE: Single copy free.

  Summary: This brochure outlines symptoms, diagnosis, and treatment of urinary tract infections (UTIs). An infection of the urinary tract commonly has the following symptoms: frequent and urgent need to urinate, painful urination, cloudy urine, lower back or abdominal pain, blood in the urine. About 80 to 90 percent of UTIs are caused by Escherichia coli bacteria, which are normally present in the rectum. Factors that may contribute to UTIs are sexual intercourse, some birth control methods, low water intake, and anatomic problems. The first step a health care provider will take to confirm a bacterial UTI is to review the symptoms and test the patient's urine. The infection should be diagnosed by a urine culture, since several other conditions, including vaginal infections, gonorrhea, chlamydia, irritable bladder, and bladder cancer, can have similar symptoms. When pain is the predominant symptom, the diagnosis may be interstitial cystitis. If the urine culture shows bacteria, the health care provider will prescribe a course of antibiotics. The brochure outlines other steps to take to treat a UTI, including drinking large amounts of water; avoiding caffeine, acid foods, spices, citrus fruits, tomatoes, alcohol, and **chocolate**; drinking cranberry juice cocktail; and trying hot water bottles or heating pads to ease cramps and soothe the pain. The brochure concludes with a section of suggestions for preventing UTIs, including drinking plenty of fluids, wiping from 'front to back' (vagina to anus) after urinating to avoid spreading bacteria, scheduling frequent bathroom breaks, drinking water before and after sex in order to ensure a good volume of urination afterward, checking the fit of a diaphragm or using another method of birth control, avoiding tight clothing and pantyhose, and wearing cotton underwear.

- **High Phosphorus Foods**

  Source: Birmingham, AL: Department of Food and Nutrition Services, University Hospital. 199x. [2 p.].

  Contact: Available from Department of Food and Nutrition Services, University Hospital. 619 South 19th Street, Birmingham, AL 35233. (205) 934-8055. Fax (205) 934-2987. PRICE: $0.65 per copy; bulk copies available; plus shipping and handling.

  Summary: Almost all foods contain some phosphorus, so the average person generally consumes more phosphorus than the body needs. Kidneys that do not function properly lose the ability to get rid of excess phosphorus. People with kidney disease can help keep their bones in the best possible condition by avoiding high phosphorus foods. This single fold brochure lists foods with the highest phosphorus, organized into six categories: dairy products, breads and cereals, dried beans and peas, meats and meat substitutes, beverages, and miscellaneous. Foods include milk, cheese, yogurt, custard, ice cream, cream soups, cream pies, cottage cheese, oatmeal, brown rice, wheat germ, raisin bran, whole wheat breads, bran cereals, bran muffins, lentils, soybeans, navy beans, lima beans, kidney beans, blackeyed peas, pinto beans, salmon, oysters, pot pies, sardines, dried beef, TV dinners, strawberry sodas, all dark colored sodas (except root beer), molasses, **chocolate**, dried fruit, nuts and seeds, and raisins and dates. The brochure is printed on cardstock and illustrated with graphics of the foods listed.

- **Are All Calories Created Equal?**

  Contact: Sugar Association, Inc., 1101 Fifteenth Street, N.W., Suite 600, Washington, DC 20005. (202) 785-1122.

  Summary: Calories are not all the same, says the Sugar Association. The human body tends to store calories from fat but not calories from carbohydrates. Because carbohydrates increase metabolism more than dietary fat, calories from carbohydrates are less fattening. Many people who claim to have a sweet tooth actually have a "fat tooth." Because carbohydrates are often found with fats (chocolate, for example, has both fat and sugar), it's not really the sugar they are craving, this brochure concludes, but the fat. Several high-carbohydrate recipes are included.

- **Celiac Sprue: Patient Resource and Information Guide**

  Source: Seattle, WA: Gluten Intolerance Group of North America. 1991. 15 p.

  Contact: Available from Gluten Intolerance Group of North America. P.O. Box 23053, Seattle, WA 98102-0353. (206) 325-6980. Fax (206) 850-2394. PRICE: $5.

  Summary: This patient resource and information guide provides basic information about celiac sprue. After an introductory section, the author discusses diagnosis, treatment options, potential long-term problems encountered by people with celiac disease, and sources of information for related disorders, including the information clearinghouses of the National Institutes of Health. The handbook presents seven recipes: xanthan gum bread, cranberry orange nut bread, easy blender mayonnaise, Mexican cornbread, 'Almost' graham crackers, picnic **chocolate** chip cookies, and apple cake. The handbook concludes with two indexes, to volumes 14 and 15 of the Gluten Intolerance Group (GIG) newsletter. A final section provides pricing information and order forms for GIG materials and membership.

- **Acne: Six Rules To Live By**

  Source: Patient Care. 33(11): 278. June 15, 1999.

  Summary: This patient information sheet provides people who have acne with information on guidelines for caring for their skin. Although acne is not caused by greasy foods and treats like **chocolate**, people who notice that certain foods seem to make acne worse should avoid them. Skin should be washed with gentle cleaners in the morning and in the evening. Astringents should be avoided unless the skin is very oily, and then, they should be used only on oily spots. Squeezing pimples will not improve a person's skin. Medications should be used according to their directions. Doctors and pharmacists may be helpful in answering questions about medications or other concerns. Remaining with the program recommended by one's physician is important because it may take more than a month for noticeable improvement.

- **Diet and Tinnitus**

  Source: London, England: Royal National Institute for Deaf People. 1998. 2 p.

  Contact: Available from RNID Helpline. P.O. Box 16464, London EC1Y 8TT, United Kingdom. 0870 60 50 123. Fax 0171-296 8199. E-mail: helpline@rnid.org.uk. Website: www.rnid.org.uk. Also available from RNID Tinnitus Helpline. Castle Cavendish Works, Norton Street, Radford, Nottingham NG7 5PN, United Kingdom. 0345 090210. Fax 0115-978 5012. E-mail: tinnitushelpline@btinternet.com. PRICE: Single copy free.

  Summary: Many people have suggested that a wide variety of foods and drinks may cause or aggravate tinnitus (noise or ringing in the ears). This fact sheet from the Royal National Institute for Deaf People (RNID) discusses the relationship between diet and tinnitus by briefly examining the evidence for cheese and **chocolate**, coffee, tea, cola, salt, tonic water, alcohol, red wine, and spirits. Historical notes are provided for some of these categories. The fact sheet recommends that readers try keeping a detailed diary of their food and beverage intake and tinnitus levels for a few days, to see whether a particular food or drink is having any effect. If a suspicious food or drink becomes apparent, the fact sheet suggests no ingesting of that item for a few days to see whether the tinnitus improves but notes that, in general, the healthier and more balanced the diet, the better. The fact sheet concludes with information on the RNID Tinnitus Helpline (in Nottingham, UK), which is also accessible online at tinnitushelpline@btinternet.com. The RNID website is at www.rnid.org.uk.

- **Heartburn: Nothing to do with the Heart**

  Source: Milwaukee, WI: International Foundation for Functional Gastrointestinal Disorders (IFFGD). 2000. [2 p.].

  Contact: Available from International Foundation for Functional Gastrointestinal Disorders (IFFGD). P.O. Box 170864, Milwaukee, WI 53217-8076. (888) 964-2001 or (414) 964-1799. E-mail: iffgd@iffgd.org. Website: www.iffgd.org. PRICE: $1.00 for nonmembers; single copy free to members.

  Summary: This brochure reviews heartburn, defined as a burning sensation in the chest behind the breastbone. The author first reviews the terminology and differentiates between heartburn and dyspepsia (pain in the upper abdomen that resembles that of a peptic ulcer), then describes how heartburn is caused. When gastric (stomach) acids escapes back from the stomach into the esophagus (gastroesophageal reflux), it irritates or damages the esophagus, resulting in heartburn. The author describes the role of the lower esophageal sphincter (LES), which acts as a gate or valve between the esophagus and stomach, and what happens when the LES is weakened or malfunctioning. The author discusses the importance of eating smaller meals and not lying down immediately after a meal, in order to prevent reflux. In addition, certain foods compromise the sphincter's ability to prevent reflux; these foods differ from person to person, but many recognize fats, onions, and **chocolate** as particularly troublesome. The author reviews other conditions (such as overweight) that can make heartburn worse and summarizes the drugs that may be used to help treat heartburn. One sidebar summarizes basic facts about GERD. The brochure concludes with a brief description of the International Foundation for Functional Gastrointestinal Disorders (IFFGD), a nonprofit education and research organization (www.iffgd.org).

- **What You Should Know About Heartburn**

  Source: Postgraduate Medicine. 101(2): 186. February 1997.

  Summary: This brief patient handout summarizes heartburn, a common problem in adults. Heartburn occurs when stomach acid backs up into the esophagus, causing pain under the breastbone. This usually happens just after a meal or when lying down or bending over. The fact sheet notes that certain foods and activities aggravate the problem and should be avoided. These include caffeinated coffee, **chocolate**, fatty red meat, pizza, tomatoes, smoking, and alcoholic beverages. Heartburn can also be made worse by excess weight or by eating within 3 hours of bedtime. The fact sheet recommends some simple lifestyle modifications, including raising the head of the bed, that may help. The fact sheet also briefly mentions diagnostic tests and drug therapy that may be used to help manage heartburn. The fact sheet concludes with a World Wide Web address for readers wishing more information.

- **Healthy Diet for Individuals with Hemochromatosis**

  Source: Richmond, BC, Canada: Canadian Hemochromatosis Society. 1997. 1 p.

  Contact: Available from Canadian Hemochromatosis Society. 272-7000 Minoru Boulevard, Richmond, BC, Canada V6Y 3Z5. (604) 279-7135. Fax (604) 279-7138. E-mail: chcts@istar.ca. PRICE: Single copy free.

  Summary: This fact sheet outlines a recommended diet for people with hemochromatosis (HH), a genetic disorder that results in an overload of iron in the body. Iron accumulates over a number of years and collects in vital organs, such as the heart, liver, and pancreas, causing damage and, in some cases, total destruction. Patients with HH can be treated successfully by regular blood withdrawals (phlebotomies), which will reduce the buildup of excess iron in the body. The fact sheet notes that a diet low in iron cannot take the place of phlebotomy, but patients with HH are nonetheless advised to minimize their intake of iron rich foods and supplements. In addition, patients must take care to replace nutrients lost through phlebotomy. The fact sheet lists enhancers that can increase the amount of iron absorbed from food, such as alcohol, organ meats, vitamin C, cooked shellfish, and foods fortified with iron. The fact sheet then lists four categories of iron inhibitors: oxalates (currents, concord grapes, figs, plums, sweet potatoes, almonds, raspberries, tomato, okra, green and wax beans, **chocolate**, cocoa, and tea), phosphates (cheese and dairy products), carbonates (sodas, soft drinks), and tannates (including tea). The least iron absorption occurs from wholemeal flour products, tea, and high fiber cereals. Although many vegetables are rich in iron, many also contain an iron inhibitor. More iron is absorbed from meat than from vegetables.

- **Diet and Dental Health**

  Source: Chicago, IL: American Academy of Pediatric Dentistry (AAPD). 199x. 2 p.

  Contact: Available from American Academy of Pediatric Dentistry. 211 East Chicago Avenue, Suite 700, Chicago, IL 60611-2616. (312) 337-2169; Fax (312) 337-6329; http://aapd.org. PRICE: Single copy free; bulk orders available.

  Summary: This fact sheet provides parents with information about food habits and preventing tooth decay in their children. Topics covered include how different types of food can cause problems for healthy teeth, the emphasis on how often a child is eating rather than what the child eats, recommended snack foods, and the dental consequences of poor nutrition. The fact sheet then lists suggestions for parents on choosing their child's snack foods; separate sections outline the benefits of **chocolate** milk and cheese. The fact sheet concludes with an address through which readers can get more information.

The NIH Search Utility

The NIH search utility allows you to search for documents on over 100 selected Web sites that comprise the NIH-WEB-SPACE. Each of these servers is "crawled" and indexed on an ongoing basis. Your search will produce a list of various documents, all of which will relate in some way to chocolate. The drawbacks of this approach are that the information is not organized by theme and that the references are often a mix of information for professionals and patients. Nevertheless, a large number of the listed Web sites provide useful background information. We can only recommend this route, therefore, for relatively rare or specific disorders, or when using highly targeted searches. To use the NIH search utility, visit the following Web page: **http://search.nih.gov/index.html**.

Additional Web Sources

A number of Web sites are available to the public that often link to government sites. These can also point you in the direction of essential information. The following is a representative sample:

- AOL: **http://search.aol.com/cat.adp?id=168&layer=&from=subcats**

- Family Village: **http://www.familyvillage.wisc.edu/specific.htm**
- Google: **http://directory.google.com/Top/Health/Conditions_and_Diseases/**
- Med Help International: **http://www.medhelp.org/HealthTopics/A.html**
- Open Directory Project: **http://dmoz.org/Health/Conditions_and_Diseases/**
- Yahoo.com: **http://dir.yahoo.com/Health/Diseases_and_Conditions/**
- WebMD®Health: **http://my.webmd.com/health_topics**

Finding Associations

There are several Internet directories that provide lists of medical associations with information on or resources relating to chocolate. By consulting all of associations listed in this chapter, you will have nearly exhausted all sources for patient associations concerned with chocolate.

The National Health Information Center (NHIC)

The National Health Information Center (NHIC) offers a free referral service to help people find organizations that provide information about chocolate. For more information, see the NHIC's Web site at **http://www.health.gov/NHIC/** or contact an information specialist by calling 1-800-336-4797.

Directory of Health Organizations

The Directory of Health Organizations, provided by the National Library of Medicine Specialized Information Services, is a comprehensive source of information on associations. The Directory of Health Organizations database can be accessed via the Internet at **http://www.sis.nlm.nih.gov/Dir/DirMain.html**. It is composed of two parts: DIRLINE and Health Hotlines.

The DIRLINE database comprises some 10,000 records of organizations, research centers, and government institutes and associations that primarily focus on health and biomedicine. To access DIRLINE directly, go to the following Web site: **http://dirline.nlm.nih.gov/**. Simply type in "chocolate" (or a synonym), and you will receive information on all relevant organizations listed in the database.

Health Hotlines directs you to toll-free numbers to over 300 organizations. You can access this database directly at **http://www.sis.nlm.nih.gov/hotlines/**. On this page, you are given the option to search by keyword or by browsing the subject list. When you have received your search results, click on the name of the organization for its description and contact information.

The Combined Health Information Database

Another comprehensive source of information on healthcare associations is the Combined Health Information Database. Using the "Detailed Search" option, you will need to limit your search to "Organizations" and "chocolate". Type the following hyperlink into your Web browser: **http://chid.nih.gov/detail/detail.html** To find associations, use the drop boxes at the bottom of the search page where "You may refine your search by." For publication date, select "All Years." Then, select your preferred language and the format option "Organization Resource Sheet." Type "chocolate" (or synonyms) into the "For these words:" box. You should check back periodically with this database since it is updated every three months.

The National Organization for Rare Disorders, Inc.

The National Organization for Rare Disorders, Inc. has prepared a Web site that provides, at no charge, lists of associations organized by health topic. You can access this database at the following Web site: **http://www.rarediseases.org/search/orgsearch.html** Type "chocolate" (or a synonym) into the search box, and click "Submit Query."

APPENDIX C. FINDING MEDICAL LIBRARIES

Overview

In this Appendix, we show you how to quickly find a medical library in your area.

Preparation

Your local public library and medical libraries have interlibrary loan programs with the National Library of Medicine (NLM), one of the largest medical collections in the world. According to the NLM, most of the literature in the general and historical collections of the National Library of Medicine is available on interlibrary loan to any library. If you would like to access NLM medical literature, then visit a library in your area that can request the publications for you.[23]

Finding a Local Medical Library

The quickest method to locate medical libraries is to use the Internet-based directory published by the National Network of Libraries of Medicine (NN/LM). This network includes 4626 members and affiliates that provide many services to librarians, health professionals, and the public. To find a library in your area, simply visit **http://nnlm.gov/members/adv.html** or call 1-800-338-7657.

Medical Libraries in the U.S. and Canada

In addition to the NN/LM, the National Library of Medicine (NLM) lists a number of libraries with reference facilities that are open to the public. The following is the NLM's list and includes hyperlinks to each library's Web site. These Web pages can provide information on hours of operation and other restrictions. The list below is a small sample of

---

[23] Adapted from the NLM: **http://www.nlm.nih.gov/psd/cas/interlibrary.html**.

libraries recommended by the National Library of Medicine (sorted alphabetically by name of the U.S. state or Canadian province where the library is located)[24]:

- **Alabama:** Health InfoNet of Jefferson County (Jefferson County Library Cooperative, Lister Hill Library of the Health Sciences), **http://www.uab.edu/infonet/**

- **Alabama:** Richard M. Scrushy Library (American Sports Medicine Institute)

- **Arizona:** Samaritan Regional Medical Center: The Learning Center (Samaritan Health System, Phoenix, Arizona), **http://www.samaritan.edu/library/bannerlibs.htm**

- **California:** Kris Kelly Health Information Center (St. Joseph Health System, Humboldt), **http://www.humboldt1.com/~kkhic/index.html**

- **California:** Community Health Library of Los Gatos, **http://www.healthlib.org/orgresources.html**

- **California:** Consumer Health Program and Services (CHIPS) (County of Los Angeles Public Library, Los Angeles County Harbor-UCLA Medical Center Library) - Carson, CA, **http://www.colapublib.org/services/chips.html**

- **California:** Gateway Health Library (Sutter Gould Medical Foundation)

- **California:** Health Library (Stanford University Medical Center), **http://www-med.stanford.edu/healthlibrary/**

- **California:** Patient Education Resource Center - Health Information and Resources (University of California, San Francisco), **http://sfghdean.ucsf.edu/barnett/PERC/default.asp**

- **California:** Redwood Health Library (Petaluma Health Care District), **http://www.phcd.org/rdwdlib.html**

- **California:** Los Gatos PlaneTree Health Library, **http://planetreesanjose.org/**

- **California:** Sutter Resource Library (Sutter Hospitals Foundation, Sacramento), **http://suttermedicalcenter.org/library/**

- **California:** Health Sciences Libraries (University of California, Davis), **http://www.lib.ucdavis.edu/healthsci/**

- **California:** ValleyCare Health Library & Ryan Comer Cancer Resource Center (ValleyCare Health System, Pleasanton), **http://gaelnet.stmarys-ca.edu/other.libs/gbal/east/vchl.html**

- **California:** Washington Community Health Resource Library (Fremont), **http://www.healthlibrary.org/**

- **Colorado:** William V. Gervasini Memorial Library (Exempla Healthcare), **http://www.saintjosephdenver.org/yourhealth/libraries/**

- **Connecticut:** Hartford Hospital Health Science Libraries (Hartford Hospital), **http://www.harthosp.org/library/**

- **Connecticut:** Healthnet: Connecticut Consumer Health Information Center (University of Connecticut Health Center, Lyman Maynard Stowe Library), **http://library.uchc.edu/departm/hnet/**

---

[24] Abstracted from **http://www.nlm.nih.gov/medlineplus/libraries.html**.

- **Connecticut:** Waterbury Hospital Health Center Library (Waterbury Hospital, Waterbury), **http://www.waterburyhospital.com/library/consumer.shtml**

- **Delaware:** Consumer Health Library (Christiana Care Health System, Eugene du Pont Preventive Medicine & Rehabilitation Institute, Wilmington), **http://www.christianacare.org/health_guide/health_guide_pmri_health_info.cfm**

- **Delaware:** Lewis B. Flinn Library (Delaware Academy of Medicine, Wilmington), **http://www.delamed.org/chls.html**

- **Georgia:** Family Resource Library (Medical College of Georgia, Augusta), **http://cmc.mcg.edu/kids_families/fam_resources/fam_res_lib/frl.htm**

- **Georgia:** Health Resource Center (Medical Center of Central Georgia, Macon), **http://www.mccg.org/hrc/hrchome.asp**

- **Hawaii:** Hawaii Medical Library: Consumer Health Information Service (Hawaii Medical Library, Honolulu), **http://hml.org/CHIS/**

- **Idaho:** DeArmond Consumer Health Library (Kootenai Medical Center, Coeur d'Alene), **http://www.nicon.org/DeArmond/index.htm**

- **Illinois:** Health Learning Center of Northwestern Memorial Hospital (Chicago), **http://www.nmh.org/health_info/hlc.html**

- **Illinois:** Medical Library (OSF Saint Francis Medical Center, Peoria), **http://www.osfsaintfrancis.org/general/library/**

- **Kentucky:** Medical Library - Services for Patients, Families, Students & the Public (Central Baptist Hospital, Lexington), **http://www.centralbap.com/education/community/library.cfm**

- **Kentucky:** University of Kentucky - Health Information Library (Chandler Medical Center, Lexington), **http://www.mc.uky.edu/PatientEd/**

- **Louisiana:** Alton Ochsner Medical Foundation Library (Alton Ochsner Medical Foundation, New Orleans), **http://www.ochsner.org/library/**

- **Louisiana:** Louisiana State University Health Sciences Center Medical Library-Shreveport, **http://lib-sh.lsuhsc.edu/**

- **Maine:** Franklin Memorial Hospital Medical Library (Franklin Memorial Hospital, Farmington), **http://www.fchn.org/fmh/lib.htm**

- **Maine:** Gerrish-True Health Sciences Library (Central Maine Medical Center, Lewiston), **http://www.cmmc.org/library/library.html**

- **Maine:** Hadley Parrot Health Science Library (Eastern Maine Healthcare, Bangor), **http://www.emh.org/hll/hpl/guide.htm**

- **Maine:** Maine Medical Center Library (Maine Medical Center, Portland), **http://www.mmc.org/library/**

- **Maine:** Parkview Hospital (Brunswick), **http://www.parkviewhospital.org/**

- **Maine:** Southern Maine Medical Center Health Sciences Library (Southern Maine Medical Center, Biddeford), **http://www.smmc.org/services/service.php3?choice=10**

- **Maine:** Stephens Memorial Hospital's Health Information Library (Western Maine Health, Norway), **http://www.wmhcc.org/Library/**

- **Manitoba, Canada:** Consumer & Patient Health Information Service (University of Manitoba Libraries), **http://www.umanitoba.ca/libraries/units/health/reference/chis.html**

- **Manitoba, Canada:** J.W. Crane Memorial Library (Deer Lodge Centre, Winnipeg), **http://www.deerlodge.mb.ca/crane_library/about.asp**

- **Maryland:** Health Information Center at the Wheaton Regional Library (Montgomery County, Dept. of Public Libraries, Wheaton Regional Library), **http://www.mont.lib.md.us/healthinfo/hic.asp**

- **Massachusetts:** Baystate Medical Center Library (Baystate Health System), **http://www.baystatehealth.com/1024/**

- **Massachusetts:** Boston University Medical Center Alumni Medical Library (Boston University Medical Center), **http://med-libwww.bu.edu/library/lib.html**

- **Massachusetts:** Lowell General Hospital Health Sciences Library (Lowell General Hospital, Lowell), **http://www.lowellgeneral.org/library/HomePageLinks/WWW.htm**

- **Massachusetts:** Paul E. Woodard Health Sciences Library (New England Baptist Hospital, Boston), **http://www.nebh.org/health_lib.asp**

- **Massachusetts:** St. Luke's Hospital Health Sciences Library (St. Luke's Hospital, Southcoast Health System, New Bedford), **http://www.southcoast.org/library/**

- **Massachusetts:** Treadwell Library Consumer Health Reference Center (Massachusetts General Hospital), **http://www.mgh.harvard.edu/library/chrcindex.html**

- **Massachusetts:** UMass HealthNet (University of Massachusetts Medical School, Worchester), **http://healthnet.umassmed.edu/**

- **Michigan:** Botsford General Hospital Library - Consumer Health (Botsford General Hospital, Library & Internet Services), **http://www.botsfordlibrary.org/consumer.htm**

- **Michigan:** Helen DeRoy Medical Library (Providence Hospital and Medical Centers), **http://www.providence-hospital.org/library/**

- **Michigan:** Marquette General Hospital - Consumer Health Library (Marquette General Hospital, Health Information Center), **http://www.mgh.org/center.html**

- **Michigan:** Patient Education Resouce Center - University of Michigan Cancer Center (University of Michigan Comprehensive Cancer Center, Ann Arbor), **http://www.cancer.med.umich.edu/learn/leares.htm**

- **Michigan:** Sladen Library & Center for Health Information Resources - Consumer Health Information (Detroit), **http://www.henryford.com/body.cfm?id=39330**

- **Montana:** Center for Health Information (St. Patrick Hospital and Health Sciences Center, Missoula)

- **National:** Consumer Health Library Directory (Medical Library Association, Consumer and Patient Health Information Section), **http://caphis.mlanet.org/directory/index.html**

- **National:** National Network of Libraries of Medicine (National Library of Medicine) - provides library services for health professionals in the United States who do not have access to a medical library, **http://nnlm.gov/**

- **National:** NN/LM List of Libraries Serving the Public (National Network of Libraries of Medicine), **http://nnlm.gov/members/**

- **Nevada:** Health Science Library, West Charleston Library (Las Vegas-Clark County Library District, Las Vegas), http://www.lvccld.org/special_collections/medical/index.htm

- **New Hampshire:** Dartmouth Biomedical Libraries (Dartmouth College Library, Hanover), http://www.dartmouth.edu/~biomed/resources.htmld/conshealth.htmld/

- **New Jersey:** Consumer Health Library (Rahway Hospital, Rahway), http://www.rahwayhospital.com/library.htm

- **New Jersey:** Dr. Walter Phillips Health Sciences Library (Englewood Hospital and Medical Center, Englewood), http://www.englewoodhospital.com/links/index.htm

- **New Jersey:** Meland Foundation (Englewood Hospital and Medical Center, Englewood), http://www.geocities.com/ResearchTriangle/9360/

- **New York:** Choices in Health Information (New York Public Library) - NLM Consumer Pilot Project participant, http://www.nypl.org/branch/health/links.html

- **New York:** Health Information Center (Upstate Medical University, State University of New York, Syracuse), http://www.upstate.edu/library/hic/

- **New York:** Health Sciences Library (Long Island Jewish Medical Center, New Hyde Park), http://www.lij.edu/library/library.html

- **New York:** ViaHealth Medical Library (Rochester General Hospital), http://www.nyam.org/library/

- **Ohio:** Consumer Health Library (Akron General Medical Center, Medical & Consumer Health Library), http://www.akrongeneral.org/hwlibrary.htm

- **Oklahoma:** The Health Information Center at Saint Francis Hospital (Saint Francis Health System, Tulsa), http://www.sfh-tulsa.com/services/healthinfo.asp

- **Oregon:** Planetree Health Resource Center (Mid-Columbia Medical Center, The Dalles), http://www.mcmc.net/phrc/

- **Pennsylvania:** Community Health Information Library (Milton S. Hershey Medical Center, Hershey), http://www.hmc.psu.edu/commhealth/

- **Pennsylvania:** Community Health Resource Library (Geisinger Medical Center, Danville), http://www.geisinger.edu/education/commlib.shtml

- **Pennsylvania:** HealthInfo Library (Moses Taylor Hospital, Scranton), http://www.mth.org/healthwellness.html

- **Pennsylvania:** Hopwood Library (University of Pittsburgh, Health Sciences Library System, Pittsburgh), http://www.hsls.pitt.edu/guides/chi/hopwood/index_html

- **Pennsylvania:** Koop Community Health Information Center (College of Physicians of Philadelphia), http://www.collphyphil.org/kooppg1.shtml

- **Pennsylvania:** Learning Resources Center - Medical Library (Susquehanna Health System, Williamsport), http://www.shscares.org/services/lrc/index.asp

- **Pennsylvania:** Medical Library (UPMC Health System, Pittsburgh), http://www.upmc.edu/passavant/library.htm

- **Quebec, Canada:** Medical Library (Montreal General Hospital), http://www.mghlib.mcgill.ca/

- **South Dakota:** Rapid City Regional Hospital Medical Library (Rapid City Regional Hospital), **http://www.rcrh.org/Services/Library/Default.asp**

- **Texas:** Houston HealthWays (Houston Academy of Medicine-Texas Medical Center Library), **http://hhw.library.tmc.edu/**

- **Washington:** Community Health Library (Kittitas Valley Community Hospital), **http://www.kvch.com/**

- **Washington:** Southwest Washington Medical Center Library (Southwest Washington Medical Center, Vancouver), **http://www.swmedicalcenter.com/body.cfm?id=72**

ONLINE GLOSSARIES

The Internet provides access to a number of free-to-use medical dictionaries. The National Library of Medicine has compiled the following list of online dictionaries:

- ADAM Medical Encyclopedia (A.D.A.M., Inc.), comprehensive medical reference: **http://www.nlm.nih.gov/medlineplus/encyclopedia.html**

- MedicineNet.com Medical Dictionary (MedicineNet, Inc.): **http://www.medterms.com/Script/Main/hp.asp**

- Merriam-Webster Medical Dictionary (Inteli-Health, Inc.): **http://www.intelihealth.com/IH/**

- Multilingual Glossary of Technical and Popular Medical Terms in Eight European Languages (European Commission) - Danish, Dutch, English, French, German, Italian, Portuguese, and Spanish: **http://allserv.rug.ac.be/~rvdstich/eugloss/welcome.html**

- On-line Medical Dictionary (CancerWEB): **http://cancerweb.ncl.ac.uk/omd/**

- Rare Diseases Terms (Office of Rare Diseases): **http://ord.aspensys.com/asp/diseases/diseases.asp**

- Technology Glossary (National Library of Medicine) - Health Care Technology: **http://www.nlm.nih.gov/nichsr/ta101/ta10108.htm**

Beyond these, MEDLINEplus contains a very patient-friendly encyclopedia covering every aspect of medicine (licensed from A.D.A.M., Inc.). The ADAM Medical Encyclopedia can be accessed at **http://www.nlm.nih.gov/medlineplus/encyclopedia.html**. ADAM is also available on commercial Web sites such as drkoop.com (**http://www.drkoop.com/**) and Web MD (**http://my.webmd.com/adam/asset/adam_disease_articles/a_to_z/a**).

Online Dictionary Directories

The following are additional online directories compiled by the National Library of Medicine, including a number of specialized medical dictionaries:

- Medical Dictionaries: Medical & Biological (World Health Organization): **http://www.who.int/hlt/virtuallibrary/English/diction.htm#Medical**

- MEL-Michigan Electronic Library List of Online Health and Medical Dictionaries (Michigan Electronic Library): **http://mel.lib.mi.us/health/health-dictionaries.html**

- Patient Education: Glossaries (DMOZ Open Directory Project): **http://dmoz.org/Health/Education/Patient_Education/Glossaries/**

- Web of Online Dictionaries (Bucknell University): **http://www.yourdictionary.com/diction5.html#medicine**

CHOCOLATE DICTIONARY

The definitions below are derived from official public sources, including the National Institutes of Health [NIH] and the European Union [EU].

Abdomen: That portion of the body that lies between the thorax and the pelvis. [NIH]

Abdominal: Having to do with the abdomen, which is the part of the body between the chest and the hips that contains the pancreas, stomach, intestines, liver, gallbladder, and other organs. [NIH]

Abdominal Pain: Sensation of discomfort, distress, or agony in the abdominal region. [NIH]

Ablation: The removal of an organ by surgery. [NIH]

Acceptor: A substance which, while normally not oxidized by oxygen or reduced by hydrogen, can be oxidized or reduced in presence of a substance which is itself undergoing oxidation or reduction. [NIH]

Acetylcholine: A neurotransmitter. Acetylcholine in vertebrates is the major transmitter at neuromuscular junctions, autonomic ganglia, parasympathetic effector junctions, a subset of sympathetic effector junctions, and at many sites in the central nervous system. It is generally not used as an administered drug because it is broken down very rapidly by cholinesterases, but it is useful in some ophthalmological applications. [NIH]

Acne: A disorder of the skin marked by inflammation of oil glands and hair glands. [NIH]

Acne Vulgaris: A chronic disorder of the pilosebaceous apparatus associated with an increase in sebum secretion. It is characterized by open comedones (blackheads), closed comedones (whiteheads), and pustular nodules. The cause is unknown, but heredity and age are predisposing factors. [NIH]

Acrylonitrile: A highly poisonous compound used widely in the manufacture of plastics, adhesives and synthetic rubber. [NIH]

Adaptability: Ability to develop some form of tolerance to conditions extremely different from those under which a living organism evolved. [NIH]

Adaptation: 1. The adjustment of an organism to its environment, or the process by which it enhances such fitness. 2. The normal ability of the eye to adjust itself to variations in the intensity of light; the adjustment to such variations. 3. The decline in the frequency of firing of a neuron, particularly of a receptor, under conditions of constant stimulation. 4. In dentistry, (a) the proper fitting of a denture, (b) the degree of proximity and interlocking of restorative material to a tooth preparation, (c) the exact adjustment of bands to teeth. 5. In microbiology, the adjustment of bacterial physiology to a new environment. [EU]

Adenosine: A nucleoside that is composed of adenine and d-ribose. Adenosine or adenosine derivatives play many important biological roles in addition to being components of DNA and RNA. Adenosine itself is a neurotransmitter. [NIH]

Adipose Tissue: Connective tissue composed of fat cells lodged in the meshes of areolar tissue. [NIH]

Adjustment: The dynamic process wherein the thoughts, feelings, behavior, and biophysiological mechanisms of the individual continually change to adjust to the environment. [NIH]

Adjuvant: A substance which aids another, such as an auxiliary remedy; in immunology, nonspecific stimulator (e.g., BCG vaccine) of the immune response. [EU]

Adrenal Cortex: The outer layer of the adrenal gland. It secretes mineralocorticoids, androgens, and glucocorticoids. [NIH]

Adrenergic: Activated by, characteristic of, or secreting epinephrine or substances with similar activity; the term is applied to those nerve fibres that liberate norepinephrine at a synapse when a nerve impulse passes, i.e., the sympathetic fibres. [EU]

Adsorption: The condensation of gases, liquids, or dissolved substances on the surfaces of solids. It includes adsorptive phenomena of bacteria and viruses as well as of tissues treated with exogenous drugs and chemicals. [NIH]

Adsorptive: It captures volatile compounds by binding them to agents such as activated carbon or adsorptive resins. [NIH]

Adverse Effect: An unwanted side effect of treatment. [NIH]

Aerosol: A solution of a drug which can be atomized into a fine mist for inhalation therapy. [EU]

Affinity: 1. Inherent likeness or relationship. 2. A special attraction for a specific element, organ, or structure. 3. Chemical affinity; the force that binds atoms in molecules; the tendency of substances to combine by chemical reaction. 4. The strength of noncovalent chemical binding between two substances as measured by the dissociation constant of the complex. 5. In immunology, a thermodynamic expression of the strength of interaction between a single antigen-binding site and a single antigenic determinant (and thus of the stereochemical compatibility between them), most accurately applied to interactions among simple, uniform antigenic determinants such as haptens. Expressed as the association constant (K litres mole -1), which, owing to the heterogeneity of affinities in a population of antibody molecules of a given specificity, actually represents an average value (mean intrinsic association constant). 6. The reciprocal of the dissociation constant. [EU]

Agar: A complex sulfated polymer of galactose units, extracted from Gelidium cartilagineum, Gracilaria confervoides, and related red algae. It is used as a gel in the preparation of solid culture media for microorganisms, as a bulk laxative, in making emulsions, and as a supporting medium for immunodiffusion and immunoelectrophoresis. [NIH]

Ageing: A physiological or morphological change in the life of an organism or its parts, generally irreversible and typically associated with a decline in growth and reproductive vigor. [NIH]

Agonist: In anatomy, a prime mover. In pharmacology, a drug that has affinity for and stimulates physiologic activity at cell receptors normally stimulated by naturally occurring substances. [EU]

Aldehydes: Organic compounds containing a carbonyl group in the form -CHO. [NIH]

Alertness: A state of readiness to detect and respond to certain specified small changes occurring at random intervals in the environment. [NIH]

Algorithms: A procedure consisting of a sequence of algebraic formulas and/or logical steps to calculate or determine a given task. [NIH]

Alimentary: Pertaining to food or nutritive material, or to the organs of digestion. [EU]

Alkaline: Having the reactions of an alkali. [EU]

Alkaloid: A member of a large group of chemicals that are made by plants and have nitrogen in them. Some alkaloids have been shown to work against cancer. [NIH]

Allergen: An antigenic substance capable of producing immediate-type hypersensitivity (allergy). [EU]

Allergic Rhinitis: Inflammation of the nasal mucous membrane associated with hay fever;

fits may be provoked by substances in the working environment. [NIH]

Alternative medicine: Practices not generally recognized by the medical community as standard or conventional medical approaches and used instead of standard treatments. Alternative medicine includes the taking of dietary supplements, megadose vitamins, and herbal preparations; the drinking of special teas; and practices such as massage therapy, magnet therapy, spiritual healing, and meditation. [NIH]

Aluminum: A metallic element that has the atomic number 13, atomic symbol Al, and atomic weight 26.98. [NIH]

Amino acid: Any organic compound containing an amino (-NH2 and a carboxyl (- COOH) group. The 20 a-amino acids listed in the accompanying table are the amino acids from which proteins are synthesized by formation of peptide bonds during ribosomal translation of messenger RNA; all except glycine, which is not optically active, have the L configuration. Other amino acids occurring in proteins, such as hydroxyproline in collagen, are formed by posttranslational enzymatic modification of amino acids residues in polypeptide chains. There are also several important amino acids, such as the neurotransmitter y-aminobutyric acid, that have no relation to proteins. Abbreviated AA. [EU]

Amino Acid Sequence: The order of amino acids as they occur in a polypeptide chain. This is referred to as the primary structure of proteins. It is of fundamental importance in determining protein conformation. [NIH]

Ammonia: A colorless alkaline gas. It is formed in the body during decomposition of organic materials during a large number of metabolically important reactions. [NIH]

Amphetamine: A powerful central nervous system stimulant and sympathomimetic. Amphetamine has multiple mechanisms of action including blocking uptake of adrenergics and dopamine, stimulation of release of monamines, and inhibiting monoamine oxidase. Amphetamine is also a drug of abuse and a psychotomimetic. The l- and the d,l-forms are included here. The l-form has less central nervous system activity but stronger cardiovascular effects. The d-form is dextroamphetamine. [NIH]

Ampulla: A sac-like enlargement of a canal or duct. [NIH]

Analgesic: An agent that alleviates pain without causing loss of consciousness. [EU]

Analog: In chemistry, a substance that is similar, but not identical, to another. [NIH]

Anaphylaxis: An acute hypersensitivity reaction due to exposure to a previously encountered antigen. The reaction may include rapidly progressing urticaria, respiratory distress, vascular collapse, systemic shock, and death. [NIH]

Anatomical: Pertaining to anatomy, or to the structure of the organism. [EU]

Anemia: A reduction in the number of circulating erythrocytes or in the quantity of hemoglobin. [NIH]

Anesthesia: A state characterized by loss of feeling or sensation. This depression of nerve function is usually the result of pharmacologic action and is induced to allow performance of surgery or other painful procedures. [NIH]

Anhydrous: Deprived or destitute of water. [EU]

Animal model: An animal with a disease either the same as or like a disease in humans. Animal models are used to study the development and progression of diseases and to test new treatments before they are given to humans. Animals with transplanted human cancers or other tissues are called xenograft models. [NIH]

Antagonism: Interference with, or inhibition of, the growth of a living organism by another living organism, due either to creation of unfavorable conditions (e. g. exhaustion of food supplies) or to production of a specific antibiotic substance (e. g. penicillin). [NIH]

Antibiotic: A drug used to treat infections caused by bacteria and other microorganisms. [NIH]

Antibodies: Immunoglobulin molecules having a specific amino acid sequence by virtue of which they interact only with the antigen that induced their synthesis in cells of the lymphoid series (especially plasma cells), or with an antigen closely related to it. [NIH]

Antibody: A type of protein made by certain white blood cells in response to a foreign substance (antigen). Each antibody can bind to only a specific antigen. The purpose of this binding is to help destroy the antigen. Antibodies can work in several ways, depending on the nature of the antigen. Some antibodies destroy antigens directly. Others make it easier for white blood cells to destroy the antigen. [NIH]

Anticarcinogenic: Pertaining to something that prevents or delays the development of cancer. [NIH]

Anticoagulant: A drug that helps prevent blood clots from forming. Also called a blood thinner. [NIH]

Antidepressant: A drug used to treat depression. [NIH]

Antigen: Any substance which is capable, under appropriate conditions, of inducing a specific immune response and of reacting with the products of that response, that is, with specific antibody or specifically sensitized T-lymphocytes, or both. Antigens may be soluble substances, such as toxins and foreign proteins, or particulate, such as bacteria and tissue cells; however, only the portion of the protein or polysaccharide molecule known as the antigenic determinant (q.v.) combines with antibody or a specific receptor on a lymphocyte. Abbreviated Ag. [EU]

Anti-infective: An agent that so acts. [EU]

Anti-Infective Agents: Substances that prevent infectious agents or organisms from spreading or kill infectious agents in order to prevent the spread of infection. [NIH]

Anti-inflammatory: Having to do with reducing inflammation. [NIH]

Anti-Inflammatory Agents: Substances that reduce or suppress inflammation. [NIH]

Antineoplastic: Inhibiting or preventing the development of neoplasms, checking the maturation and proliferation of malignant cells. [EU]

Antineoplastic Agents: Substances that inhibit or prevent the proliferation of neoplasms. [NIH]

Antioxidant: A substance that prevents damage caused by free radicals. Free radicals are highly reactive chemicals that often contain oxygen. They are produced when molecules are split to give products that have unpaired electrons. This process is called oxidation. [NIH]

Antipyretic: An agent that relieves or reduces fever. Called also antifebrile, antithermic and febrifuge. [EU]

Antitussive: An agent that relieves or prevents cough. [EU]

Anus: The opening of the rectum to the outside of the body. [NIH]

Anxiety: Persistent feeling of dread, apprehension, and impending disaster. [NIH]

Apolipoproteins: The protein components of lipoproteins which remain after the lipids to which the proteins are bound have been removed. They play an important role in lipid transport and metabolism. [NIH]

Apoptosis: One of the two mechanisms by which cell death occurs (the other being the pathological process of necrosis). Apoptosis is the mechanism responsible for the physiological deletion of cells and appears to be intrinsically programmed. It is characterized by distinctive morphologic changes in the nucleus and cytoplasm, chromatin cleavage at regularly spaced sites, and the endonucleolytic cleavage of genomic DNA (DNA fragmentation) at internucleosomal sites. This mode of cell death serves as a balance to mitosis in regulating the size of animal tissues and in mediating pathologic processes associated with tumor growth. [NIH]

Applicability: A list of the commodities to which the candidate method can be applied as presented or with minor modifications. [NIH]

Approximate: Approximal [EU]

Aqueous: Having to do with water. [NIH]

Arachidonate 15-Lipoxygenase: An enzyme that catalyzes the oxidation of arachidonic acid to yield 15-hydroperoxyarachidonate (15-HPETE) which is rapidly converted to 15-hydroxy-5,8,11,13-eicosatetraenoate (15-HETE). The 15-hydroperoxides are preferentially formed in neutrophils and lymphocytes. EC 1.13.11.33. [NIH]

Arachidonate Lipoxygenases: Enzymes catalyzing the oxidation of arachidonic acid to hydroperoxyarachidonates (HPETES). These products are then rapidly converted by a peroxidase to hydroxyeicosatetraenoic acids (HETES). The positional specificity of the enzyme reaction varies from tissue to tissue. The final lipoxygenase pathway leads to the leukotrienes. EC 1.13.11.- . [NIH]

Arachidonic Acid: An unsaturated, essential fatty acid. It is found in animal and human fat as well as in the liver, brain, and glandular organs, and is a constituent of animal phosphatides. It is formed by the synthesis from dietary linoleic acid and is a precursor in the biosynthesis of prostaglandins, thromboxanes, and leukotrienes. [NIH]

Arginine: An essential amino acid that is physiologically active in the L-form. [NIH]

Argon: A noble gas with the atomic symbol Ar, atomic number 18, and atomic weight 39.948. It is used in fluorescent tubes and wherever an inert atmosphere is desired and nitrogen cannot be used. [NIH]

Aromatic: Having a spicy odour. [EU]

Arterial: Pertaining to an artery or to the arteries. [EU]

Arteries: The vessels carrying blood away from the heart. [NIH]

Arterioles: The smallest divisions of the arteries located between the muscular arteries and the capillaries. [NIH]

Ascorbic Acid: A six carbon compound related to glucose. It is found naturally in citrus fruits and many vegetables. Ascorbic acid is an essential nutrient in human diets, and necessary to maintain connective tissue and bone. Its biologically active form, vitamin C, functions as a reducing agent and coenzyme in several metabolic pathways. Vitamin C is considered an antioxidant. [NIH]

Aspartame: Flavoring agent sweeter than sugar, metabolized as phenylalanine and aspartic acid. [NIH]

Aspartate: A synthetic amino acid. [NIH]

Aspartic: The naturally occurring substance is L-aspartic acid. One of the acidic-amino-acids is obtained by the hydrolysis of proteins. [NIH]

Aspartic Acid: One of the non-essential amino acids commonly occurring in the L-form. It is found in animals and plants, especially in sugar cane and sugar beets. It may be a neurotransmitter. [NIH]

Aspiration: The act of inhaling. [NIH]

Aspirin: A drug that reduces pain, fever, inflammation, and blood clotting. Aspirin belongs to the family of drugs called nonsteroidal anti-inflammatory agents. It is also being studied in cancer prevention. [NIH]

Assay: Determination of the amount of a particular constituent of a mixture, or of the biological or pharmacological potency of a drug. [EU]

Atmospheric Pressure: The pressure at any point in an atmosphere due solely to the weight of the atmospheric gases above the point concerned. [NIH]

Atypical: Irregular; not conformable to the type; in microbiology, applied specifically to strains of unusual type. [EU]

Aura: A subjective sensation or motor phenomenon that precedes and marks the of a paroxysmal attack, such as an epileptic attack on set. [EU]

Autonomic: Self-controlling; functionally independent. [EU]

Autonomic Nervous System: The enteric, parasympathetic, and sympathetic nervous systems taken together. Generally speaking, the autonomic nervous system regulates the internal environment during both peaceful activity and physical or emotional stress. Autonomic activity is controlled and integrated by the central nervous system, especially the hypothalamus and the solitary nucleus, which receive information relayed from visceral afferents; these and related central and sensory structures are sometimes (but not here) considered to be part of the autonomic nervous system itself. [NIH]

Bacteria: Unicellular prokaryotic microorganisms which generally possess rigid cell walls, multiply by cell division, and exhibit three principal forms: round or coccal, rodlike or bacillary, and spiral or spirochetal. [NIH]

Bacteriophage: A virus whose host is a bacterial cell; A virus that exclusively infects bacteria. It generally has a protein coat surrounding the genome (DNA or RNA). One of the coliphages most extensively studied is the lambda phage, which is also one of the most important. [NIH]

Bacterium: Microscopic organism which may have a spherical, rod-like, or spiral unicellular or non-cellular body. Bacteria usually reproduce through asexual processes. [NIH]

Barium: An element of the alkaline earth group of metals. It has an atomic symbol Ba, atomic number 56, and atomic weight 138. All of its acid-soluble salts are poisonous. [NIH]

Base: In chemistry, the nonacid part of a salt; a substance that combines with acids to form salts; a substance that dissociates to give hydroxide ions in aqueous solutions; a substance whose molecule or ion can combine with a proton (hydrogen ion); a substance capable of donating a pair of electrons (to an acid) for the formation of a coordinate covalent bond. [EU]

Baths: The immersion or washing of the body or any of its parts in water or other medium for cleansing or medical treatment. It includes bathing for personal hygiene as well as for medical purposes with the addition of therapeutic agents, such as alkalines, antiseptics, oil, etc. [NIH]

Beer: An alcoholic beverage usually made from malted cereal grain (as barley), flavored with hops, and brewed by slow fermentation. [NIH]

Benign: Not cancerous; does not invade nearby tissue or spread to other parts of the body. [NIH]

Beta-Endorphin: A peptide consisting of amino acid sequence 61-91 of the endogenous pituitary hormone beta-lipotropin. The first four amino acids show a common tetrapeptide sequence with methionine- and leucine enkephalin. The compound shows opiate-like activity. Injection of beta-endorphin induces a profound analgesia of the whole body for several hours. This action is reversed after administration of naloxone. [NIH]

Bile: An emulsifying agent produced in the liver and secreted into the duodenum. Its composition includes bile acids and salts, cholesterol, and electrolytes. It aids digestion of fats in the duodenum. [NIH]

Bile Acids: Acids made by the liver that work with bile to break down fats. [NIH]

Biliary: Having to do with the liver, bile ducts, and/or gallbladder. [NIH]

Biliary Tract: The gallbladder and its ducts. [NIH]

Bioavailability: The degree to which a drug or other substance becomes available to the target tissue after administration. [EU]

Bioavailable: The ability of a drug or other substance to be absorbed and used by the body. Orally bioavailable means that a drug or other substance that is taken by mouth can be absorbed and used by the body. [NIH]

Biogenic Amines: A group of naturally occurring amines derived by enzymatic decarboxylation of the natural amino acids. Many have powerful physiological effects (e.g., histamine, serotonin, epinephrine, tyramine). Those derived from aromatic amino acids, and also their synthetic analogs (e.g., amphetamine), are of use in pharmacology. [NIH]

Biomarkers: Substances sometimes found in an increased amount in the blood, other body fluids, or tissues and that may suggest the presence of some types of cancer. Biomarkers include CA 125 (ovarian cancer), CA 15-3 (breast cancer), CEA (ovarian, lung, breast, pancreas, and GI tract cancers), and PSA (prostate cancer). Also called tumor markers. [NIH]

Biopsy: Removal and pathologic examination of specimens in the form of small pieces of tissue from the living body. [NIH]

Biopsy specimen: Tissue removed from the body and examined under a microscope to determine whether disease is present. [NIH]

Biotechnology: Body of knowledge related to the use of organisms, cells or cell-derived constituents for the purpose of developing products which are technically, scientifically and clinically useful. Alteration of biologic function at the molecular level (i.e., genetic engineering) is a central focus; laboratory methods used include transfection and cloning technologies, sequence and structure analysis algorithms, computer databases, and gene and protein structure function analysis and prediction. [NIH]

Biotransformation: The chemical alteration of an exogenous substance by or in a biological system. The alteration may inactivate the compound or it may result in the production of an active metabolite of an inactive parent compound. The alteration may be either non-synthetic (oxidation-reduction, hydrolysis) or synthetic (glucuronide formation, sulfate conjugation, acetylation, methylation). This also includes metabolic detoxication and clearance. [NIH]

Biotype: A group of individuals having the same genotype. [NIH]

Bladder: The organ that stores urine. [NIH]

Bloating: Fullness or swelling in the abdomen that often occurs after meals. [NIH]

Blood Coagulation: The process of the interaction of blood coagulation factors that results in an insoluble fibrin clot. [NIH]

Blood pressure: The pressure of blood against the walls of a blood vessel or heart chamber. Unless there is reference to another location, such as the pulmonary artery or one of the heart chambers, it refers to the pressure in the systemic arteries, as measured, for example, in the forearm. [NIH]

Blood vessel: A tube in the body through which blood circulates. Blood vessels include a network of arteries, arterioles, capillaries, venules, and veins. [NIH]

Body Fluids: Liquid components of living organisms. [NIH]

Body Mass Index: One of the anthropometric measures of body mass; it has the highest correlation with skinfold thickness or body density. [NIH]

Body Regions: Anatomical areas of the body. [NIH]

Bowel: The long tube-shaped organ in the abdomen that completes the process of digestion. There is both a small and a large bowel. Also called the intestine. [NIH]

Bowel Movement: Body wastes passed through the rectum and anus. [NIH]

Bradykinin: A nonapeptide messenger that is enzymatically produced from kallidin in the blood where it is a potent but short-lived agent of arteriolar dilation and increased capillary permeability. Bradykinin is also released from mast cells during asthma attacks, from gut walls as a gastrointestinal vasodilator, from damaged tissues as a pain signal, and may be a neurotransmitter. [NIH]

Branch: Most commonly used for branches of nerves, but applied also to other structures. [NIH]

Breakdown: A physical, metal, or nervous collapse. [NIH]

Bronchi: The larger air passages of the lungs arising from the terminal bifurcation of the trachea. [NIH]

Bronchial: Pertaining to one or more bronchi. [EU]

Buffers: A chemical system that functions to control the levels of specific ions in solution. When the level of hydrogen ion in solution is controlled the system is called a pH buffer. [NIH]

Bupropion: A unicyclic, aminoketone antidepressant. The mechanism of its therapeutic actions is not well understood, but it does appear to block dopamine uptake. The hydrochloride is available as an aid to smoking cessation treatment. [NIH]

Cacao: A tree of the family Sterculiaceae (or Byttneriaceae), usually Theobroma cacao, or its seeds, which after fermentation and roasting, yield cocoa and chocolate. [NIH]

Caffeine: A methylxanthine naturally occurring in some beverages and also used as a pharmacological agent. Caffeine's most notable pharmacological effect is as a central nervous system stimulant, increasing alertness and producing agitation. It also relaxes smooth muscle, stimulates cardiac muscle, stimulates diuresis, and appears to be useful in the treatment of some types of headache. Several cellular actions of caffeine have been observed, but it is not entirely clear how each contributes to its pharmacological profile. Among the most important are inhibition of cyclic nucleotide phosphodiesterases, antagonism of adenosine receptors, and modulation of intracellular calcium handling. [NIH]

Calcium: A basic element found in nearly all organized tissues. It is a member of the alkaline earth family of metals with the atomic symbol Ca, atomic number 20, and atomic weight 40. Calcium is the most abundant mineral in the body and combines with phosphorus to form calcium phosphate in the bones and teeth. It is essential for the normal functioning of nerves and muscles and plays a role in blood coagulation (as factor IV) and in many enzymatic processes. [NIH]

Calcium Carbonate: Carbonic acid calcium salt ($CaCO_3$). An odorless, tasteless powder or crystal that occurs in nature. It is used therapeutically as a phosphate buffer in hemodialysis patients and as a calcium supplement. [NIH]

Calcium Compounds: Inorganic compounds that contain calcium as an integral part of the molecule. [NIH]

Calcium Gluconate: The calcium salt of gluconic acid. The compound has a variety of uses, including its use as a calcium replenisher in hypocalcemic states. [NIH]

Calcium Hydroxide: $Ca(OH)_2$. A white powder that has many therapeutic uses. Because of its ability to stimulate mineralization, it is found in many dental formulations. [NIH]

Calcium Oxalate: The calcium salt of oxalic acid, occurring in the urine as crystals and in certain calculi. [NIH]

Calciuria: The presence of calcium in the urine. [EU]

Calculi: An abnormal concretion occurring mostly in the urinary and biliary tracts, usually composed of mineral salts. Also called stones. [NIH]

Calculus I: An abnormal concretion occurring within the animal body and usually composed of mineral salts. [EU]

Cannabis: The hemp plant Cannabis sativa. Products prepared from the dried flowering tops of the plant include marijuana, hashish, bhang, and ganja. [NIH]

Capillary: Any one of the minute vessels that connect the arterioles and venules, forming a network in nearly all parts of the body. Their walls act as semipermeable membranes for the interchange of various substances, including fluids, between the blood and tissue fluid; called also vas capillare. [EU]

Capillary Fragility: The lack of resistance, or susceptibility, of capillaries to damage or disruption under conditions of increased stress. [NIH]

Capsules: Hard or soft soluble containers used for the oral administration of medicine. [NIH]

Carbohydrate: An aldehyde or ketone derivative of a polyhydric alcohol, particularly of the pentahydric and hexahydric alcohols. They are so named because the hydrogen and oxygen are usually in the proportion to form water, $(CH_2O)n$. The most important carbohydrates are the starches, sugars, celluloses, and gums. They are classified into mono-, di-, tri-, poly- and heterosaccharides. [EU]

Cardiac: Having to do with the heart. [NIH]

Cardiovascular: Having to do with the heart and blood vessels. [NIH]

Carotene: The general name for a group of pigments found in green, yellow, and leafy vegetables, and yellow fruits. The pigments are fat-soluble, unsaturated aliphatic hydrocarbons functioning as provitamins and are converted to vitamin A through enzymatic processes in the intestinal wall. [NIH]

Case report: A detailed report of the diagnosis, treatment, and follow-up of an individual patient. Case reports also contain some demographic information about the patient (for example, age, gender, ethnic origin). [NIH]

Case series: A group or series of case reports involving patients who were given similar treatment. Reports of case series usually contain detailed information about the individual patients. This includes demographic information (for example, age, gender, ethnic origin) and information on diagnosis, treatment, response to treatment, and follow-up after treatment. [NIH]

Catechin: Extracted from Uncaria gambier, Acacia catechu and other plants; it stabilizes collagen and is therefore used in tanning and dyeing; it prevents capillary fragility and abnormal permeability, but was formerly used as an antidiarrheal. [NIH]

Catecholamine: A group of chemical substances manufactured by the adrenal medulla and secreted during physiological stress. [NIH]

Catheter: A flexible tube used to deliver fluids into or withdraw fluids from the body. [NIH]

Causal: Pertaining to a cause; directed against a cause. [EU]

Celiac Disease: A disease characterized by intestinal malabsorption and precipitated by gluten-containing foods. The intestinal mucosa shows loss of villous structure. [NIH]

Cell: The individual unit that makes up all of the tissues of the body. All living things are made up of one or more cells. [NIH]

Cell Aggregation: The phenomenon by which dissociated cells intermixed in vitro tend to group themselves with cells of their own type. [NIH]

Cell Death: The termination of the cell's ability to carry out vital functions such as metabolism, growth, reproduction, responsiveness, and adaptability. [NIH]

Cell Division: The fission of a cell. [NIH]

Cellobiose: A disaccharide consisting of two glucose units in beta (1-4) glycosidic linkage. Obtained from the partial hydrolysis of cellulose. [NIH]

Cellulose: A polysaccharide with glucose units linked as in cellobiose. It is the chief constituent of plant fibers, cotton being the purest natural form of the substance. As a raw material, it forms the basis for many derivatives used in chromatography, ion exchange materials, explosives manufacturing, and pharmaceutical preparations. [NIH]

Central Nervous System: The main information-processing organs of the nervous system, consisting of the brain, spinal cord, and meninges. [NIH]

Central Nervous System Infections: Pathogenic infections of the brain, spinal cord, and meninges. DNA virus infections; RNA virus infections; bacterial infections; mycoplasma infections; Spirochaetales infections; fungal infections; protozoan infections; helminthiasis; and prion diseases may involve the central nervous system as a primary or secondary process. [NIH]

Character: In current usage, approximately equivalent to personality. The sum of the relatively fixed personality traits and habitual modes of response of an individual. [NIH]

Chin: The anatomical frontal portion of the mandible, also known as the mentum, that contains the line of fusion of the two separate halves of the mandible (symphysis menti). This line of fusion divides inferiorly to enclose a triangular area called the mental protuberance. On each side, inferior to the second premolar tooth, is the mental foramen for the passage of blood vessels and a nerve. [NIH]

Cholecystography: Radiography of the gallbladder after ingestion of a contrast medium. [NIH]

Cholesterol: The principal sterol of all higher animals, distributed in body tissues, especially the brain and spinal cord, and in animal fats and oils. [NIH]

Cholesterol Esters: Fatty acid esters of cholesterol which constitute about two-thirds of the cholesterol in the plasma. The accumulation of cholesterol esters in the arterial intima is a characteristic feature of atherosclerosis. [NIH]

Cholinergic: Resembling acetylcholine in pharmacological action; stimulated by or releasing acetylcholine or a related compound. [EU]

Chromatin: The material of chromosomes. It is a complex of DNA, histones, and nonhistone proteins (chromosomal proteins, non-histone) found within the nucleus of a cell. [NIH]

Chromosomal: Pertaining to chromosomes. [EU]

Chronic: A disease or condition that persists or progresses over a long period of time. [NIH]

Chylomicrons: A class of lipoproteins that carry dietary cholesterol and triglycerides from the small intestines to the tissues. [NIH]

Cirrhosis: A type of chronic, progressive liver disease. [NIH]

Citrus: Any tree or shrub of the Rue family or the fruit of these plants. [NIH]

Clamp: A u-shaped steel rod used with a pin or wire for skeletal traction in the treatment of certain fractures. [NIH]

Claviceps: A genus of ascomycetous fungi, family Clavicipitaceae, order Hypocreales, parasitic on various grasses. The sclerotia contain several toxic alkaloids. Claviceps purpurea on rye causes ergotism. [NIH]

Clear cell carcinoma: A rare type of tumor of the female genital tract in which the inside of the cells looks clear when viewed under a microscope. [NIH]

Clinical Medicine: The study and practice of medicine by direct examination of the patient. [NIH]

Clinical trial: A research study that tests how well new medical treatments or other interventions work in people. Each study is designed to test new methods of screening, prevention, diagnosis, or treatment of a disease. [NIH]

Cloning: The production of a number of genetically identical individuals; in genetic engineering, a process for the efficient replication of a geat number of identical DNA molecules. [NIH]

Cochlear: Of or pertaining to the cochlea. [EU]

Cochlear Diseases: Diseases of the cochlea, the part of the inner ear that is concerned with hearing. [NIH]

Cod Liver Oil: Oil obtained from fresh livers of the cod family, Gadidae. It is a source of vitamins A and D. [NIH]

Codeine: An opioid analgesic related to morphine but with less potent analgesic properties and mild sedative effects. It also acts centrally to suppress cough. [NIH]

Coenzyme: An organic nonprotein molecule, frequently a phosphorylated derivative of a water-soluble vitamin, that binds with the protein molecule (apoenzyme) to form the active enzyme (holoenzyme). [EU]

Cofactor: A substance, microorganism or environmental factor that activates or enhances the action of another entity such as a disease-causing agent. [NIH]

Colic: Paroxysms of pain. This condition usually occurs in the abdominal region but may occur in other body regions as well. [NIH]

Colitis: Inflammation of the colon. [NIH]

Collagen: A polypeptide substance comprising about one third of the total protein in mammalian organisms. It is the main constituent of skin, connective tissue, and the organic substance of bones and teeth. Different forms of collagen are produced in the body but all consist of three alpha-polypeptide chains arranged in a triple helix. Collagen is differentiated from other fibrous proteins, such as elastin, by the content of proline, hydroxyproline, and hydroxylysine; by the absence of tryptophan; and particularly by the high content of polar groups which are responsible for its swelling properties. [NIH]

Collapse: 1. A state of extreme prostration and depression, with failure of circulation. 2. Abnormal falling in of the walls of any part of organ. [EU]

Colloidal: Of the nature of a colloid. [EU]

Colon: The long, coiled, tubelike organ that removes water from digested food. The remaining material, solid waste called stool, moves through the colon to the rectum and leaves the body through the anus. [NIH]

Complement: A term originally used to refer to the heat-labile factor in serum that causes immune cytolysis, the lysis of antibody-coated cells, and now referring to the entire functionally related system comprising at least 20 distinct serum proteins that is the effector not only of immune cytolysis but also of other biologic functions. Complement activation occurs by two different sequences, the classic and alternative pathways. The proteins of the classic pathway are termed 'components of complement' and are designated by the symbols C1 through C9. C1 is a calcium-dependent complex of three distinct proteins C1q, C1r and C1s. The proteins of the alternative pathway (collectively referred to as the properdin system) and complement regulatory proteins are known by semisystematic or trivial names. Fragments resulting from proteolytic cleavage of complement proteins are designated with lower-case letter suffixes, e.g., C3a. Inactivated fragments may be designated with the suffix 'i', e.g. C3bi. Activated components or complexes with biological activity are designated by a bar over the symbol e.g. C1 or C4b,2a. The classic pathway is activated by the binding of C1 to classic pathway activators, primarily antigen-antibody complexes containing IgM, IgG1, IgG3; C1q binds to a single IgM molecule or two adjacent IgG molecules. The alternative pathway can be activated by IgA immune complexes and also by nonimmunologic materials including bacterial endotoxins, microbial polysaccharides, and cell walls. Activation of the classic pathway triggers an enzymatic cascade involving C1, C4, C2 and C3; activation of the alternative pathway triggers a cascade involving C3 and factors B, D and P. Both result in the cleavage of C5 and the formation of the membrane attack complex. Complement activation also results in the formation of many biologically active complement fragments that act as anaphylatoxins, opsonins, or chemotactic factors. [EU]

Complementary and alternative medicine: CAM. Forms of treatment that are used in addition to (complementary) or instead of (alternative) standard treatments. These practices are not considered standard medical approaches. CAM includes dietary supplements, megadose vitamins, herbal preparations, special teas, massage therapy, magnet therapy, spiritual healing, and meditation. [NIH]

Complementary medicine: Practices not generally recognized by the medical community as standard or conventional medical approaches and used to enhance or complement the standard treatments. Complementary medicine includes the taking of dietary supplements, megadose vitamins, and herbal preparations; the drinking of special teas; and practices such as massage therapy, magnet therapy, spiritual healing, and meditation. [NIH]

Computational Biology: A field of biology concerned with the development of techniques for the collection and manipulation of biological data, and the use of such data to make biological discoveries or predictions. This field encompasses all computational methods and theories applicable to molecular biology and areas of computer-based techniques for solving biological problems including manipulation of models and datasets. [NIH]

Concentric: Having a common center of curvature or symmetry. [NIH]

Concomitant: Accompanying; accessory; joined with another. [EU]

Concretion: Minute, hard, yellow masses found in the palpebral conjunctivae of elderly people or following chronic conjunctivitis, composed of the products of cellular degeneration retained in the depressions and tubular recesses in the conjunctiva. [NIH]

Condiments: Aromatic substances added to food before or after cooking to enhance its flavor. These are usually of vegetable origin. [NIH]

Condoms: A sheath that is worn over the penis during sexual behavior in order to prevent pregnancy or spread of sexually transmitted disease. [NIH]

Conduction: The transfer of sound waves, heat, nervous impulses, or electricity. [EU]

Cone: One of the special retinal receptor elements which are presumed to be primarily concerned with perception of light and color stimuli when the eye is adapted to light. [NIH]

Conjugated: Acting or operating as if joined; simultaneous. [EU]

Connective Tissue: Tissue that supports and binds other tissues. It consists of connective tissue cells embedded in a large amount of extracellular matrix. [NIH]

Connective Tissue: Tissue that supports and binds other tissues. It consists of connective tissue cells embedded in a large amount of extracellular matrix. [NIH]

Consciousness: Sense of awareness of self and of the environment. [NIH]

Constipation: Infrequent or difficult evacuation of feces. [NIH]

Consumption: Pulmonary tuberculosis. [NIH]

Contamination: The soiling or pollution by inferior material, as by the introduction of organisms into a wound, or sewage into a stream. [EU]

Continuum: An area over which the vegetation or animal population is of constantly changing composition so that homogeneous, separate communities cannot be distinguished. [NIH]

Contraindications: Any factor or sign that it is unwise to pursue a certain kind of action or treatment, e. g. giving a general anesthetic to a person with pneumonia. [NIH]

Contrast Media: Substances used in radiography that allow visualization of certain tissues. [NIH]

Contrast medium: A substance that is introduced into or around a structure and, because of the difference in absorption of x-rays by the contrast medium and the surrounding tissues, allows radiographic visualization of the structure. [EU]

Corneum: The superficial layer of the epidermis containing keratinized cells. [NIH]

Coronary: Encircling in the manner of a crown; a term applied to vessels; nerves, ligaments, etc. The term usually denotes the arteries that supply the heart muscle and, by extension, a pathologic involvement of them. [EU]

Coronary Disease: Disorder of cardiac function due to an imbalance between myocardial function and the capacity of the coronary vessels to supply sufficient flow for normal function. It is a form of myocardial ischemia (insufficient blood supply to the heart muscle) caused by a decreased capacity of the coronary vessels. [NIH]

Coronary heart disease: A type of heart disease caused by narrowing of the coronary arteries that feed the heart, which needs a constant supply of oxygen and nutrients carried by the blood in the coronary arteries. When the coronary arteries become narrowed or clogged by fat and cholesterol deposits and cannot supply enough blood to the heart, CHD results. [NIH]

Coronary Thrombosis: Presence of a thrombus in a coronary artery, often causing a myocardial infarction. [NIH]

Coronary Vessels: The veins and arteries of the heart. [NIH]

Corpus: The body of the uterus. [NIH]

Corpus Luteum: The yellow glandular mass formed in the ovary by an ovarian follicle that has ruptured and discharged its ovum [NIH]

Cranial: Pertaining to the cranium, or to the anterior (in animals) or superior (in humans) end of the body. [EU]

Cranial Nerves: Twelve pairs of nerves that carry general afferent, visceral afferent, special afferent, somatic efferent, and autonomic efferent fibers. [NIH]

Craniocerebral Trauma: Traumatic injuries involving the cranium and intracranial structures (i.e., brain; cranial nerves; meninges; and other structures). Injuries may be classified by whether or not the skull is penetrated (i.e., penetrating vs. nonpenetrating) or whether there is an associated hemorrhage. [NIH]

Cross-pollination: The pollination of a biotype with pollen from one or more different biotypes. [NIH]

Crystallization: The formation of crystals; conversion to a crystalline form. [EU]

Culture Media: Any liquid or solid preparation made specifically for the growth, storage, or transport of microorganisms or other types of cells. The variety of media that exist allow for the culturing of specific microorganisms and cell types, such as differential media, selective media, test media, and defined media. Solid media consist of liquid media that have been solidified with an agent such as agar or gelatin. [NIH]

Cyclic: Pertaining to or occurring in a cycle or cycles; the term is applied to chemical compounds that contain a ring of atoms in the nucleus. [EU]

Cyst: A sac or capsule filled with fluid. [NIH]

Cyst Fluid: Liquid material found in epithelial-lined closed cavities or sacs. [NIH]

Cystitis: Inflammation of the urinary bladder. [EU]

Cytoplasm: The protoplasm of a cell exclusive of that of the nucleus; it consists of a continuous aqueous solution (cytosol) and the organelles and inclusions suspended in it (phaneroplasm), and is the site of most of the chemical activities of the cell. [EU]

Cytotoxicity: Quality of being capable of producing a specific toxic action upon cells of special organs. [NIH]

Dairy Products: Raw and processed or manufactured milk and milk-derived products. These are usually from cows (bovine) but are also from goats, sheep, reindeer, and water buffalo. [NIH]

Decarboxylation: The removal of a carboxyl group, usually in the form of carbon dioxide, from a chemical compound. [NIH]

Decompression: Decompression external to the body, most often the slow lessening of external pressure on the whole body (especially in caisson workers, deep sea divers, and persons who ascend to great heights) to prevent decompression sickness. It includes also sudden accidental decompression, but not surgical (local) decompression or decompression applied through body openings. [NIH]

Dehydration: The condition that results from excessive loss of body water. [NIH]

Deletion: A genetic rearrangement through loss of segments of DNA (chromosomes), bringing sequences, which are normally separated, into close proximity. [NIH]

Dementia: An acquired organic mental disorder with loss of intellectual abilities of sufficient severity to interfere with social or occupational functioning. The dysfunction is multifaceted and involves memory, behavior, personality, judgment, attention, spatial relations, language, abstract thought, and other executive functions. The intellectual decline is usually progressive, and initially spares the level of consciousness. [NIH]

Density: The logarithm to the base 10 of the opacity of an exposed and processed film. [NIH]

Dental Caries: Localized destruction of the tooth surface initiated by decalcification of the enamel followed by enzymatic lysis of organic structures and leading to cavity formation. If left unchecked, the cavity may penetrate the enamel and dentin and reach the pulp. The three most prominent theories used to explain the etiology of the disase are that acids produced by bacteria lead to decalcification; that micro-organisms destroy the enamel protein; or that keratolytic micro-organisms produce chelates that lead to decalcification. [NIH]

Dental Plaque: A film that attaches to teeth, often causing dental caries and gingivitis. It is composed of mucins, secreted from salivary glands, and microorganisms. [NIH]

Dentures: An appliance used as an artificial or prosthetic replacement for missing teeth and adjacent tissues. It does not include crowns, dental abutments, nor artificial teeth. [NIH]

Dermal: Pertaining to or coming from the skin. [NIH]

Dermatitis: Any inflammation of the skin. [NIH]

Dermatology: A medical specialty concerned with the skin, its structure, functions, diseases, and treatment. [NIH]

Dermis: A layer of vascular connective tissue underneath the epidermis. The surface of the dermis contains sensitive papillae. Embedded in or beneath the dermis are sweat glands, hair follicles, and sebaceous glands. [NIH]

DES: Diethylstilbestrol. A synthetic hormone that was prescribed from the early 1940s until 1971 to help women with complications of pregnancy. DES has been linked to an increased risk of clear cell carcinoma of the vagina in daughters of women who used DES. DES may also increase the risk of breast cancer in women who used DES. [NIH]

Desiccation: Removal of moisture from a substance (chemical, food, tissue, etc.). [NIH]

Deuterium: Deuterium. The stable isotope of hydrogen. It has one neutron and one proton in the nucleus. [NIH]

Developed Countries: Countries that have reached a level of economic achievement through an increase of production, per capita income and consumption, and utilization of natural and human resources. [NIH]

Developing Countries: Countries in the process of change directed toward economic growth, that is, an increase in production, per capita consumption, and income. The process of economic growth involves better utilization of natural and human resources, which results in a change in the social, political, and economic structures. [NIH]

Dextromethorphan: The d-isomer of the codeine analog of levorphanol. Dextromethorphan shows high affinity binding to several regions of the brain, including the medullary cough center. This compound is a NMDA receptor antagonist (receptors, N-methyl-D-aspartate) and acts as a non-competitive channel blocker. It is used widely as an antitussive agent, and is also used to study the involvement of glutamate receptors in neurotoxicity. [NIH]

Diagnostic procedure: A method used to identify a disease. [NIH]

Diaphragm: The musculofibrous partition that separates the thoracic cavity from the abdominal cavity. Contraction of the diaphragm increases the volume of the thoracic cavity aiding inspiration. [NIH]

Diarrhea: Passage of excessively liquid or excessively frequent stools. [NIH]

Diastolic: Of or pertaining to the diastole. [EU]

Dietary Fats: Fats present in food, especially in animal products such as meat, meat products, butter, ghee. They are present in lower amounts in nuts, seeds, and avocados. [NIH]

Digestion: The process of breakdown of food for metabolism and use by the body. [NIH]

Digestive system: The organs that take in food and turn it into products that the body can use to stay healthy. Waste products the body cannot use leave the body through bowel movements. The digestive system includes the salivary glands, mouth, esophagus, stomach, liver, pancreas, gallbladder, small and large intestines, and rectum. [NIH]

Digestive tract: The organs through which food passes when food is eaten. These organs are the mouth, esophagus, stomach, small and large intestines, and rectum. [NIH]

Dimethyl: A volatile metabolite of the amino acid methionine. [NIH]

Diploid: Having two sets of chromosomes. [NIH]

Direct: 1. Straight; in a straight line. 2. Performed immediately and without the intervention of subsidiary means. [EU]

Discrete: Made up of separate parts or characterized by lesions which do not become blended; not running together; separate. [NIH]

Dispenser: Glass, metal or plastic shell fitted with valve from which a pressurized formulation is dispensed; an instrument for atomizing. [NIH]

Disposition: A tendency either physical or mental toward certain diseases. [EU]

Dissociation: 1. The act of separating or state of being separated. 2. The separation of a molecule into two or more fragments (atoms, molecules, ions, or free radicals) produced by the absorption of light or thermal energy or by solvation. 3. In psychology, a defense mechanism in which a group of mental processes are segregated from the rest of a person's mental activity in order to avoid emotional distress, as in the dissociative disorders (q.v.), or in which an idea or object is segregated from its emotional significance; in the first sense it is roughly equivalent to splitting, in the second, to isolation. 4. A defect of mental integration in which one or more groups of mental processes become separated off from normal consciousness and, thus separated, function as a unitary whole. [EU]

Distal: Remote; farther from any point of reference; opposed to proximal. In dentistry, used to designate a position on the dental arch farther from the median line of the jaw. [EU]

Diuresis: Increased excretion of urine. [EU]

Diving: An activity in which the organism plunges into water. It includes scuba and bell diving. Diving as natural behavior of animals goes here, as well as diving in decompression experiments with humans or animals. [NIH]

Dopamine: An endogenous catecholamine and prominent neurotransmitter in several systems of the brain. In the synthesis of catecholamines from tyrosine, it is the immediate precursor to norepinephrine and epinephrine. Dopamine is a major transmitter in the extrapyramidal system of the brain, and important in regulating movement. A family of dopaminergic receptor subtypes mediate its action. Dopamine is used pharmacologically for its direct (beta adrenergic agonist) and indirect (adrenergic releasing) sympathomimetic effects including its actions as an inotropic agent and as a renal vasodilator. [NIH]

Dormancy: The period when an organism (i. e., a virus or a bacterium) is in the body but not producing any ill effects. [NIH]

Double-blind: Pertaining to a clinical trial or other experiment in which neither the subject nor the person administering treatment knows which treatment any particular subject is receiving. [EU]

Drive: A state of internal activity of an organism that is a necessary condition before a given stimulus will elicit a class of responses; e.g., a certain level of hunger (drive) must be present before food will elicit an eating response. [NIH]

Drug Tolerance: Progressive diminution of the susceptibility of a human or animal to the effects of a drug, resulting from its continued administration. It should be differentiated from drug resistance wherein an organism, disease, or tissue fails to respond to the intended effectiveness of a chemical or drug. It should also be differentiated from maximum tolerated dose and no-observed-adverse-effect level. [NIH]

Duct: A tube through which body fluids pass. [NIH]

Duodenum: The first part of the small intestine. [NIH]

Dyes: Chemical substances that are used to stain and color other materials. The coloring may or may not be permanent. Dyes can also be used as therapeutic agents and test reagents in medicine and scientific research. [NIH]

Dyspepsia: Impaired digestion, especially after eating. [NIH]

Eating Disorders: A group of disorders characterized by physiological and psychological disturbances in appetite or food intake. [NIH]

Eczema: A pruritic papulovesicular dermatitis occurring as a reaction to many endogenous and exogenous agents (Dorland, 27th ed). [NIH]

Efficacy: The extent to which a specific intervention, procedure, regimen, or service produces a beneficial result under ideal conditions. Ideally, the determination of efficacy is based on the results of a randomized control trial. [NIH]

Elastic: Susceptible of resisting and recovering from stretching, compression or distortion applied by a force. [EU]

Electrode: Component of the pacing system which is at the distal end of the lead. It is the interface with living cardiac tissue across which the stimulus is transmitted. [NIH]

Electrolyte: A substance that dissociates into ions when fused or in solution, and thus becomes capable of conducting electricity; an ionic solute. [EU]

Electrophoresis: An electrochemical process in which macromolecules or colloidal particles with a net electric charge migrate in a solution under the influence of an electric current. [NIH]

Emollient: Softening or soothing; called also malactic. [EU]

Empirical: A treatment based on an assumed diagnosis, prior to receiving confirmatory laboratory test results. [NIH]

Emulsion: A preparation of one liquid distributed in small globules throughout the body of a second liquid. The dispersed liquid is the discontinuous phase, and the dispersion medium is the continuous phase. When oil is the dispersed liquid and an aqueous solution is the continuous phase, it is known as an oil-in-water emulsion, whereas when water or aqueous solution is the dispersed phase and oil or oleaginous substance is the continuous phase, it is known as a water-in-oil emulsion. Pharmaceutical emulsions for which official standards have been promulgated include cod liver oil emulsion, cod liver oil emulsion with malt, liquid petrolatum emulsion, and phenolphthalein in liquid petrolatum emulsion. [EU]

Enamel: A very hard whitish substance which covers the dentine of the anatomical crown of a tooth. [NIH]

Encapsulated: Confined to a specific, localized area and surrounded by a thin layer of tissue. [NIH]

Endemic: Present or usually prevalent in a population or geographical area at all times; said of a disease or agent. Called also endemial. [EU]

Endocrine Glands: Ductless glands that secrete substances which are released directly into the circulation and which influence metabolism and other body functions. [NIH]

Endogenous: Produced inside an organism or cell. The opposite is external (exogenous) production. [NIH]

Endometrial: Having to do with the endometrium (the layer of tissue that lines the uterus). [NIH]

Endometriosis: A condition in which tissue more or less perfectly resembling the uterine mucous membrane (the endometrium) and containing typical endometrial granular and stromal elements occurs aberrantly in various locations in the pelvic cavity. [NIH]

Endometrium: The layer of tissue that lines the uterus. [NIH]

Endoscope: A thin, lighted tube used to look at tissues inside the body. [NIH]

Endoscopic: A technique where a lateral-view endoscope is passed orally to the duodenum for visualization of the ampulla of Vater. [NIH]

Endothelial cell: The main type of cell found in the inside lining of blood vessels, lymph vessels, and the heart. [NIH]

Endothelium: A layer of epithelium that lines the heart, blood vessels (endothelium, vascular), lymph vessels (endothelium, lymphatic), and the serous cavities of the body. [NIH]

Endothelium-derived: Small molecule that diffuses to the adjacent muscle layer and relaxes it. [NIH]

Endotoxic: Of, relating to, or acting as an endotoxin (= a heat-stable toxin, associated with the outer membranes of certain gram-negative bacteria. Endotoxins are not secreted and are released only when the cells are disrupted). [EU]

Enhancer: Transcriptional element in the virus genome. [NIH]

Enkephalin: A natural opiate painkiller, in the hypothalamus. [NIH]

Environmental Health: The science of controlling or modifying those conditions, influences, or forces surrounding man which relate to promoting, establishing, and maintaining health. [NIH]

Enzymatic: Phase where enzyme cuts the precursor protein. [NIH]

Enzyme: A protein that speeds up chemical reactions in the body. [NIH]

Enzyme Inhibitors: Compounds or agents that combine with an enzyme in such a manner as to prevent the normal substrate-enzyme combination and the catalytic reaction. [NIH]

Epidemic: Occurring suddenly in numbers clearly in excess of normal expectancy; said especially of infectious diseases but applied also to any disease, injury, or other health-related event occurring in such outbreaks. [EU]

Epidemiological: Relating to, or involving epidemiology. [EU]

Epidermis: Nonvascular layer of the skin. It is made up, from within outward, of five layers: 1) basal layer (stratum basale epidermidis); 2) spinous layer (stratum spinosum epidermidis); 3) granular layer (stratum granulosum epidermidis); 4) clear layer (stratum lucidum epidermidis); and 5) horny layer (stratum corneum epidermidis). [NIH]

Epigastric: Having to do with the upper middle area of the abdomen. [NIH]

Epinephrine: The active sympathomimetic hormone from the adrenal medulla in most species. It stimulates both the alpha- and beta- adrenergic systems, causes systemic vasoconstriction and gastrointestinal relaxation, stimulates the heart, and dilates bronchi and cerebral vessels. It is used in asthma and cardiac failure and to delay absorption of local anesthetics. [NIH]

Epithelial: Refers to the cells that line the internal and external surfaces of the body. [NIH]

Epithelial Cells: Cells that line the inner and outer surfaces of the body. [NIH]

Epithelium: One or more layers of epithelial cells, supported by the basal lamina, which covers the inner or outer surfaces of the body. [NIH]

Erectile: The inability to get or maintain an erection for satisfactory sexual intercourse. Also called impotence. [NIH]

Erection: The condition of being made rigid and elevated; as erectile tissue when filled with blood. [EU]

Ergot: Cataract due to ergot poisoning caused by eating of rye cereals contaminated by a fungus. [NIH]

Erythema: Redness of the skin produced by congestion of the capillaries. This condition may result from a variety of causes. [NIH]

Erythritol: A four-carbon sugar that is found in algae, fungi, and lichens. It is twice as sweet as sucrose and can be used as a coronary vasodilator. [NIH]

Esophageal: Having to do with the esophagus, the muscular tube through which food passes from the throat to the stomach. [NIH]

Esophageal Varices: Stretched veins in the esophagus that occur when the liver is not working properly. If the veins burst, the bleeding can cause death. [NIH]

Esophagus: The muscular tube through which food passes from the throat to the stomach. [NIH]

Ethanol: A clear, colorless liquid rapidly absorbed from the gastrointestinal tract and distributed throughout the body. It has bactericidal activity and is used often as a topical disinfectant. It is widely used as a solvent and preservative in pharmaceutical preparations as well as serving as the primary ingredient in alcoholic beverages. [NIH]

Ether: One of a class of organic compounds in which any two organic radicals are attached directly to a single oxygen atom. [NIH]

Evacuation: An emptying, as of the bowels. [EU]

Excipient: Any more or less inert substance added to a prescription in order to confer a suitable consistency or form to the drug; a vehicle. [EU]

Excitability: Property of a cardiac cell whereby, when the cell is depolarized to a critical level (called threshold), the membrane becomes permeable and a regenerative inward current causes an action potential. [NIH]

Exocrine: Secreting outwardly, via a duct. [EU]

Exogenous: Developed or originating outside the organism, as exogenous disease. [EU]

Extender: Any of several colloidal substances of high molecular weight, used as a blood or plasma substitute in transfusion for increasing the volume of the circulating blood. [NIH]

Extracellular: Outside a cell or cells. [EU]

Extracorporeal: Situated or occurring outside the body. [EU]

Extraction: The process or act of pulling or drawing out. [EU]

Extrapyramidal: Outside of the pyramidal tracts. [EU]

Exudate: Material, such as fluid, cells, or cellular debris, which has escaped from blood vessels and has been deposited in tissues or on tissue surfaces, usually as a result of inflammation. An exudate, in contrast to a transudate, is characterized by a high content of protein, cells, or solid materials derived from cells. [EU]

Facial: Of or pertaining to the face. [EU]

Family Planning: Programs or services designed to assist the family in controlling reproduction by either improving or diminishing fertility. [NIH]

Fat: Total lipids including phospholipids. [NIH]

Fat Substitutes: Compounds used in food or in food preparation to replace dietary fats. They may be carbohydrate-, protein-, or fat-based. Fat substitutes are usually lower in calories but provide the same texture as fats. [NIH]

Fatigue: The state of weariness following a period of exertion, mental or physical, characterized by a decreased capacity for work and reduced efficiency to respond to stimuli. [NIH]

Fatty acids: A major component of fats that are used by the body for energy and tissue development. [NIH]

Febrile: Pertaining to or characterized by fever. [EU]

Feces: The excrement discharged from the intestines, consisting of bacteria, cells exfoliated from the intestines, secretions, chiefly of the liver, and a small amount of food residue. [EU]

Fermentation: An enzyme-induced chemical change in organic compounds that takes place in the absence of oxygen. The change usually results in the production of ethanol or lactic acid, and the production of energy. [NIH]

Fibrosis: Any pathological condition where fibrous connective tissue invades any organ, usually as a consequence of inflammation or other injury. [NIH]

Filler: An inactive substance used to make a product bigger or easier to handle. For example, fillers are often used to make pills or capsules because the amount of active drug is too small to be handled conveniently. [NIH]

Fish Products: Food products manufactured from fish (e.g., fish flour, fish meal). [NIH]

Flatus: Gas passed through the rectum. [NIH]

Flavoring Agents: Substances added to foods and medicine to improve the quality of taste. [NIH]

Fluorine: A nonmetallic, diatomic gas that is a trace element and member of the halogen family. It is used in dentistry as flouride to prevent dental caries. [NIH]

Flushing: A transient reddening of the face that may be due to fever, certain drugs, exertion, stress, or a disease process. [NIH]

Folate: A B-complex vitamin that is being studied as a cancer prevention agent. Also called folic acid. [NIH]

Fold: A plication or doubling of various parts of the body. [NIH]

Folic Acid: N-(4-(((2-Amino-1,4-dihydro-4-oxo-6-pteridinyl)methyl)amino)benzoyl)-L-glutamic acid. A member of the vitamin B family that stimulates the hematopoietic system. It is present in the liver and kidney and is found in mushrooms, spinach, yeast, green leaves, and grasses. Folic acid is used in the treatment and prevention of folate deficiencies and megaloblastic anemia. [NIH]

Food Additives: Substances which are of little or no nutritive value, but are used in the processing or storage of foods or animal feed, especially in the developed countries; includes antioxidants, food preservatives, food coloring agents, flavoring agents, anti-infective agents (both plain and local), vehicles, excipients and other similarly used substances. Many of the same substances are pharmaceutic aids when added to pharmaceuticals rather than to foods. [NIH]

Food Chain: The sequence of transfers of matter and energy from organism to organism in the form of food. Food chains intertwine locally into a food web because most organisms consume more than one type of animal or plant. Plants, which convert solar energy to food by photosynthesis, are the primary food source. In a predator chain, a plant-eating animal is eaten by a larger animal. In a parasite chain, a smaller organism consumes part of a larger host and may itself be parasitized by smaller organisms. In a saprophytic chain, microorganisms live on dead organic matter. [NIH]

Food Contamination: The presence in food of harmful, unpalatable, or otherwise objectionable foreign substances, e.g. chemicals, microorganisms or diluents, before, during, or after processing or storage. [NIH]

Food Habits: Acquired or learned food preferences. [NIH]

Food Handling: Any aspect of the operations in the preparation, transport, storage, packaging, wrapping, exposure for sale, service, or delivery of food. [NIH]

Food Preferences: The selection of one food over another. [NIH]

Food Preservatives: Substances capable of inhibiting, retarding or arresting the process of fermentation, acidification or other deterioration of foods. [NIH]

Food Technology: The application of knowledge to the food industry. [NIH]

Forearm: The part between the elbow and the wrist. [NIH]

Formulary: A book containing a list of pharmaceutical products with their formulas and means of preparation. [NIH]

Frameshift: A type of mutation which causes out-of-phase transcription of the base sequence; such mutations arise from the addition or delection of nucleotide(s) in numbers other than 3 or multiples of 3. [NIH]

Frameshift Mutation: A type of mutation in which a number of nucleotides not divisible by three is deleted from or inserted into a coding sequence, thereby causing an alteration in the reading frame of the entire sequence downstream of the mutation. These mutations may be induced by certain types of mutagens or may occur spontaneously. [NIH]

Free Radicals: Highly reactive molecules with an unsatisfied electron valence pair. Free radicals are produced in both normal and pathological processes. They are proven or suspected agents of tissue damage in a wide variety of circumstances including radiation, damage from environment chemicals, and aging. Natural and pharmacological prevention of free radical damage is being actively investigated. [NIH]

Friction: Surface resistance to the relative motion of one body against the rubbing, sliding, rolling, or flowing of another with which it is in contact. [NIH]

Fructose: A type of sugar found in many fruits and vegetables and in honey. Fructose is used to sweeten some diet foods. It is considered a nutritive sweetener because it has calories. [NIH]

Fungi: A kingdom of eukaryotic, heterotrophic organisms that live as saprobes or parasites, including mushrooms, yeasts, smuts, molds, etc. They reproduce either sexually or asexually, and have life cycles that range from simple to complex. Filamentous fungi refer to those that grow as multicelluar colonies (mushrooms and molds). [NIH]

Fungus: A general term used to denote a group of eukaryotic protists, including mushrooms, yeasts, rusts, moulds, smuts, etc., which are characterized by the absence of chlorophyll and by the presence of a rigid cell wall composed of chitin, mannans, and sometimes cellulose. They are usually of simple morphological form or show some reversible cellular specialization, such as the formation of pseudoparenchymatous tissue in the fruiting body of a mushroom. The dimorphic fungi grow, according to environmental conditions, as moulds or yeasts. [EU]

Gallate: Antioxidant present in tea. [NIH]

Gallbladder: The pear-shaped organ that sits below the liver. Bile is concentrated and stored in the gallbladder. [NIH]

Gallic Acid: A colorless or slightly yellow crystalline compound obtained from nutgalls. It is used in photography, pharmaceuticals, and as an analytical reagent. [NIH]

Gamma irradiation: A type of radiation therapy that uses gamma radiation. Gamma radiation is a type of high-energy radiation that is different from x-rays. [NIH]

Ganglia: Clusters of multipolar neurons surrounded by a capsule of loosely organized connective tissue located outside the central nervous system. [NIH]

Gas: Air that comes from normal breakdown of food. The gases are passed out of the body through the rectum (flatus) or the mouth (burp). [NIH]

Gastric: Having to do with the stomach. [NIH]

Gastric Juices: Liquids produced in the stomach to help break down food and kill bacteria. [NIH]

Gastric Mucosa: Surface epithelium in the stomach that invaginates into the lamina propria, forming gastric pits. Tubular glands, characteristic of each region of the stomach (cardiac, gastric, and pyloric), empty into the gastric pits. The gastric mucosa is made up of several different kinds of cells. [NIH]

Gastroesophageal Reflux: Reflux of gastric juice and/or duodenal contents (bile acids, pancreatic juice) into the distal esophagus, commonly due to incompetence of the lower esophageal sphincter. Gastric regurgitation is an extension of this process with entry of fluid into the pharynx or mouth. [NIH]

Gastrointestinal: Refers to the stomach and intestines. [NIH]

Gastrointestinal tract: The stomach and intestines. [NIH]

Gelatin: A product formed from skin, white connective tissue, or bone collagen. It is used as a protein food adjuvant, plasma substitute, hemostatic, suspending agent in pharmaceutical preparations, and in the manufacturing of capsules and suppositories. [NIH]

Gels: Colloids with a solid continuous phase and liquid as the dispersed phase; gels may be unstable when, due to temperature or other cause, the solid phase liquifies; the resulting colloid is called a sol. [NIH]

Gene: The functional and physical unit of heredity passed from parent to offspring. Genes are pieces of DNA, and most genes contain the information for making a specific protein. [NIH]

Genetics: The biological science that deals with the phenomena and mechanisms of heredity. [NIH]

Genital: Pertaining to the genitalia. [EU]

Genitourinary: Pertaining to the genital and urinary organs; urogenital; urinosexual. [EU]

Gingivitis: Inflammation of the gingivae. Gingivitis associated with bony changes is referred to as periodontitis. Called also oulitis and ulitis. [EU]

Gland: An organ that produces and releases one or more substances for use in the body. Some glands produce fluids that affect tissues or organs. Others produce hormones or participate in blood production. [NIH]

Glomerular: Pertaining to or of the nature of a glomerulus, especially a renal glomerulus. [EU]

Glucose: D-Glucose. A primary source of energy for living organisms. It is naturally occurring and is found in fruits and other parts of plants in its free state. It is used therapeutically in fluid and nutrient replacement. [NIH]

Glutamate: Excitatory neurotransmitter of the brain. [NIH]

Glutamic Acid: A non-essential amino acid naturally occurring in the L-form. Glutamic acid (glutamate) is the most common excitatory neurotransmitter in the central nervous system. [NIH]

Gluten: The protein of wheat and other grains which gives to the dough its tough elastic character. [EU]

Glycerol: A trihydroxy sugar alcohol that is an intermediate in carbohydrate and lipid metabolism. It is used as a solvent, emollient, pharmaceutical agent, and sweetening agent. [NIH]

Glycine: A non-essential amino acid. It is found primarily in gelatin and silk fibroin and used therapeutically as a nutrient. It is also a fast inhibitory neurotransmitter. [NIH]

Goats: Any of numerous agile, hollow-horned ruminants of the genus Capra, closely related to the sheep. [NIH]

Gonorrhea: Acute infectious disease characterized by primary invasion of the urogenital tract. The etiologic agent, Neisseria gonorrhoeae, was isolated by Neisser in 1879. [NIH]

Governing Board: The group in which legal authority is vested for the control of health-related institutions and organizations. [NIH]

Grade: The grade of a tumor depends on how abnormal the cancer cells look under a microscope and how quickly the tumor is likely to grow and spread. Grading systems are different for each type of cancer. [NIH]

Gram-negative: Losing the stain or decolorized by alcohol in Gram's method of staining, a primary characteristic of bacteria having a cell wall composed of a thin layer of peptidoglycan covered by an outer membrane of lipoprotein and lipopolysaccharide. [EU]

Gram-Negative Bacteria: Bacteria which lose crystal violet stain but are stained pink when treated by Gram's method. [NIH]

Grasses: A large family, Gramineae, of narrow-leaved herbaceous monocots. Many grasses produce highly allergenic pollens and are hosts to cattle parasites and toxic fungi. [NIH]

Growth: The progressive development of a living being or part of an organism from its earliest stage to maturity. [NIH]

Guanylate Cyclase: An enzyme that catalyzes the conversion of GTP to 3',5'-cyclic GMP and pyrophosphate. It also acts on ITP and dGTP. (From Enzyme Nomenclature, 1992) EC 4.6.1.2. [NIH]

Gum Arabic: Powdered exudate from various Acacia species, especially A. senegal (Leguminosae). It forms mucilage or syrup in water. Gum arabic is used as a suspending agent, excipient, and emulsifier in foods and pharmaceuticals. [NIH]

Habitual: Of the nature of a habit; according to habit; established by or repeated by force of habit, customary. [EU]

Hair follicles: Shafts or openings on the surface of the skin through which hair grows. [NIH]

Haploid: An organism with one basic chromosome set, symbolized by n; the normal condition of gametes in diploids. [NIH]

Hay Fever: A seasonal variety of allergic rhinitis, marked by acute conjunctivitis with lacrimation and itching, regarded as an allergic condition triggered by specific allergens. [NIH]

Headache: Pain in the cranial region that may occur as an isolated and benign symptom or as a manifestation of a wide variety of conditions including subarachnoid hemorrhage; craniocerebral trauma; central nervous system infections; intracranial hypertension; and other disorders. In general, recurrent headaches that are not associated with a primary disease process are referred to as headache disorders (e.g., migraine). [NIH]

Headache Disorders: Common conditions characterized by persistent or recurrent headaches. Headache syndrome classification systems may be based on etiology (e.g., vascular headache, post-traumatic headaches, etc.), temporal pattern (e.g., cluster headache, paroxysmal hemicrania, etc.), and precipitating factors (e.g., cough headache). [NIH]

Health Behavior: Behaviors expressed by individuals to protect, maintain or promote their health status. For example, proper diet, and appropriate exercise are activities perceived to influence health status. Life style is closely associated with health behavior and factors influencing life style are socioeconomic, educational, and cultural. [NIH]

Health Status: The level of health of the individual, group, or population as subjectively assessed by the individual or by more objective measures. [NIH]

Heartburn: Substernal pain or burning sensation, usually associated with regurgitation of gastric juice into the esophagus. [NIH]

Hematology: A subspecialty of internal medicine concerned with morphology, physiology, and pathology of the blood and blood-forming tissues. [NIH]

Hematuria: Presence of blood in the urine. [NIH]

Heme: The color-furnishing portion of hemoglobin. It is found free in tissues and as the prosthetic group in many hemeproteins. [NIH]

Hemochromatosis: A disease that occurs when the body absorbs too much iron. The body stores the excess iron in the liver, pancreas, and other organs. May cause cirrhosis of the liver. Also called iron overload disease. [NIH]

Hemodialysis: The use of a machine to clean wastes from the blood after the kidneys have failed. The blood travels through tubes to a dialyzer, which removes wastes and extra fluid. The cleaned blood then flows through another set of tubes back into the body. [NIH]

Hemorrhage: Bleeding or escape of blood from a vessel. [NIH]

Hemorrhoids: Varicosities of the hemorrhoidal venous plexuses. [NIH]

Heredity: 1. The genetic transmission of a particular quality or trait from parent to offspring. 2. The genetic constitution of an individual. [EU]

Herpes: Any inflammatory skin disease caused by a herpesvirus and characterized by the formation of clusters of small vesicles. When used alone, the term may refer to herpes simplex or to herpes zoster. [EU]

Herpes Zoster: Acute vesicular inflammation. [NIH]

Heterogenic: Derived from a different source or species. Also called heterogenous. [NIH]

Heterogenous: Derived from a different source or species. Also called heterogenic. [NIH]

Heterotrophic: Pertaining to organisms that are consumers and dependent on other organisms for their source of energy (food). [NIH]

Histamine: 1H-Imidazole-4-ethanamine. A depressor amine derived by enzymatic decarboxylation of histidine. It is a powerful stimulant of gastric secretion, a constrictor of bronchial smooth muscle, a vasodilator, and also a centrally acting neurotransmitter. [NIH]

Homogeneous: Consisting of or composed of similar elements or ingredients; of a uniform quality throughout. [EU]

Hormone: A substance in the body that regulates certain organs. Hormones such as gastrin help in breaking down food. Some hormones come from cells in the stomach and small intestine. [NIH]

Horny layer: The superficial layer of the epidermis containing keratinized cells. [NIH]

Host: Any animal that receives a transplanted graft. [NIH]

Hybrid: Cross fertilization between two varieties or, more usually, two species of vines, see also crossing. [NIH]

Hydration: Combining with water. [NIH]

Hydrogen: The first chemical element in the periodic table. It has the atomic symbol H, atomic number 1, and atomic weight 1. It exists, under normal conditions, as a colorless, odorless, tasteless, diatomic gas. Hydrogen ions are protons. Besides the common H1 isotope, hydrogen exists as the stable isotope deuterium and the unstable, radioactive isotope tritium. [NIH]

Hydrogen Peroxide: A strong oxidizing agent used in aqueous solution as a ripening agent, bleach, and topical anti-infective. It is relatively unstable and solutions deteriorate over time unless stabilized by the addition of acetanilide or similar organic materials. [NIH]

Hydrogenation: Specific method of reduction in which hydrogen is added to a substance by the direct use of gaseous hydrogen. [NIH]

Hydrolysis: The process of cleaving a chemical compound by the addition of a molecule of water. [NIH]

Hydrophilic: Readily absorbing moisture; hygroscopic; having strongly polar groups that readily interact with water. [EU]

Hydrophobic: Not readily absorbing water, or being adversely affected by water, as a hydrophobic colloid. [EU]

Hydroxyproline: A hydroxylated form of the imino acid proline. A deficiency in ascorbic acid can result in impaired hydroxyproline formation. [NIH]

Hyperbaric: Characterized by greater than normal pressure or weight; applied to gases under greater than atmospheric pressure, as hyperbaric oxygen, or to a solution of greater specific gravity than another taken as a standard of reference. [EU]

Hyperbaric oxygen: Oxygen that is at an atmospheric pressure higher than the pressure at sea level. Breathing hyperbaric oxygen to enhance the effectiveness of radiation therapy is being studied. [NIH]

Hyperoxaluria: Excretion of an excessive amount of oxalate in the urine. [NIH]

Hypersensitivity: Altered reactivity to an antigen, which can result in pathologic reactions upon subsequent exposure to that particular antigen. [NIH]

Hypertension: Persistently high arterial blood pressure. Currently accepted threshold levels are 140 mm Hg systolic and 90 mm Hg diastolic pressure. [NIH]

Hypodermic: Applied or administered beneath the skin. [EU]

Ice Cream: A frozen dairy food made from cream or butterfat, milk, sugar, and flavorings. Frozen custard and French-type ice creams also contain eggs. [NIH]

Id: The part of the personality structure which harbors the unconscious instinctive desires and strivings of the individual. [NIH]

Immersion: The placing of a body or a part thereof into a liquid. [NIH]

Immune function: Production and action of cells that fight disease or infection. [NIH]

Immune response: The activity of the immune system against foreign substances (antigens). [NIH]

Immunity: Nonsusceptibility to the invasive or pathogenic effects of foreign microorganisms or to the toxic effect of antigenic substances. [NIH]

Immunodiffusion: Technique involving the diffusion of antigen or antibody through a semisolid medium, usually agar or agarose gel, with the result being a precipitin reaction. [NIH]

Immunoelectrophoresis: A technique that combines protein electrophoresis and double immunodiffusion. In this procedure proteins are first separated by gel electrophoresis (usually agarose), then made visible by immunodiffusion of specific antibodies. A distinct elliptical precipitin arc results for each protein detectable by the antisera. [NIH]

Immunogenic: Producing immunity; evoking an immune response. [EU]

Impairment: In the context of health experience, an impairment is any loss or abnormality of psychological, physiological, or anatomical structure or function. [NIH]

Impotence: The inability to perform sexual intercourse. [NIH]

In vitro: In the laboratory (outside the body). The opposite of in vivo (in the body). [NIH]

In vivo: In the body. The opposite of in vitro (outside the body or in the laboratory). [NIH]

Incision: A cut made in the body during surgery. [NIH]

Incompetence: Physical or mental inadequacy or insufficiency. [EU]

Indicative: That indicates; that points out more or less exactly; that reveals fairly clearly. [EU]

Indigestion: Poor digestion. Symptoms include heartburn, nausea, bloating, and gas. Also called dyspepsia. [NIH]

Infarction: A pathological process consisting of a sudden insufficient blood supply to an area, which results in necrosis of that area. It is usually caused by a thrombus, an embolus, or a vascular torsion. [NIH]

Infection: 1. Invasion and multiplication of microorganisms in body tissues, which may be clinically unapparent or result in local cellular injury due to competitive metabolism, toxins, intracellular replication, or antigen-antibody response. The infection may remain localized, subclinical, and temporary if the body's defensive mechanisms are effective. A local infection may persist and spread by extension to become an acute, subacute, or chronic clinical infection or disease state. A local infection may also become systemic when the microorganisms gain access to the lymphatic or vascular system. 2. An infectious disease. [EU]

Inflammation: A pathological process characterized by injury or destruction of tissues caused by a variety of cytologic and chemical reactions. It is usually manifested by typical signs of pain, heat, redness, swelling, and loss of function. [NIH]

Inflammatory bowel disease: A general term that refers to the inflammation of the colon and rectum. Inflammatory bowel disease includes ulcerative colitis and Crohn's disease. [NIH]

Infusion: A method of putting fluids, including drugs, into the bloodstream. Also called intravenous infusion. [NIH]

Ingestion: Taking into the body by mouth [NIH]

Inhalation: The drawing of air or other substances into the lungs. [EU]

Inotropic: Affecting the force or energy of muscular contractions. [EU]

Insomnia: Difficulty in going to sleep or getting enough sleep. [NIH]

Intermittent: Occurring at separated intervals; having periods of cessation of activity. [EU]

Internal Medicine: A medical specialty concerned with the diagnosis and treatment of diseases of the internal organ systems of adults. [NIH]

Interstitial: Pertaining to or situated between parts or in the interspaces of a tissue. [EU]

Intestinal: Having to do with the intestines. [NIH]

Intestinal Mucosa: The surface lining of the intestines where the cells absorb nutrients. [NIH]

Intestine: A long, tube-shaped organ in the abdomen that completes the process of digestion. There is both a large intestine and a small intestine. Also called the bowel. [NIH]

Intracellular: Inside a cell. [NIH]

Intracranial Hypertension: Increased pressure within the cranial vault. This may result from several conditions, including hydrocephalus; brain edema; intracranial masses; severe systemic hypertension; pseudotumor cerebri; and other disorders. [NIH]

Intrinsic: Situated entirely within or pertaining exclusively to a part. [EU]

Inulin: A starch found in the tubers and roots of many plants. Since it is hydrolyzable to fructose, it is classified as a fructosan. It has been used in physiologic investigation for determination of the rate of glomerular function. [NIH]

Invasive: 1. Having the quality of invasiveness. 2. Involving puncture or incision of the skin or insertion of an instrument or foreign material into the body; said of diagnostic techniques. [EU]

Invert sugar: Subjected to chemical inversion : inverted. [EU]

Ionization: 1. Any process by which a neutral atom gains or loses electrons, thus acquiring a net charge, as the dissociation of a substance in solution into ions or ion production by the passage of radioactive particles. 2. Iontophoresis. [EU]

Ions: An atom or group of atoms that have a positive or negative electric charge due to a gain (negative charge) or loss (positive charge) of one or more dectrons. Atoms with a positive charge are known as cations; those with a negative charge are anions. [NIH]

Iron Compounds: Inorganic compounds that contain iron as an integral part of the molecule. [NIH]

Irradiation: The use of high-energy radiation from x-rays, neutrons, and other sources to kill cancer cells and shrink tumors. Radiation may come from a machine outside the body (external-beam radiation therapy) or from materials called radioisotopes. Radioisotopes produce radiation and can be placed in or near the tumor or in the area near cancer cells. This type of radiation treatment is called internal radiation therapy, implant radiation, interstitial radiation, or brachytherapy. Systemic radiation therapy uses a radioactive substance, such as a radiolabeled monoclonal antibody, that circulates throughout the body. Irradiation is also called radiation therapy, radiotherapy, and x-ray therapy. [NIH]

Juniper: A slow growing coniferous evergreen tree or shrub, genus Juniperus. The Juniper is cultivated for its berries, which take up to three years to ripen. The resinous, sweetly flavored berries are borne only by the female juniper, and can be found in various stages of ripeness on the same plant. [NIH]

Kava: Dried rhizome and roots of Piper methysticum, a shrub native to Oceania and known for its anti-anxiety and sedative properties. Heavy usage results in some adverse effects. It contains alkaloids, lactones, kawain, methysticin, mucilage, starch, and yangonin. Kava is also the name of the pungent beverage prepared from the plant's roots. [NIH]

Kb: A measure of the length of DNA fragments, 1 Kb = 1000 base pairs. The largest DNA fragments are up to 50 kilobases long. [NIH]

Kidney Disease: Any one of several chronic conditions that are caused by damage to the cells of the kidney. People who have had diabetes for a long time may have kidney damage. Also called nephropathy. [NIH]

Kidney Pelvis: The flattened, funnel-shaped expansion connecting the ureter to the kidney calices. [NIH]

Kidney stone: A stone that develops from crystals that form in urine and build up on the inner surfaces of the kidney, in the renal pelvis, or in the ureters. [NIH]

Kinetics: The study of rate dynamics in chemical or physical systems. [NIH]

Krypton: A noble gas that is found in the atmosphere. It has the atomic symbol Kr, atomic number 36, atomic weight 83.80, and has been used in electric bulbs. [NIH]

Lactose Intolerance: The disease state resulting from the absence of lactase enzyme in the musocal cells of the gastrointestinal tract, and therefore an inability to break down the disaccharide lactose in milk for absorption from the gastrointestinal tract. It is manifested by indigestion of a mild nature to severe diarrhea. It may be due to inborn defect genetically conditioned or may be acquired. [NIH]

Large Intestine: The part of the intestine that goes from the cecum to the rectum. The large intestine absorbs water from stool and changes it from a liquid to a solid form. The large intestine is 5 feet long and includes the appendix, cecum, colon, and rectum. Also called colon. [NIH]

Latent: Phoria which occurs at one distance or another and which usually has no troublesome effect. [NIH]

Latex Allergy: Hypersensitivity to products containing processed natural rubber latex such as rubber gloves, condoms, catheters, dental dams, balloons, and sporting equipment. Both T-cell mediated (delayed hypersensitivity) and IgE antibody-mediated (immediate hypersensitivity) allergic responses are possible. Delayed hypersensitivity results from exposure to antioxidants present in the rubber; immediate hypersensitivity results from exposure to a latex protein. [NIH]

Laxative: An agent that acts to promote evacuation of the bowel; a cathartic or purgative. [EU]

Lenses: Pieces of glass or other transparent materials used for magnification or increased visual acuity. [NIH]

Leucine: An essential branched-chain amino acid important for hemoglobin formation. [NIH]

Levorphanol: A narcotic analgesic that may be habit-forming. It is nearly as effective orally as by injection. [NIH]

Libido: The psychic drive or energy associated with sexual instinct in the broad sense (pleasure and love-object seeking). It may also connote the psychic energy associated with instincts in general that motivate behavior. [NIH]

Library Services: Services offered to the library user. They include reference and circulation. [NIH]

Lichens: Any of a group of plants formed by a mutual combination of an alga and a fungus. [NIH]

Life cycle: The successive stages through which an organism passes from fertilized ovum or spore to the fertilized ovum or spore of the next generation. [NIH]

Ligaments: Shiny, flexible bands of fibrous tissue connecting together articular extremities of bones. They are pliant, tough, and inextensile. [NIH]

Linkages: The tendency of two or more genes in the same chromosome to remain together from one generation to the next more frequently than expected according to the law of independent assortment. [NIH]

Lipid: Fat. [NIH]

Lipid A: Lipid A is the biologically active component of lipopolysaccharides. It shows strong endotoxic activity and exhibits immunogenic properties. [NIH]

Lipid Peroxidation: Peroxidase catalyzed oxidation of lipids using hydrogen peroxide as an electron acceptor. [NIH]

Lipid Peroxides: Peroxides produced in the presence of a free radical by the oxidation of unsaturated fatty acids in the cell in the presence of molecular oxygen. The formation of lipid peroxides results in the destruction of the original lipid leading to the loss of integrity of the membranes. They therefore cause a variety of toxic effects in vivo and their formation is considered a pathological process in biological systems. Their formation can be inhibited by antioxidants, such as vitamin E, structural separation or low oxygen tension. [NIH]

Lipophilic: Having an affinity for fat; pertaining to or characterized by lipophilia. [EU]

Lipopolysaccharides: Substance consisting of polysaccharide and lipid. [NIH]

Lipoprotein: Any of the lipid-protein complexes in which lipids are transported in the blood; lipoprotein particles consist of a spherical hydrophobic core of triglycerides or cholesterol esters surrounded by an amphipathic monolayer of phospholipids, cholesterol, and apolipoproteins; the four principal classes are high-density, low-density, and very-low-density lipoproteins and chylomicrons. [EU]

Lipoxygenase: An enzyme of the oxidoreductase class that catalyzes reactions between linoleate and other fatty acids and oxygen to form hydroperoxy-fatty acid derivatives. Related enzymes in this class include the arachidonate lipoxygenases, arachidonate 5-lipoxygenase, arachidonate 12-lipoxygenase, and arachidonate 15-lipoxygenase. EC 1.13.11.12. [NIH]

Liquor: 1. A liquid, especially an aqueous solution containing a medicinal substance. 2. A general term used in anatomical nomenclature for certain fluids of the body. [EU]

Lithotripsy: The destruction of a calculus of the kidney, ureter, bladder, or gallbladder by physical forces, including crushing with a lithotriptor through a catheter. Focused percutaneous ultrasound and focused hydraulic shock waves may be used without surgery. Lithotripsy does not include the dissolving of stones by acids or litholysis. Lithotripsy by laser is laser lithotripsy. [NIH]

Liver: A large, glandular organ located in the upper abdomen. The liver cleanses the blood and aids in digestion by secreting bile. [NIH]

Localization: The process of determining or marking the location or site of a lesion or disease. May also refer to the process of keeping a lesion or disease in a specific location or site. [NIH]

Localized: Cancer which has not metastasized yet. [NIH]

Locomotion: Movement or the ability to move from one place or another. It can refer to humans, vertebrate or invertebrate animals, and microorganisms. [NIH]

Low-density lipoprotein: Lipoprotein that contains most of the cholesterol in the blood. LDL carries cholesterol to the tissues of the body, including the arteries. A high level of LDL increases the risk of heart disease. LDL typically contains 60 to 70 percent of the total serum cholesterol and both are directly correlated with CHD risk. [NIH]

Lower Esophageal Sphincter: The muscle between the esophagus and stomach. When a person swallows, this muscle relaxes to let food pass from the esophagus to the stomach. It stays closed at other times to keep stomach contents from flowing back into the esophagus. [NIH]

Lubricants: Oily or slippery substances. [NIH]

Lubrication: The application of a substance to diminish friction between two surfaces. It may refer to oils, greases, and similar substances for the lubrication of medical equipment but it can be used for the application of substances to tissue to reduce friction, such as lotions for skin and vaginal lubricants. [NIH]

Lymph: The almost colorless fluid that travels through the lymphatic system and carries cells that help fight infection and disease. [NIH]

Lymphatic: The tissues and organs, including the bone marrow, spleen, thymus, and lymph nodes, that produce and store cells that fight infection and disease. [NIH]

Lymphocyte: A white blood cell. Lymphocytes have a number of roles in the immune system, including the production of antibodies and other substances that fight infection and diseases. [NIH]

Malabsorption: Impaired intestinal absorption of nutrients. [EU]

Malignant: Cancerous; a growth with a tendency to invade and destroy nearby tissue and spread to other parts of the body. [NIH]

Malondialdehyde: The dialdehyde of malonic acid. [NIH]

Meat: The edible portions of any animal used for food including domestic mammals (the major ones being cattle, swine, and sheep) along with poultry, fish, shellfish, and game. [NIH]

Mediate: Indirect; accomplished by the aid of an intervening medium. [EU]

Medicament: A medicinal substance or agent. [EU]

MEDLINE: An online database of MEDLARS, the computerized bibliographic Medical Literature Analysis and Retrieval System of the National Library of Medicine. [NIH]

Medullary: Pertaining to the marrow or to any medulla; resembling marrow. [EU]

Megaloblastic: A large abnormal red blood cell appearing in the blood in pernicious anaemia. [EU]

Melanin: The substance that gives the skin its color. [NIH]

Membrane: A very thin layer of tissue that covers a surface. [NIH]

Memory: Complex mental function having four distinct phases: (1) memorizing or learning, (2) retention, (3) recall, and (4) recognition. Clinically, it is usually subdivided into immediate, recent, and remote memory. [NIH]

Menstrual Cycle: The period of the regularly recurring physiologic changes in the endometrium occurring during the reproductive period in human females and some primates and culminating in partial sloughing of the endometrium (menstruation). [NIH]

Menstruation: The normal physiologic discharge through the vagina of blood and mucosal tissues from the nonpregnant uterus. [NIH]

Mental: Pertaining to the mind; psychic. 2. (L. mentum chin) pertaining to the chin. [EU]

Mental Disorders: Psychiatric illness or diseases manifested by breakdowns in the adaptational process expressed primarily as abnormalities of thought, feeling, and behavior producing either distress or impairment of function. [NIH]

Mental Processes: Conceptual functions or thinking in all its forms. [NIH]

Metabolite: Any substance produced by metabolism or by a metabolic process. [EU]

Methionine: A sulfur containing essential amino acid that is important in many body functions. It is a chelating agent for heavy metals. [NIH]

MI: Myocardial infarction. Gross necrosis of the myocardium as a result of interruption of the blood supply to the area; it is almost always caused by atherosclerosis of the coronary arteries, upon which coronary thrombosis is usually superimposed. [NIH]

Micelle: A colloid particle formed by an aggregation of small molecules. [EU]

Microbe: An organism which cannot be observed with the naked eye; e. g. unicellular animals, lower algae, lower fungi, bacteria. [NIH]

Microbiological: Pertaining to microbiology : the science that deals with microorganisms, including algae, bacteria, fungi, protozoa and viruses. [EU]

Microbiology: The study of microorganisms such as fungi, bacteria, algae, archaea, and viruses. [NIH]

Microgram: A unit of mass (weight) of the metric system, being one-millionth of a gram (10-6 gm.) or one one-thousandth of a milligram (10-3 mg.). [EU]

Microorganism: An organism that can be seen only through a microscope. Microorganisms include bacteria, protozoa, algae, and fungi. Although viruses are not considered living organisms, they are sometimes classified as microorganisms. [NIH]

Migration: The systematic movement of genes between populations of the same species, geographic race, or variety. [NIH]

Milligram: A measure of weight. A milligram is approximately 450,000-times smaller than a pound and 28,000-times smaller than an ounce. [NIH]

Mineralization: The action of mineralizing; the state of being mineralized. [EU]

Mitosis: A method of indirect cell division by means of which the two daughter nuclei normally receive identical complements of the number of chromosomes of the somatic cells of the species. [NIH]

Modification: A change in an organism, or in a process in an organism, that is acquired from its own activity or environment. [NIH]

Molasses: The syrup remaining after sugar is crystallized out of sugar cane or sugar beet juice. It is also used in animal feed, and in a fermented form, is used to make industrial ethyl alcohol and alcoholic beverages. [NIH]

Molecular: Of, pertaining to, or composed of molecules : a very small mass of matter. [EU]

Molecule: A chemical made up of two or more atoms. The atoms in a molecule can be the same (an oxygen molecule has two oxygen atoms) or different (a water molecule has two hydrogen atoms and one oxygen atom). Biological molecules, such as proteins and DNA, can be made up of many thousands of atoms. [NIH]

Mood Disorders: Those disorders that have a disturbance in mood as their predominant feature. [NIH]

Morphine: The principal alkaloid in opium and the prototype opiate analgesic and narcotic. Morphine has widespread effects in the central nervous system and on smooth muscle. [NIH]

Morphological: Relating to the configuration or the structure of live organs. [NIH]

Morphology: The science of the form and structure of organisms (plants, animals, and other forms of life). [NIH]

Motion Sickness: Sickness caused by motion, as sea sickness, train sickness, car sickness, and air sickness. [NIH]

Mucins: A secretion containing mucopolysaccharides and protein that is the chief constituent of mucus. [NIH]

Myocardial Ischemia: A disorder of cardiac function caused by insufficient blood flow to the muscle tissue of the heart. The decreased blood flow may be due to narrowing of the coronary arteries (coronary arteriosclerosis), to obstruction by a thrombus (coronary thrombosis), or less commonly, to diffuse narrowing of arterioles and other small vessels within the heart. Severe interruption of the blood supply to the myocardial tissue may result in necrosis of cardiac muscle (myocardial infarction). [NIH]

Myocardium: The muscle tissue of the heart composed of striated, involuntary muscle known as cardiac muscle. [NIH]

Naloxone: A specific opiate antagonist that has no agonist activity. It is a competitive antagonist at mu, delta, and kappa opioid receptors. [NIH]

Narcosis: A general and nonspecific reversible depression of neuronal excitability, produced by a number of physical and chemical aspects, usually resulting in stupor. [NIH]

Narcotic: 1. Pertaining to or producing narcosis. 2. An agent that produces insensibility or stupor, applied especially to the opioids, i.e. to any natural or synthetic drug that has morphine-like actions. [EU]

Nausea: An unpleasant sensation in the stomach usually accompanied by the urge to vomit. Common causes are early pregnancy, sea and motion sickness, emotional stress, intense pain, food poisoning, and various enteroviruses. [NIH]

NCI: National Cancer Institute. NCI, part of the National Institutes of Health of the United States Department of Health and Human Services, is the federal government's principal agency for cancer research. NCI conducts, coordinates, and funds cancer research, training, health information dissemination, and other programs with respect to the cause, diagnosis, prevention, and treatment of cancer. Access the NCI Web site at http://cancer.gov. [NIH]

Need: A state of tension or dissatisfaction felt by an individual that impels him to action toward a goal he believes will satisfy the impulse. [NIH]

Neon: Neon. A noble gas with the atomic symbol Ne, atomic number 10, and atomic weight 20.18. It is found in the earth's crust and atmosphere as an inert, odorless gas and is used in vacuum tubes and incandescent lamps. [NIH]

Neoplasms: New abnormal growth of tissue. Malignant neoplasms show a greater degree of anaplasia and have the properties of invasion and metastasis, compared to benign neoplasms. [NIH]

Nephrolithiasis: Kidney stones. [NIH]

Nephropathy: Disease of the kidneys. [EU]

Nerve: A cordlike structure of nervous tissue that connects parts of the nervous system with other tissues of the body and conveys nervous impulses to, or away from, these tissues. [NIH]

Nervous System: The entire nerve apparatus composed of the brain, spinal cord, nerves and ganglia. [NIH]

Nervous System Diseases: Diseases of the central and peripheral nervous system. This includes disorders of the brain, spinal cord, cranial nerves, peripheral nerves, nerve roots, autonomic nervous system, neuromuscular junction, and muscle. [NIH]

Neuromuscular: Pertaining to muscles and nerves. [EU]

Neuromuscular Junction: The synapse between a neuron and a muscle. [NIH]

Neuronal: Pertaining to a neuron or neurons (= conducting cells of the nervous system). [EU]

Neurons: The basic cellular units of nervous tissue. Each neuron consists of a body, an axon, and dendrites. Their purpose is to receive, conduct, and transmit impulses in the nervous system. [NIH]

Neurotoxicity: The tendency of some treatments to cause damage to the nervous system. [NIH]

Neurotransmitter: Any of a group of substances that are released on excitation from the axon terminal of a presynaptic neuron of the central or peripheral nervous system and travel across the synaptic cleft to either excite or inhibit the target cell. Among the many substances that have the properties of a neurotransmitter are acetylcholine, norepinephrine, epinephrine, dopamine, glycine, y-aminobutyrate, glutamic acid, substance P, enkephalins, endorphins, and serotonin. [EU]

Nicotine: Nicotine is highly toxic alkaloid. It is the prototypical agonist at nicotinic cholinergic receptors where it dramatically stimulates neurons and ultimately blocks synaptic transmission. Nicotine is also important medically because of its presence in tobacco smoke. [NIH]

Nitric Oxide: A free radical gas produced endogenously by a variety of mammalian cells. It is synthesized from arginine by a complex reaction, catalyzed by nitric oxide synthase. Nitric oxide is endothelium-derived relaxing factor. It is released by the vascular endothelium and mediates the relaxation induced by some vasodilators such as acetylcholine and bradykinin. It also inhibits platelet aggregation, induces disaggregation of aggregated platelets, and inhibits platelet adhesion to the vascular endothelium. Nitric oxide activates cytosolic guanylate cyclase and thus elevates intracellular levels of cyclic GMP. [NIH]

Nitrogen: An element with the atomic symbol N, atomic number 7, and atomic weight 14. Nitrogen exists as a diatomic gas and makes up about 78% of the earth's atmosphere by volume. It is a constituent of proteins and nucleic acids and found in all living cells. [NIH]

Noble Gases: Gases which are members of the zero group of the periodic system. These gases generally do not react chemically. [NIH]

Norepinephrine: Precursor of epinephrine that is secreted by the adrenal medulla and is a widespread central and autonomic neurotransmitter. Norepinephrine is the principal transmitter of most postganglionic sympathetic fibers and of the diffuse projection system in the brain arising from the locus ceruleus. It is also found in plants and is used pharmacologically as a sympathomimetic. [NIH]

Nuclei: A body of specialized protoplasm found in nearly all cells and containing the chromosomes. [NIH]

Nucleic acid: Either of two types of macromolecule (DNA or RNA) formed by polymerization of nucleotides. Nucleic acids are found in all living cells and contain the information (genetic code) for the transfer of genetic information from one generation to the next. [NIH]

Nucleus: A body of specialized protoplasm found in nearly all cells and containing the chromosomes. [NIH]

Nutritive Value: An indication of the contribution of a food to the nutrient content of the diet. This value depends on the quantity of a food which is digested and absorbed and the amounts of the essential nutrients (protein, fat, carbohydrate, minerals, vitamins) which it contains. This value can be affected by soil and growing conditions, handling and storage, and processing. [NIH]

Odour: A volatile emanation that is perceived by the sense of smell. [EU]

Opacity: Degree of density (area most dense taken for reading). [NIH]

Opiate: A remedy containing or derived from opium; also any drug that induces sleep. [EU]

Oral Health: The optimal state of the mouth and normal functioning of the organs of the mouth without evidence of disease. [NIH]

Orbit: One of the two cavities in the skull which contains an eyeball. Each eye is located in a bony socket or orbit. [NIH]

Organoleptic: Of, relating to, or involving the employment of the sense organs; used especially of subjective testing (as of flavor, odor, appearance) of food and drug products. [NIH]

Osteoporosis: Reduction of bone mass without alteration in the composition of bone, leading to fractures. Primary osteoporosis can be of two major types: postmenopausal osteoporosis and age-related (or senile) osteoporosis. [NIH]

Ovarian Follicle: Spheroidal cell aggregation in the ovary containing an ovum. It consists of an external fibro-vascular coat, an internal coat of nucleated cells, and a transparent, albuminous fluid in which the ovum is suspended. [NIH]

Ovary: Either of the paired glands in the female that produce the female germ cells and secrete some of the female sex hormones. [NIH]

Overweight: An excess of body weight but not necessarily body fat; a body mass index of 25 to 29.9 kg/m2. [NIH]

Ovum: A female germ cell extruded from the ovary at ovulation. [NIH]

Oxalate: A chemical that combines with calcium in urine to form the most common type of kidney stone (calcium oxalate stone). [NIH]

Oxalic Acid: A strong dicarboxylic acid occurring in many plants and vegetables. It is produced in the body by metabolism of glyoxylic acid or ascorbic acid. It is not metabolized but excreted in the urine. It is used as an analytical reagent and general reducing agent. [NIH]

Oxidation: The act of oxidizing or state of being oxidized. Chemically it consists in the increase of positive charges on an atom or the loss of negative charges. Most biological oxidations are accomplished by the removal of a pair of hydrogen atoms (dehydrogenation) from a molecule. Such oxidations must be accompanied by reduction of an acceptor molecule. Univalent o. indicates loss of one electron; divalent o., the loss of two electrons. [EU]

Oxidative Stress: A disturbance in the prooxidant-antioxidant balance in favor of the former, leading to potential damage. Indicators of oxidative stress include damaged DNA bases, protein oxidation products, and lipid peroxidation products (Sies, Oxidative Stress, 1991, pxv-xvi). [NIH]

Oxygenase: Enzyme which breaks down heme, the iron-containing oxygen-carrying constituent of the red blood cells. [NIH]

Palmitic Acid: A common saturated fatty acid found in fats and waxes including olive oil, palm oil, and body lipids. [NIH]

Pancreas: A mixed exocrine and endocrine gland situated transversely across the posterior abdominal wall in the epigastric and hypochondriac regions. The endocrine portion is comprised of the Islets of Langerhans, while the exocrine portion is a compound acinar gland that secretes digestive enzymes. [NIH]

Pancreatic: Having to do with the pancreas. [NIH]

Pancreatic Juice: The fluid containing digestive enzymes secreted by the pancreas in response to food in the duodenum. [NIH]

Parasite: An animal or a plant that lives on or in an organism of another species and gets at least some of its nutrition from that other organism. [NIH]

Paroxysmal: Recurring in paroxysms (= spasms or seizures). [EU]

Patch: A piece of material used to cover or protect a wound, an injured part, etc.: a patch over the eye. [NIH]

Pathogenesis: The cellular events and reactions that occur in the development of disease. [NIH]

Pathologic: 1. Indicative of or caused by a morbid condition. 2. Pertaining to pathology (= branch of medicine that treats the essential nature of the disease, especially the structural and functional changes in tissues and organs of the body caused by the disease). [EU]

Pathologic Processes: The abnormal mechanisms and forms involved in the dysfunctions of tissues and organs. [NIH]

Pathologies: The study of abnormality, especially the study of diseases. [NIH]

Patient Education: The teaching or training of patients concerning their own health needs. [NIH]

Pelvic: Pertaining to the pelvis. [EU]

Pelvis: The lower part of the abdomen, located between the hip bones. [NIH]

Pepsin: An enzyme made in the stomach that breaks down proteins. [NIH]

Pepsin A: Formed from pig pepsinogen by cleavage of one peptide bond. The enzyme is a single polypeptide chain and is inhibited by methyl 2-diaazoacetamidohexanoate. It cleaves peptides preferentially at the carbonyl linkages of phenylalanine or leucine and acts as the principal digestive enzyme of gastric juice. [NIH]

Peptic: Pertaining to pepsin or to digestion; related to the action of gastric juices. [EU]

Peptic Ulcer: Ulcer that occurs in those portions of the alimentary tract which come into contact with gastric juice containing pepsin and acid. It occurs when the amount of acid and pepsin is sufficient to overcome the gastric mucosal barrier. [NIH]

Peptic Ulcer Hemorrhage: Bleeding from a peptic ulcer. [NIH]

Peptide: Any compound consisting of two or more amino acids, the building blocks of proteins. Peptides are combined to make proteins. [NIH]

Perception: The ability quickly and accurately to recognize similarities and differences among presented objects, whether these be pairs of words, pairs of number series, or multiple sets of these or other symbols such as geometric figures. [NIH]

Percutaneous: Performed through the skin, as injection of radiopacque material in radiological examination, or the removal of tissue for biopsy accomplished by a needle. [EU]

Perennial: Lasting through the year of for several years. [EU]

Peripheral Nervous System: The nervous system outside of the brain and spinal cord. The peripheral nervous system has autonomic and somatic divisions. The autonomic nervous system includes the enteric, parasympathetic, and sympathetic subdivisions. The somatic nervous system includes the cranial and spinal nerves and their ganglia and the peripheral sensory receptors. [NIH]

Petrolatum: A colloidal system of semisolid hydrocarbons obtained from petroleum. It is used as an ointment base, topical protectant, and lubricant. [NIH]

Petroleum: Naturally occurring complex liquid hydrocarbons which, after distillation, yield combustible fuels, petrochemicals, and lubricants. [NIH]

Pharmaceutic Aids: Substances which are of little or no therapeutic value, but are necessary in the manufacture, compounding, storage, etc., of pharmaceutical preparations or drug dosage forms. They include solvents, diluting agents, and suspending agents, and emulsifying agents. Also, antioxidants; preservatives, pharmaceutical; dyes (coloring agents); flavoring agents; vehicles; excipients; ointment bases. [NIH]

Pharmaceutical Preparations: Drugs intended for human or veterinary use, presented in their finished dosage form. Included here are materials used in the preparation and/or formulation of the finished dosage form. [NIH]

Pharmacists: Those persons legally qualified by education and training to engage in the practice of pharmacy. [NIH]

Pharmacogenetics: A branch of genetics which deals with the genetic components of variability in individual responses to and metabolism (biotransformation) of drugs. [NIH]

Pharmacologic: Pertaining to pharmacology or to the properties and reactions of drugs. [EU]

Pharynx: The hollow tube about 5 inches long that starts behind the nose and ends at the top of the trachea (windpipe) and esophagus (the tube that goes to the stomach). [NIH]

Phenolphthalein: An acid-base indicator which is colorless in acid solution, but turns pink to red as the solution becomes alkaline. It is used medicinally as a cathartic. [NIH]

Phenylalanine: An aromatic amino acid that is essential in the animal diet. It is a precursor of melanin, dopamine, noradrenalin, and thyroxine. [NIH]

Phlebotomy: The letting of blood from a vein. Although it is one of the techniques used in drawing blood to be used in diagnostic procedures, in modern medicine, it is used commonly in the treatment of erythrocytosis, hemochromocytosis, polycythemia vera, and porphyria cutanea tarda. Its historical counterpart is bloodletting. (From Cecil Textbook of Medicine, 19th ed & Wintrobe's Clinical Hematology, 9th ed) Venipuncture is not only for the letting of blood from a vein but also br the injecting of a drug into the vein for diagnostic analysis. [NIH]

Phosphates: Inorganic salts of phosphoric acid. [NIH]

Phospholipids: Lipids containing one or more phosphate groups, particularly those derived from either glycerol (phosphoglycerides; glycerophospholipids) or sphingosine (sphingolipids). They are polar lipids that are of great importance for the structure and function of cell membranes and are the most abundant of membrane lipids, although not stored in large amounts in the system. [NIH]

Phosphorus: A non-metallic element that is found in the blood, muscles, nevers, bones, and teeth, and is a component of adenosine triphosphate (ATP; the primary energy source for the body's cells.) [NIH]

Physical Examination: Systematic and thorough inspection of the patient for physical signs of disease or abnormality. [NIH]

Physiologic: Having to do with the functions of the body. When used in the phrase "physiologic age," it refers to an age assigned by general health, as opposed to calendar age. [NIH]

Physiology: The science that deals with the life processes and functions of organismus, their cells, tissues, and organs. [NIH]

Pigments: Any normal or abnormal coloring matter in plants, animals, or micro-organisms. [NIH]

Pilot study: The initial study examining a new method or treatment. [NIH]

Pitch: The subjective awareness of the frequency or spectral distribution of a sound. [NIH]

Placenta: A highly vascular fetal organ through which the fetus absorbs oxygen and other nutrients and excretes carbon dioxide and other wastes. It begins to form about the eighth day of gestation when the blastocyst adheres to the decidua. [NIH]

Plant Oils: Oils derived from plants or plant products. [NIH]

Plants: Multicellular, eukaryotic life forms of the kingdom Plantae. They are characterized by a mainly photosynthetic mode of nutrition; essentially unlimited growth at localized regions of cell divisions (meristems); cellulose within cells providing rigidity; the absence of organs of locomotion; absense of nervous and sensory systems; and an alteration of haploid and diploid generations. [NIH]

Plaque: A clear zone in a bacterial culture grown on an agar plate caused by localized destruction of bacterial cells by a bacteriophage. The concentration of infective virus in a fluid can be estimated by applying the fluid to a culture and counting the number of. [NIH]

Plasma: The clear, yellowish, fluid part of the blood that carries the blood cells. The proteins that form blood clots are in plasma. [NIH]

Plasmid: An autonomously replicating, extra-chromosomal DNA molecule found in many bacteria. Plasmids are widely used as carriers of cloned genes. [NIH]

Plasticity: In an individual or a population, the capacity for adaptation: a) through gene changes (genetic plasticity) or b) through internal physiological modifications in response to changes of environment (physiological plasticity). [NIH]

Platelet Aggregation: The attachment of platelets to one another. This clumping together can be induced by a number of agents (e.g., thrombin, collagen) and is part of the mechanism leading to the formation of a thrombus. [NIH]

Platelets: A type of blood cell that helps prevent bleeding by causing blood clots to form. Also called thrombocytes. [NIH]

Pneumonia: Inflammation of the lungs. [NIH]

Poisoning: A condition or physical state produced by the ingestion, injection or inhalation of, or exposure to a deleterious agent. [NIH]

Pollen: The male fertilizing element of flowering plants analogous to sperm in animals. It is released from the anthers as yellow dust, to be carried by insect or other vectors, including wind, to the ovary (stigma) of other flowers to produce the embryo enclosed by the seed. The pollens of many plants are allergenic. [NIH]

Polyesters: Polymers of organic acids and alcohols, with ester linkages--usually polyethylene terephthalate; can be cured into hard plastic, films or tapes, or fibers which can be woven into fabrics, meshes or velours. [NIH]

Polyethylene: A vinyl polymer made from ethylene. It can be branched or linear. Branched or low-density polyethylene is tough and pliable but not to the same degree as linear polyethylene. Linear or high-density polyethylene has a greater hardness and tensile strength. Polyethylene is used in a variety of products, including implants and prostheses. [NIH]

Polymers: Compounds formed by the joining of smaller, usually repeating, units linked by covalent bonds. These compounds often form large macromolecules (e.g., polypeptides, proteins, plastics). [NIH]

Polymorphic: Occurring in several or many forms; appearing in different forms at different stages of development. [EU]

Polysaccharide: A type of carbohydrate. It contains sugar molecules that are linked together chemically. [NIH]

Polyunsaturated fat: An unsaturated fat found in greatest amounts in foods derived from plants, including safflower, sunflower, corn, and soybean oils. [NIH]

Porphyria: A group of disorders characterized by the excessive production of porphyrins or their precursors that arises from abnormalities in the regulation of the porphyrin-heme pathway. The porphyrias are usually divided into three broad groups, erythropoietic, hepatic, and erythrohepatic, according to the major sites of abnormal porphyrin synthesis. [NIH]

Porphyria Cutanea Tarda: A form of hepatic porphyria (porphyria, hepatic) characterized by photosensitivity resulting in bullae that rupture easily to form shallow ulcers. This condition occurs in two forms: a sporadic, nonfamilial form that begins in middle age and has normal amounts of uroporphyrinogen decarboxylase with diminished activity in the liver; and a familial form in which there is an autosomal dominant inherited deficiency of uroporphyrinogen decarboxylase in the liver and red blood cells. [NIH]

Posterior: Situated in back of, or in the back part of, or affecting the back or dorsal surface of the body. In lower animals, it refers to the caudal end of the body. [EU]

Postmenopausal: Refers to the time after menopause. Menopause is the time in a woman's life when menstrual periods stop permanently; also called "change of life." [NIH]

Postprandial: Occurring after dinner, or after a meal; postcibal. [EU]

Potassium: An element that is in the alkali group of metals. It has an atomic symbol K, atomic number 19, and atomic weight 39.10. It is the chief cation in the intracellular fluid of muscle and other cells. Potassium ion is a strong electrolyte and it plays a significant role in the regulation of fluid volume and maintenance of the water-electrolyte balance. [NIH]

Practice Guidelines: Directions or principles presenting current or future rules of policy for the health care practitioner to assist him in patient care decisions regarding diagnosis, therapy, or related clinical circumstances. The guidelines may be developed by government agencies at any level, institutions, professional societies, governing boards, or by the convening of expert panels. The guidelines form a basis for the evaluation of all aspects of health care and delivery. [NIH]

Precursor: Something that precedes. In biological processes, a substance from which another, usually more active or mature substance is formed. In clinical medicine, a sign or symptom that heralds another. [EU]

Premenstrual: Occurring before menstruation. [EU]

Premenstrual Syndrome: A syndrome occurring most often during the last week of the menstrual cycle and ending soon after the onset of menses. Some of the symptoms are emotional instability, insomnia, headache, nausea, vomiting, abdominal distension, and painful breasts. [NIH]

Progeny: The offspring produced in any generation. [NIH]

Progesterone: Pregn-4-ene-3,20-dione. The principal progestational hormone of the body, secreted by the corpus luteum, adrenal cortex, and placenta. Its chief function is to prepare the uterus for the reception and development of the fertilized ovum. It acts as an antiovulatory agent when administered on days 5-25 of the menstrual cycle. [NIH]

Progression: Increase in the size of a tumor or spread of cancer in the body. [NIH]

Progressive: Advancing; going forward; going from bad to worse; increasing in scope or severity. [EU]

Prone: Having the front portion of the body downwards. [NIH]

Prophylaxis: An attempt to prevent disease. [NIH]

Propylene Glycol: A clear, colorless, viscous organic solvent and diluent used in pharmaceutical preparations. [NIH]

Prostaglandin: Any of a group of components derived from unsaturated 20-carbon fatty acids, primarily arachidonic acid, via the cyclooxygenase pathway that are extremely potent mediators of a diverse group of physiologic processes. The abbreviation for prostaglandin is PG; specific compounds are designated by adding one of the letters A through I to indicate the type of substituents found on the hydrocarbon skeleton and a subscript (1, 2 or 3) to indicate the number of double bonds in the hydrocarbon skeleton e.g., PGE2. The predominant naturally occurring prostaglandins all have two double bonds and are synthesized from arachidonic acid (5,8,11,14-eicosatetraenoic acid) by the pathway shown in the illustration. The 1 series and 3 series are produced by the same pathway with fatty acids having one fewer double bond (8,11,14-eicosatrienoic acid or one more double bond (5,8,11,14,17-eicosapentaenoic acid) than arachidonic acid. The subscript a or ß indicates the configuration at C-9 (a denotes a substituent below the plane of the ring, ß, above the plane). The naturally occurring PGF's have the a configuration, e.g., PGF2a. All of the prostaglandins act by binding to specific cell-surface receptors causing an increase in the level of the intracellular second messenger cyclic AMP (and in some cases cyclic GMP also). The effect produced by the cyclic AMP increase depends on the specific cell type. In some cases there is also a positive feedback effect. Increased cyclic AMP increases prostaglandin synthesis leading to further increases in cyclic AMP. [EU]

Prostaglandins A: (13E,15S)-15-Hydroxy-9-oxoprosta-10,13-dien-1-oic acid (PGA(1)); (5Z,13E,15S)-15-hydroxy-9-oxoprosta-5,10,13-trien-1-oic acid (PGA(2)); (5Z,13E,15S,17Z)-15-hydroxy-9-oxoprosta-5,10,13,17-tetraen-1-oic acid (PGA(3)). A group of naturally occurring secondary prostaglandins derived from PGE. PGA(1) and PGA(2) as well as their 19-hydroxy derivatives are found in many organs and tissues. [NIH]

Prostate: A gland in males that surrounds the neck of the bladder and the urethra. It secretes a substance that liquifies coagulated semen. It is situated in the pelvic cavity behind the lower part of the pubic symphysis, above the deep layer of the triangular ligament, and rests upon the rectum. [NIH]

Protease: Proteinase (= any enzyme that catalyses the splitting of interior peptide bonds in a protein). [EU]

Protein C: A vitamin-K dependent zymogen present in the blood, which, upon activation by thrombin and thrombomodulin exerts anticoagulant properties by inactivating factors Va and VIIIa at the rate-limiting steps of thrombin formation. [NIH]

Protein S: The vitamin K-dependent cofactor of activated protein C. Together with protein C, it inhibits the action of factors VIIIa and Va. A deficiency in protein S can lead to recurrent venous and arterial thrombosis. [NIH]

Proteins: Polymers of amino acids linked by peptide bonds. The specific sequence of amino acids determines the shape and function of the protein. [NIH]

Protons: Stable elementary particles having the smallest known positive charge, found in the nuclei of all elements. The proton mass is less than that of a neutron. A proton is the nucleus of the light hydrogen atom, i.e., the hydrogen ion. [NIH]

Protozoa: A subkingdom consisting of unicellular organisms that are the simplest in the animal kingdom. Most are free living. They range in size from submicroscopic to macroscopic. Protozoa are divided into seven phyla: Sarcomastigophora, Labyrinthomorpha, Apicomplexa, Microspora, Ascetospora, Myxozoa, and Ciliophora. [NIH]

Pruritic: Pertaining to or characterized by pruritus. [EU]

Psychiatry: The medical science that deals with the origin, diagnosis, prevention, and treatment of mental disorders. [NIH]

Psychic: Pertaining to the psyche or to the mind; mental. [EU]

Psychology: The science dealing with the study of mental processes and behavior in man and animals. [NIH]

Public Policy: A course or method of action selected, usually by a government, from among alternatives to guide and determine present and future decisions. [NIH]

Pulmonary: Relating to the lungs. [NIH]

Pulmonary Artery: The short wide vessel arising from the conus arteriosus of the right ventricle and conveying unaerated blood to the lungs. [NIH]

Purifying: Respiratory equipment whose function is to remove contaminants from otherwise wholesome air. [NIH]

Pustular: Pertaining to or of the nature of a pustule; consisting of pustules (= a visible collection of pus within or beneath the epidermis). [EU]

Race: A population within a species which exhibits general similarities within itself, but is both discontinuous and distinct from other populations of that species, though not sufficiently so as to achieve the status of a taxon. [NIH]

Radiation: Emission or propagation of electromagnetic energy (waves/rays), or the waves/rays themselves; a stream of electromagnetic particles (electrons, neutrons, protons, alpha particles) or a mixture of these. The most common source is the sun. [NIH]

Radiation therapy: The use of high-energy radiation from x-rays, gamma rays, neutrons, and other sources to kill cancer cells and shrink tumors. Radiation may come from a machine outside the body (external-beam radiation therapy), or it may come from radioactive material placed in the body in the area near cancer cells (internal radiation therapy, implant radiation, or brachytherapy). Systemic radiation therapy uses a radioactive substance, such as a radiolabeled monoclonal antibody, that circulates throughout the body. Also called radiotherapy. [NIH]

Radioactive: Giving off radiation. [NIH]

Radium: A radioactive element of the alkaline earth series of metals. It has the atomic symbol Ra, atomic number 88, and atomic weight 226. Radium is the product of the disintegration of uranium and is present in pitchblende and all ores containing uranium. It is used clinically as a source of beta and gamma-rays in radiotherapy, particularly brachytherapy. [NIH]

Radius: The lateral bone of the forearm. [NIH]

Radon: A naturally radioactive element with atomic symbol Rn, atomic number 86, and atomic weight 222. It is a member of the noble gas family and released during the decay of radium and found in soil. There is a link between exposure to radon and lung cancer. [NIH]

Randomized: Describes an experiment or clinical trial in which animal or human subjects are assigned by chance to separate groups that compare different treatments. [NIH]

Reagent: A substance employed to produce a chemical reaction so as to detect, measure, produce, etc., other substances. [EU]

Reagin: The antibody-like substances responsible for allergic phenomena; part of the gamma globulin fraction of serum [NIH]

Receptor: A molecule inside or on the surface of a cell that binds to a specific substance and causes a specific physiologic effect in the cell. [NIH]

Recombinant: A cell or an individual with a new combination of genes not found together in either parent; usually applied to linked genes. [EU]

Rectum: The last 8 to 10 inches of the large intestine. [NIH]

Recurrence: The return of a sign, symptom, or disease after a remission. [NIH]

Red blood cells: RBCs. Cells that carry oxygen to all parts of the body. Also called erythrocytes. [NIH]

Refer: To send or direct for treatment, aid, information, de decision. [NIH]

Reflux: The term used when liquid backs up into the esophagus from the stomach. [NIH]

Regeneration: The natural renewal of a structure, as of a lost tissue or part. [EU]

Regimen: A treatment plan that specifies the dosage, the schedule, and the duration of treatment. [NIH]

Regurgitation: A backward flowing, as the casting up of undigested food, or the backward flowing of blood into the heart, or between the chambers of the heart when a valve is incompetent. [EU]

Remission: A decrease in or disappearance of signs and symptoms of cancer. In partial remission, some, but not all, signs and symptoms of cancer have disappeared. In complete remission, all signs and symptoms of cancer have disappeared, although there still may be cancer in the body. [NIH]

Renal pelvis: The area at the center of the kidney. Urine collects here and is funneled into the ureter, the tube that connects the kidney to the bladder. [NIH]

Retina: The ten-layered nervous tissue membrane of the eye. It is continuous with the optic nerve and receives images of external objects and transmits visual impulses to the brain. Its outer surface is in contact with the choroid and the inner surface with the vitreous body. The outer-most layer is pigmented, whereas the inner nine layers are transparent. [NIH]

Retinal: 1. Pertaining to the retina. 2. The aldehyde of retinol, derived by the oxidative enzymatic splitting of absorbed dietary carotene, and having vitamin A activity. In the retina, retinal combines with opsins to form visual pigments. One isomer, 11-cis retinal combines with opsin in the rods (scotopsin) to form rhodopsin, or visual purple. Another, all-trans retinal (trans-r.); visual yellow; xanthopsin) results from the bleaching of rhodopsin by light, in which the 11-cis form is converted to the all-trans form. Retinal also combines with opsins in the cones (photopsins) to form the three pigments responsible for colour vision. Called also retinal, and retinene1. [EU]

Reversion: A return to the original condition, e. g. the reappearance of the normal or wild type in previously mutated cells, tissues, or organisms. [NIH]

Rhamnose: A methylpentose whose L- isomer is found naturally in many plant glycosides and some gram-negative bacterial lipopolysaccharides. [NIH]

Ribosome: A granule of protein and RNA, synthesized in the nucleolus and found in the cytoplasm of cells. Ribosomes are the main sites of protein synthesis. Messenger RNA attaches to them and there receives molecules of transfer RNA bearing amino acids. [NIH]

Rigidity: Stiffness or inflexibility, chiefly that which is abnormal or morbid; rigor. [EU]

Risk factor: A habit, trait, condition, or genetic alteration that increases a person's chance of developing a disease. [NIH]

Rod: A reception for vision, located in the retina. [NIH]

Rubber: A high-molecular-weight polymeric elastomer derived from the milk juice (latex) of Hevea brasiliensis and other trees. It is a substance that can be stretched at room temperature to atleast twice its original length and after releasing the stress, retractrapidly, and recover its original dimensions fully. Synthetic rubber is made from many different chemicals, including styrene, acrylonitrile, ethylene, propylene, and isoprene. [NIH]

Rye: A hardy grain crop, Secale cereale, grown in northern climates. It is the most frequent host to ergot (claviceps), the toxic fungus. Its hybrid with wheat is triticale, another grain. [NIH]

Saccharin: Flavoring agent and non-nutritive sweetener. [NIH]

Salicylate: Non-steroidal anti-inflammatory drugs. [NIH]

Salicylic: A tuberculosis drug. [NIH]

Salicylic Acids: Derivatives and salts of salicylic acid. [NIH]

Saliva: The clear, viscous fluid secreted by the salivary glands and mucous glands of the mouth. It contains mucins, water, organic salts, and ptylin. [NIH]

Salivary: The duct that convey saliva to the mouth. [NIH]

Salivary glands: Glands in the mouth that produce saliva. [NIH]

Satiation: Full gratification of a need or desire followed by a state of relative insensitivity to that particular need or desire. [NIH]

Saturated fat: A type of fat found in greatest amounts in foods from animals, such as fatty cuts of meat, poultry with the skin, whole-milk dairy products, lard, and in some vegetable oils, including coconut, palm kernel, and palm oils. Saturated fat raises blood cholesterol more than anything else eaten. On a Step I Diet, no more than 8 to 10 percent of total calories should come from saturated fat, and in the Step II Diet, less than 7 percent of the day's total calories should come from saturated fat. [NIH]

Sclerotherapy: Treatment of varicose veins, hemorrhoids, gastric and esophageal varices, and peptic ulcer hemorrhage by injection or infusion of chemical agents which cause localized thrombosis and eventual fibrosis and obliteration of the vessels. [NIH]

Screening: Checking for disease when there are no symptoms. [NIH]

Seafood: Marine fish and shellfish used as food or suitable for food. (Webster, 3d ed) shellfish and fish products are more specific types of seafood. [NIH]

Sebaceous: Gland that secretes sebum [NIH]

Sebaceous gland: Gland that secretes sebum [NIH]

Sebum: The oily substance secreted by sebaceous glands. It is composed of keratin, fat, and cellular debris. [NIH]

Secretion: 1. The process of elaborating a specific product as a result of the activity of a gland; this activity may range from separating a specific substance of the blood to the elaboration of a new chemical substance. 2. Any substance produced by secretion. [EU]

Sedative: 1. Allaying activity and excitement. 2. An agent that allays excitement. [EU]

Senile: Relating or belonging to old age; characteristic of old age; resulting from infirmity of old age. [NIH]

Sensor: A device designed to respond to physical stimuli such as temperature, light, magnetism or movement and transmit resulting impulses for interpretation, recording, movement, or operating control. [NIH]

Serotonin: A biochemical messenger and regulator, synthesized from the essential amino acid L-tryptophan. In humans it is found primarily in the central nervous system, gastrointestinal tract, and blood platelets. Serotonin mediates several important physiological functions including neurotransmission, gastrointestinal motility, hemostasis, and cardiovascular integrity. Multiple receptor families (receptors, serotonin) explain the broad physiological actions and distribution of this biochemical mediator. [NIH]

Serum: The clear liquid part of the blood that remains after blood cells and clotting proteins have been removed. [NIH]

Shock: The general bodily disturbance following a severe injury; an emotional or moral upset occasioned by some disturbing or unexpected experience; disruption of the circulation, which can upset all body functions: sometimes referred to as circulatory shock. [NIH]

Side effect: A consequence other than the one(s) for which an agent or measure is used, as the adverse effects produced by a drug, especially on a tissue or organ system other than the one sought to be benefited by its administration. [EU]

Skeletal: Having to do with the skeleton (boney part of the body). [NIH]

Skeleton: The framework that supports the soft tissues of vertebrate animals and protects many of their internal organs. The skeletons of vertebrates are made of bone and/or cartilage. [NIH]

Skull: The skeleton of the head including the bones of the face and the bones enclosing the brain. [NIH]

Small intestine: The part of the digestive tract that is located between the stomach and the large intestine. [NIH]

Smoking Cessation: Discontinuation of the habit of smoking, the inhaling and exhaling of tobacco smoke. [NIH]

Smooth muscle: Muscle that performs automatic tasks, such as constricting blood vessels. [NIH]

Sodium: An element that is a member of the alkali group of metals. It has the atomic symbol Na, atomic number 11, and atomic weight 23. With a valence of 1, it has a strong affinity for oxygen and other nonmetallic elements. Sodium provides the chief cation of the extracellular body fluids. Its salts are the most widely used in medicine. (From Dorland, 27th ed) Physiologically the sodium ion plays a major role in blood pressure regulation, maintenance of fluid volume, and electrolyte balance. [NIH]

Sodium Bicarbonate: A white, crystalline powder that is commonly used as a pH buffering agent, an electrolyte replenisher, systemic alkalizer and in topical cleansing solutions. [NIH]

Soft tissue: Refers to muscle, fat, fibrous tissue, blood vessels, or other supporting tissue of the body. [NIH]

Solvent: 1. Dissolving; effecting a solution. 2. A liquid that dissolves or that is capable of dissolving; the component of a solution that is present in greater amount. [EU]

Sorbitol: A polyhydric alcohol with about half the sweetness of sucrose. Sorbitol occurs naturally and is also produced synthetically from glucose. It was formerly used as a diuretic and may still be used as a laxative and in irrigating solutions for some surgical procedures. It is also used in many manufacturing processes, as a pharmaceutical aid, and in several research applications. [NIH]

Sound wave: An alteration of properties of an elastic medium, such as pressure, particle displacement, or density, that propagates through the medium, or a superposition of such alterations. [NIH]

Soybean Oil: Oil from soybean or soybean plant. [NIH]

Specialist: In medicine, one who concentrates on 1 special branch of medical science. [NIH]

Species: A taxonomic category subordinate to a genus (or subgenus) and superior to a subspecies or variety, composed of individuals possessing common characters distinguishing them from other categories of individuals of the same taxonomic level. In taxonomic nomenclature, species are designated by the genus name followed by a Latin or Latinized adjective or noun. [EU]

Specificity: Degree of selectivity shown by an antibody with respect to the number and types of antigens with which the antibody combines, as well as with respect to the rates and the extents of these reactions. [NIH]

Spectrometer: An apparatus for determining spectra; measures quantities such as wavelengths and relative amplitudes of components. [NIH]

Sphincter: A ringlike band of muscle fibres that constricts a passage or closes a natural orifice; called also musculus sphincter. [EU]

Spices: The dried seeds, bark, root, stems, buds, leaves, or fruit of aromatic plants used to season food. [NIH]

Spinal cord: The main trunk or bundle of nerves running down the spine through holes in the spinal bone (the vertebrae) from the brain to the level of the lower back. [NIH]

Spinous: Like a spine or thorn in shape; having spines. [NIH]

Sporadic: Neither endemic nor epidemic; occurring occasionally in a random or isolated manner. [EU]

Sprue: A non febrile tropical disease of uncertain origin. [NIH]

Sputum: The material expelled from the respiratory passages by coughing or clearing the throat. [NIH]

Stabilization: The creation of a stable state. [EU]

Stabilizer: A device for maintaining constant X-ray tube voltage or current. [NIH]

Standardize: To compare with or conform to a standard; to establish standards. [EU]

Staphylococcal Food Poisoning: Poisoning by staphylococcal toxins present in contaminated food. [NIH]

Steady state: Dynamic equilibrium. [EU]

Steel: A tough, malleable, iron-based alloy containing up to, but no more than, two percent carbon and often other metals. It is used in medicine and dentistry in implants and instrumentation. [NIH]

Sterilization: The destroying of all forms of life, especially microorganisms, by heat, chemical, or other means. [NIH]

Stimulant: 1. Producing stimulation; especially producing stimulation by causing tension on muscle fibre through the nervous tissue. 2. An agent or remedy that produces stimulation. [EU]

Stimulus: That which can elicit or evoke action (response) in a muscle, nerve, gland or other excitable issue, or cause an augmenting action upon any function or metabolic process. [NIH]

Stomach: An organ of digestion situated in the left upper quadrant of the abdomen between the termination of the esophagus and the beginning of the duodenum. [NIH]

Stool: The waste matter discharged in a bowel movement; feces. [NIH]

Stress: Forcibly exerted influence; pressure. Any condition or situation that causes strain or tension. Stress may be either physical or psychologic, or both. [NIH]

Stroke: Sudden loss of function of part of the brain because of loss of blood flow. Stroke may be caused by a clot (thrombosis) or rupture (hemorrhage) of a blood vessel to the brain. [NIH]

Stromal: Large, veil-like cell in the bone marrow. [NIH]

Struvite: A type of kidney stone caused by infection. [NIH]

Stupor: Partial or nearly complete unconsciousness, manifested by the subject's responding only to vigorous stimulation. Also, in psychiatry, a disorder marked by reduced responsiveness. [EU]

Styrene: A colorless, toxic liquid with a strong aromatic odor. It is used to make rubbers, polymers and copolymers, and polystyrene plastics. [NIH]

Subacute: Somewhat acute; between acute and chronic. [EU]

Subarachnoid: Situated or occurring between the arachnoid and the pia mater. [EU]

Subclinical: Without clinical manifestations; said of the early stage(s) of an infection or other disease or abnormality before symptoms and signs become apparent or detectable by clinical examination or laboratory tests, or of a very mild form of an infection or other disease or abnormality. [EU]

Subspecies: A category intermediate in rank between species and variety, based on a smaller number of correlated characters than are used to differentiate species and generally conditioned by geographical and/or ecological occurrence. [NIH]

Substrate: A substance upon which an enzyme acts. [EU]

Suction: The removal of secretions, gas or fluid from hollow or tubular organs or cavities by means of a tube and a device that acts on negative pressure. [NIH]

Superoxide: Derivative of molecular oxygen that can damage cells. [NIH]

Supplementation: Adding nutrients to the diet. [NIH]

Suppositories: A small cone-shaped medicament having cocoa butter or gelatin at its basis and usually intended for the treatment of local conditions in the rectum. [NIH]

Suppression: A conscious exclusion of disapproved desire contrary with repression, in which the process of exclusion is not conscious. [NIH]

Surfactant: A fat-containing protein in the respiratory passages which reduces the surface tension of pulmonary fluids and contributes to the elastic properties of pulmonary tissue. [NIH]

Suspensions: Colloids with liquid continuous phase and solid dispersed phase; the term is used loosely also for solid-in-gas (aerosol) and other colloidal systems; water-insoluble drugs may be given as suspensions. [NIH]

Sweat: The fluid excreted by the sweat glands. It consists of water containing sodium chloride, phosphate, urea, ammonia, and other waste products. [NIH]

Sweat Glands: Sweat-producing structures that are embedded in the dermis. Each gland consists of a single tube, a coiled body, and a superficial duct. [NIH]

Sympathomimetic: 1. Mimicking the effects of impulses conveyed by adrenergic postganglionic fibres of the sympathetic nervous system. 2. An agent that produces effects similar to those of impulses conveyed by adrenergic postganglionic fibres of the sympathetic nervous system. Called also adrenergic. [EU]

Symptomatic: Having to do with symptoms, which are signs of a condition or disease. [NIH]

Synaptic: Pertaining to or affecting a synapse (= site of functional apposition between neurons, at which an impulse is transmitted from one neuron to another by electrical or chemical means); pertaining to synapsis (= pairing off in point-for-point association of homologous chromosomes from the male and female pronuclei during the early prophase of meiosis). [EU]

Synaptic Transmission: The communication from a neuron to a target (neuron, muscle, or secretory cell) across a synapse. In chemical synaptic transmission, the presynaptic neuron releases a neurotransmitter that diffuses across the synaptic cleft and binds to specific synaptic receptors. These activated receptors modulate ion channels and/or second-messenger systems to influence the postsynaptic cell. Electrical transmission is less common in the nervous system, and, as in other tissues, is mediated by gap junctions. [NIH]

Synchronism: Occurring at the same time. [NIH]

Systemic: Affecting the entire body. [NIH]

Systolic: Indicating the maximum arterial pressure during contraction of the left ventricle of the heart. [EU]

Tetracycline: An antibiotic originally produced by Streptomyces viridifaciens, but used mostly in synthetic form. It is an inhibitor of aminoacyl-tRNA binding during protein synthesis. [NIH]

Thermal: Pertaining to or characterized by heat. [EU]

Thoracic: Having to do with the chest. [NIH]

Thorax: A part of the trunk between the neck and the abdomen; the chest. [NIH]

Threshold: For a specified sensory modality (e. g. light, sound, vibration), the lowest level (absolute threshold) or smallest difference (difference threshold, difference limen) or intensity of the stimulus discernible in prescribed conditions of stimulation. [NIH]

Thrombin: An enzyme formed from prothrombin that converts fibrinogen to fibrin. (Dorland, 27th ed) EC 3.4.21.5. [NIH]

Thrombomodulin: A cell surface glycoprotein of endothelial cells that binds thrombin and serves as a cofactor in the activation of protein C and its regulation of blood coagulation. [NIH]

Thrombosis: The formation or presence of a blood clot inside a blood vessel. [NIH]

Thrombus: An aggregation of blood factors, primarily platelets and fibrin with entrapment of cellular elements, frequently causing vascular obstruction at the point of its formation. Some authorities thus differentiate thrombus formation from simple coagulation or clot formation. [EU]

Thyroid: A gland located near the windpipe (trachea) that produces thyroid hormone, which helps regulate growth and metabolism. [NIH]

Tinnitus: Sounds that are perceived in the absence of any external noise source which may take the form of buzzing, ringing, clicking, pulsations, and other noises. Objective tinnitus refers to noises generated from within the ear or adjacent structures that can be heard by other individuals. The term subjective tinnitus is used when the sound is audible only to the affected individual. Tinnitus may occur as a manifestation of cochlear diseases; vestibulocochlear nerve diseases; intracranial hypertension; craniocerebral trauma; and other conditions. [NIH]

Tissue: A group or layer of cells that are alike in type and work together to perform a specific function. [NIH]

Tolerance: 1. The ability to endure unusually large doses of a drug or toxin. 2. Acquired drug tolerance; a decreasing response to repeated constant doses of a drug or the need for increasing doses to maintain a constant response. [EU]

Tone: 1. The normal degree of vigour and tension; in muscle, the resistance to passive elongation or stretch; tonus. 2. A particular quality of sound or of voice. 3. To make permanent, or to change, the colour of silver stain by chemical treatment, usually with a heavy metal. [EU]

Tonic: 1. Producing and restoring the normal tone. 2. Characterized by continuous tension. 3. A term formerly used for a class of medicinal preparations believed to have the power of restoring normal tone to tissue. [EU]

Topical: On the surface of the body. [NIH]

Toxic: Having to do with poison or something harmful to the body. Toxic substances usually cause unwanted side effects. [NIH]

Toxicity: The quality of being poisonous, especially the degree of virulence of a toxic microbe or of a poison. [EU]

Toxicology: The science concerned with the detection, chemical composition, and pharmacologic action of toxic substances or poisons and the treatment and prevention of toxic manifestations. [NIH]

Toxin: A poison; frequently used to refer specifically to a protein produced by some higher plants, certain animals, and pathogenic bacteria, which is highly toxic for other living organisms. Such substances are differentiated from the simple chemical poisons and the vegetable alkaloids by their high molecular weight and antigenicity. [EU]

Trace element: Substance or element essential to plant or animal life, but present in extremely small amounts. [NIH]

Trachea: The cartilaginous and membranous tube descending from the larynx and branching into the right and left main bronchi. [NIH]

Traction: The act of pulling. [NIH]

Transcriptase: An enzyme which catalyses the synthesis of a complementary mRNA molecule from a DNA template in the presence of a mixture of the four ribonucleotides (ATP, UTP, GTP and CTP). [NIH]

Transdermal: Entering through the dermis, or skin, as in administration of a drug applied to the skin in ointment or patch form. [EU]

Transfection: The uptake of naked or purified DNA into cells, usually eukaryotic. It is analogous to bacterial transformation. [NIH]

Transfusion: The infusion of components of blood or whole blood into the bloodstream. The blood may be donated from another person, or it may have been taken from the person earlier and stored until needed. [NIH]

Translation: The process whereby the genetic information present in the linear sequence of ribonucleotides in mRNA is converted into a corresponding sequence of amino acids in a protein. It occurs on the ribosome and is unidirectional. [NIH]

Transmitter: A chemical substance which effects the passage of nerve impulses from one cell to the other at the synapse. [NIH]

Trees: Woody, usually tall, perennial higher plants (Angiosperms, Gymnosperms, and some Pterophyta) having usually a main stem and numerous branches. [NIH]

Triglyceride: A lipid carried through the blood stream to tissues. Most of the body's fat tissue is in the form of triglycerides, stored for use as energy. Triglycerides are obtained primarily from fat in foods. [NIH]

Tumor marker: A substance sometimes found in an increased amount in the blood, other body fluids, or tissues and which may mean that a certain type of cancer is in the body. Examples of tumor markers include CA 125 (ovarian cancer), CA 15-3 (breast cancer), CEA (ovarian, lung, breast, pancreas, and gastrointestinal tract cancers), and PSA (prostate cancer). Also called biomarker. [NIH]

Tumor model: A type of animal model which can be used to study the development and progression of diseases and to test new treatments before they are given to humans. Animals with transplanted human cancers or other tissues are called xenograft models. [NIH]

Typhimurium: Microbial assay which measures his-his+ reversion by chemicals which cause base substitutions or frameshift mutations in the genome of this organism. [NIH]

Tyramine: An indirect sympathomimetic. Tyramine does not directly activate adrenergic receptors, but it can serve as a substrate for adrenergic uptake systems and monoamine oxidase so it prolongs the actions of adrenergic transmitters. It also provokes transmitter release from adrenergic terminals. Tyramine may be a neurotransmitter in some invertebrate nervous systems. [NIH]

Tyrosine: A non-essential amino acid. In animals it is synthesized from phenylalanine. It is also the precursor of epinephrine, thyroid hormones, and melanin. [NIH]

Unconscious: Experience which was once conscious, but was subsequently rejected, as the "personal unconscious". [NIH]

Ureter: One of a pair of thick-walled tubes that transports urine from the kidney pelvis to the bladder. [NIH]

Urethra: The tube through which urine leaves the body. It empties urine from the bladder. [NIH]

Urethritis: Inflammation of the urethra. [EU]

Uric: A kidney stone that may result from a diet high in animal protein. When the body breaks down this protein, uric acid levels rise and can form stones. [NIH]

Urinary: Having to do with urine or the organs of the body that produce and get rid of urine. [NIH]

Urinary tract: The organs of the body that produce and discharge urine. These include the kidneys, ureters, bladder, and urethra. [NIH]

Urinary tract infection: An illness caused by harmful bacteria growing in the urinary tract. [NIH]

Urinate: To release urine from the bladder to the outside. [NIH]

Urine: Fluid containing water and waste products. Urine is made by the kidneys, stored in the bladder, and leaves the body through the urethra. [NIH]

Urogenital: Pertaining to the urinary and genital apparatus; genitourinary. [EU]

Urologist: A doctor who specializes in diseases of the urinary organs in females and the urinary and sex organs in males. [NIH]

Urticaria: A vascular reaction of the skin characterized by erythema and wheal formation due to localized increase of vascular permeability. The causative mechanism may be allergy, infection, or stress. [NIH]

Uterus: The small, hollow, pear-shaped organ in a woman's pelvis. This is the organ in which a fetus develops. Also called the womb. [NIH]

Vaccines: Suspensions of killed or attenuated microorganisms (bacteria, viruses, fungi, protozoa, or rickettsiae), antigenic proteins derived from them, or synthetic constructs, administered for the prevention, amelioration, or treatment of infectious and other diseases. [NIH]

Vagina: The muscular canal extending from the uterus to the exterior of the body. Also called the birth canal. [NIH]

Vaginal: Of or having to do with the vagina, the birth canal. [NIH]

Varicose: The common ulcer in the lower third of the leg or near the ankle. [NIH]

Varicose vein: An abnormal swelling and tortuosity especially of the superficial veins of the legs. [EU]

Vascular: Pertaining to blood vessels or indicative of a copious blood supply. [EU]

Vasodilator: An agent that widens blood vessels. [NIH]

Vein: Vessel-carrying blood from various parts of the body to the heart. [NIH]

Venous: Of or pertaining to the veins. [EU]

Ventricle: One of the two pumping chambers of the heart. The right ventricle receives oxygen-poor blood from the right atrium and pumps it to the lungs through the pulmonary artery. The left ventricle receives oxygen-rich blood from the left atrium and pumps it to the body through the aorta. [NIH]

Venules: The minute vessels that collect blood from the capillary plexuses and join together to form veins. [NIH]

Vesicular: 1. Composed of or relating to small, saclike bodies. 2. Pertaining to or made up of vesicles on the skin. [EU]

Vestibulocochlear Nerve: The 8th cranial nerve. The vestibulocochlear nerve has a cochlear part (cochlear nerve) which is concerned with hearing and a vestibular part (vestibular nerve) which mediates the sense of balance and head position. The fibers of the cochlear nerve originate from neurons of the spiral ganglion and project to the cochlear nuclei (cochlear nucleus). The fibers of the vestibular nerve arise from neurons of Scarpa's ganglion and project to the vestibular nuclei. [NIH]

Vestibulocochlear Nerve Diseases: Diseases of the vestibular and/or cochlear (acoustic) nerves, which join to form the vestibulocochlear nerve. Vestibular neuritis, cochlear neuritis, and acoustic neuromas are relatively common conditions that affect these nerves. Clinical manifestations vary with which nerve is primarily affected, and include hearing loss, vertigo, and tinnitus. [NIH]

Veterinary Medicine: The medical science concerned with the prevention, diagnosis, and treatment of diseases in animals. [NIH]

Vial: A small bottle. [EU]

Video Recording: The storing or preserving of video signals for television to be played back later via a transmitter or receiver. Recordings may be made on magnetic tape or discs (videodisc recording). [NIH]

Videodisc Recording: The storing of visual and usually sound signals on discs for later reproduction on a television screen or monitor. [NIH]

Villous: Of a surface, covered with villi. [NIH]

Virulence: The degree of pathogenicity within a group or species of microorganisms or viruses as indicated by case fatality rates and/or the ability of the organism to invade the tissues of the host. [NIH]

Virus: Submicroscopic organism that causes infectious disease. In cancer therapy, some viruses may be made into vaccines that help the body build an immune response to, and kill, tumor cells. [NIH]

Viscosity: A physical property of fluids that determines the internal resistance to shear forces. [EU]

Vitro: Descriptive of an event or enzyme reaction under experimental investigation occurring outside a living organism. Parts of an organism or microorganism are used together with artificial substrates and/or conditions. [NIH]

Vivo: Outside of or removed from the body of a living organism. [NIH]

Weight Gain: Increase in body weight over existing weight. [NIH]

Wetting Agents: A surfactant that renders a surface wettable by water or enhances the spreading of water over the surface; used in foods and cosmetics; important in contrast media; also with contact lenses, dentures, and some prostheses. Synonyms: humectants; hydrating agents. [NIH]

White blood cell: A type of cell in the immune system that helps the body fight infection and disease. White blood cells include lymphocytes, granulocytes, macrophages, and others. [NIH]

Windpipe: A rigid tube, 10 cm long, extending from the cricoid cartilage to the upper border of the fifth thoracic vertebra. [NIH]

Xanthine: An urinary calculus. [NIH]

Xanthine Alkaloids: Alkaloids, which contain xanthine as their nitrogenous base. [NIH]

Xenograft: The cells of one species transplanted to another species. [NIH]

Xenon: A noble gas with the atomic symbol Xe, atomic number 54, and atomic weight 131.30. It is found in the earth's atmosphere and has been used as an anesthetic. [NIH]

X-ray: High-energy radiation used in low doses to diagnose diseases and in high doses to treat cancer. [NIH]

Yeasts: A general term for single-celled rounded fungi that reproduce by budding. Brewers' and bakers' yeasts are Saccharomyces cerevisiae; therapeutic dried yeast is dried yeast. [NIH]

Zymogen: Inactive form of an enzyme which can then be converted to the active form, usually by excision of a polypeptide, e. g. trypsinogen is the zymogen of trypsin. [NIH]

INDEX

Printed in the United States
134142LV00001B/33/A